Birmingham Metropolitan College
Matthew Boulton Campus

Library Resource Centre

Standard Loan	Telephone for renewals: **0121 446 4545 ext. 8036**
This is a 4 week loan and must be returned by the latest date shown below	

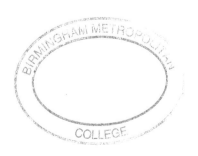

The Invisalign System

The Invisalign System

Orhan C. Tuncay, DMD
Professor and Chairman
Department of Orthodontics
School of Dentistry
Temple University
Philadelphia, Pennsylvania

Quintessence Publishing Co, Ltd
London, Berlin, Chicago, Tokyo, Barcelona, Beijing,
Istanbul, Milan, Moscow, Mumbai, Paris,
Prague, São Paulo, and Warsaw

British Library Cataloging in Publication Data
  1. Orthodontics, Corrective 2. Orthodontic appliances
  3. Orthodontics – Diagnosis
  I. Tuncay, Orhan C.
  617.6'43'00284

ISBN-10: 1850971277

© 2006 Quintessence Publishing Co, Ltd

Quintessence Publishing Co, Ltd
Grafton Road
New Malden
Surrey KT3 3AB
United Kingdom
www.quintpub.co.uk

ISBN-10: 1-85097-127-7
ISBN-13: 978-1-85097-127-6
Printed in Germany

Table of Contents

SECTION I—HISTORY OF THE CONCEPT

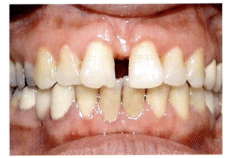 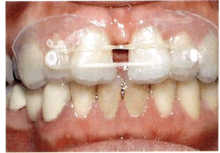 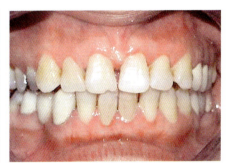

SECTION II—MODELING IN THE INVISALIGN SYSTEM

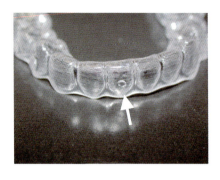 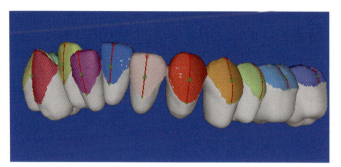

SECTION III—PERFORMANCE CHARACTERISTICS OF THE INVISALIGN SYSTEM

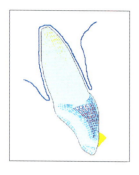 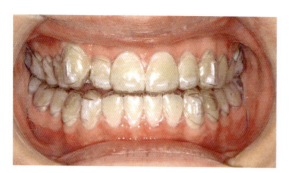

SECTION IV—CLINICAL CONSIDERATIONS IN USING THE INVISALIGN SYSTEM

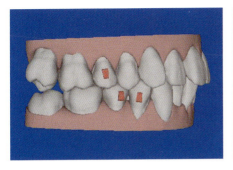 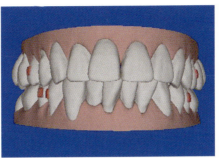 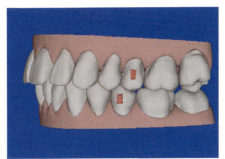

SECTION V—OFFICE DESIGN AND TECHNOLOGY

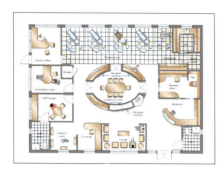

Preface

The long-awaited paradigm shift in orthodontics arrived with the introduction of the Invisalign System. This unique treatment approach has been instrumental in removing the ever-present shroud of mystery surrounding orthodontics by allowing both dental practitioner and patient to develop a visual understanding of orthodontic tooth movement. In this way, it has founded a culture of true and attainable visual treatment objectives. Moreover, the esthetic and practical advantages of the system have extended orthodontic services to a greater population.

The Invisalign System is multilingual. Its spoken languages are image acquisition, software (ClinCheck), and the Invisalign aligner. The dialects are the generation of forces, attachment designs, and response of periodontal tissues to the forces generated by the aligner. The regional accents were born through the various applications of ClinCheck, spectrum of cases treated, attachment preferences, and instructions to patients. The adoption of the Invisalign System into a practice, however, is a language unto itself. It has its roots in two different tongues: biology and technology. To be fluent in all of these languages and dialects, the clinician must know the root of the language and how the dialects have been derived.

This book, the first to be written about the Invisalign System, was compiled as an educational tool for all of the languages, dialects, and accents spoken in the world of Invisalign. It is not a how-to manual. Instead, it is designed to expose the clinician to behind-the-scene elements of customization that underlie the production of Invisalign aligners. Equipped with such information, the clinician will better understand the nature of tooth movement with the Invisalign System.

Our deepest gratitude goes to the authors from Align Technology. These individuals took precious time from their daily schedules to write about the inner workings of their operation. The Invisalign System is primarily company driven; therefore, it is their contribution that makes this textbook possible. In particular, Dr Trang Duong's indefatigability in collecting chapters from Align Technology authors is greatly appreciated. We gratefully acknowledge the monumental commitment of Align Technology, through the leadership of Amir Abolfathi, to this project. Finally, we thank Jonathan S. Simmons, whose efforts in the editing, organization, and overall preparation of the manuscript have been invaluable.

Contributors

Marc B. Ackerman, DMD
Associate Professor
Department of Orthodontics
School of Dentistry
Temple University
Philadelphia, Pennsylvania

Andrew Beers, PhD
Director of Engineering Systems
Align Technology, Inc

Robert L. Boyd, DDS
Professor and Chairman
Department of Orthodontics
School of Dentistry
University of the Pacific
San Francisco, California

Heng Cao, PhD
Research and Development Engineer
Align Technology, Inc

Jihua Cheng, PhD
Algorithm Specialist
Align Technology, Inc

David Chenin, DDS
Orthodontist Resident
Department of Orthodontics
School of Dentistry
University of the Pacific
San Francisco, California

Craig Crawford, DDS
Orthodontist
Align Technology, Inc

Mitra Derakhshan, DDS
Clinical Manager of European
  Operations
Align Technology, Inc

Trang Duong, DDS
Senior Staff Orthodontist
Align Technology, Inc

Robert Fry, DDS
Private Practice in Orthodontics
Olathe, Kansas

Paul-Georg Jost-Brinkmann,
  Prof Dr Med Dent
Senior Lecturer
Department of Dentofacial
  Orthopedics and Orthodontics
University Hospital Charité
Humboldt University of Berlin
Berlin, Germany

Agnes A. Kan
Architect
Philadelphia, Pennsylvania

Srinivas Kaza
Product Engineer
Align Technology, Inc

Peter Knopp
Senior Manager and Product
  Engineer
Align Technology, Inc

Eric Kuo, DDS
Director of Product Development
Align Technology, Inc

Marc S. Lemchen, DMD
Private Practice in Orthodontics
New York, New York

Chunha Li, PhD
Manager of Materials Research
Align Technology, Inc

Vadim Matov, PhD
Senior Alogrithm Specialist
Align Technology, Inc

Rainer-Reginald Miethke,
  Prof Dr Med Dent
Professor and Chairman
Department of Dentofacial
  Orthopedics and Orthodontics
University Hospital Charité
Humboldt University of Berlin
Berlin, Germany

Ross Miller, DDS
Private Practice in Orthodontics
Sunnyvale, California

Henry I. Nahoum, DDS
Professor
Department of Orthodontics
School of Dentistry
Loma Linda University
Loma Linda, California

C. Van Nguyen, DDS
Private Practice in Orthodontics
Houston, Texas

David E. Paquette, DDS
Private Practice in Orthodontics
Charlotte, North Carolina

John M. Powers, PhD
Professor of Oral Biomaterials
Director, Houston Biomaterials
  Research Center
University of Texas Dental Branch at
  Houston
Houston, Texas

John Sheridan, DDS
Professor
School of Dentistry
Louisiana State University Health
  Sciences Center
Baton Rouge, Louisiana

Associate Professor
Department of Orthodontics
Jacksonville University
Jacksonville, Florida

Rene Sterental, DDS
Staff Orthodontist
Align Technology, Inc

Robert Tricca, PhD
Director of Product Development
Align Technology, Inc

Andrew Trosien, DDS
Consulting Orthodontist
Align Technology, Inc

Orhan C. Tuncay, DMD
Professor and Chairman
Department of Orthodontics
School of Dentistry
Temple University
Philadelphia, Pennsylvania

Kent Verdis
Manufacturing Process Engineer
Align Technology, Inc

SECTION I

HISTORY OF THE CONCEPT

chapter 1

THE DENTAL CONTOUR APPLIANCE: A HISTORICAL REVIEW

by
Henry I. Nahoum, DDS

Background and Process of Thermoforming

Although thermoplastic sheets were manufactured as far back as 1896,[1] plastic sheet forming, or thermoforming, was not well known before 1950. This process shapes a plastic product by applying air pressure or vacuum to a heat-softened sheet. On occasion, pressurized steam or hot oil has been used instead of air pressure.

As pressure-forming machines improved—for example, by combining the heating and forming processes on a single machine—the development of materials advanced concurrently. Acrylics and styrene were developed in the 1930s. Ethyl cellulose, polyethylene, the vinyls, oriented styrene, cellulose acetate, and cellulose acetate butyrate followed quickly. There is a plethora of calendered plastics available for different uses (eg, packaging, food trays, accessories). Sheet feeding and roll feeding are available in various sizes. The material varies from 0.001 to 0.375 inches in thickness (0.025 to 9.12 mm).[2] Today, machines are highly automated and can be precisely controlled with computers.

When a piece of thermoplastic is heated to temperatures between 250°F and 450°F, depending on the plastic, it will become soft enough that it can be formed over a surface either mechanically or by positive air pressure. Unlike casting and injection molding, which require a three-dimensional mold, a two-dimensional surface is all that is required for thermoforming: the surface becomes the mold. Vacuum forming is the simplest type of pressure forming since it uses atmospheric air pressure.

When the plastic is held over the mold and allowed to cool, the plastic will retain the exact shape of the mold. With the proper equipment and the appropriate material, the finest details can be duplicated on the mold side of the plastic, like an impression. The side away from the mold is less distinct. The final product is thinner than the original sheet because the plastic stretches during the forming process.

In 1959, an industrial-grade vacuum former, produced by The Tronomatic Machine Manufacturing Company of New York, was used to make appliances that could be used to maintain or change contours[3] (Fig 1-1). This was a novel way to fabricate dental appliances that were suitable for various procedures in orthodontics, periodontics, restorative dentistry, dental surgery, and for other purposes in dental practice.

The dental contour appliance is made by a drape-forming method in which the heated plastic is clamped and pushed or allowed to drape over a plaster cast.[1] The sheet is sealed at the edges of the mold and then vacuum is applied, forcing the sheet to adapt to the surface of the model (Fig 1-2).

To ensure that the maximum vacuum pressure (28 inches Hg) is obtained, an auxiliary tank is evacuated before the process begins. The vacuum pump is kept on through-

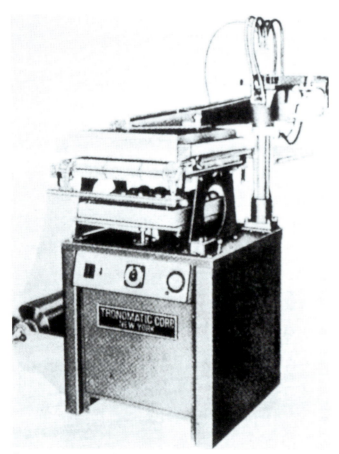

FIG 1-1 A commercial vacuum former.

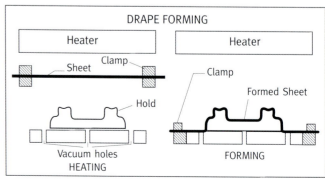

FIG 1-2 The vacuum-forming process. (After Butzko and Stratton.[1])

FIG 1-3 A clear plastic vacuum-formed maxillary appliance (*left*), and an opaque vinyl vacuum-formed mandibular appliance (*right*). Note the excellent detail in both appliances.

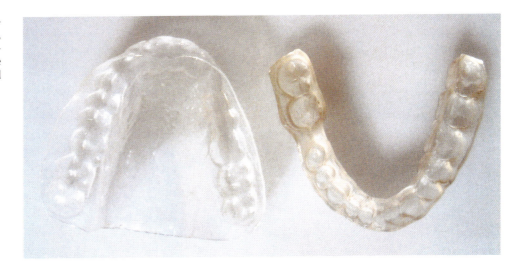

out the process so that both the vacuum pump and the tank operate simultaneously. The negative atmospheric pressure created by the combination of the evacuation tank and the pump ensured excellent draping of plastic over the plaster cast. Atmospheric pressure equivalent to approximately 14 psi molds the plastic instantaneously. Excellent detail is achieved with acetates, vinyl, styrene, polyethylene, and butyrate, in clear, translucent, opaque, or colored films and sheets (Fig 1-3). Positive air pressure can also be used, but this is not necessary for these plastics. Small vacuum-forming machines that use a vacuum-cleaner motor do not achieve this level of efficiency.

Rationale for Material Selection

Plastics differ in their characteristics. The selection of the material to be used in producing a dental contour appliance depends on such factors as the length of time that the appliance is to be used, the thickness of the material, and the purpose of the appliance. For nightguards, a hard material may be used, whereas for orthodontic purposes a soft, resilient plastic is desired. In all cases, it is necessary for the material to be inert, nontoxic, odorless, tasteless, and unaffected by the chemicals of the body. It should have a minimum of water absorption and it must not warp. In addition, molding qualities must be good or excellent. After the appliance is molded, it is washed in a mild alkaline solution or detergent to remove any surface impurities and excess plasticizer.

Orthodontic Applications

It is readily apparent that this contour appliance can be used as an immediate retainer, to prevent teeth from moving, following orthodontic treatment. If clear plastic is used, the result is a cosmetically innocuous appliance that can be worn all the time. Each dental arch is treated independently.

This type of appliance can also be fabricated to move teeth. Anterior spaces can be closed and minor rotations can be corrected. To do this, a plaster cast is made of the dentition, and the teeth are numbered for identification. The teeth that require correction are sawed off the cast with a fine jeweler's saw or fissure bur, as is done for a Kesling rubber positioner[4] (Fig 1-4). The teeth are then repositioned on the model and held in the corrected positions with pink baseplate wax (Fig 1-5). The contour appliance is vacuum formed over the altered model. Since the forming process is instantaneous, the teeth that are held by the baseplate wax do not move because the plastic will mold before the wax melts (Figs 1-6a and 1-6b). After the mold cools, the excess plastic is trimmed with a razor, and the appliance is removed from the cast. Final trimming is done with a fine scissors. The appliance is then cleaned and inserted in the mouth.

Several appliances can be made on the altered cast, which is used over and over. A hole may be made in the center of the base of the cast to assist in the vacuum-forming process. After the appliance is made and trimmed, compressed air directed into the hole helps in removing the appliance.

Movement of teeth occurs as a result of the pressure exerted on the irregular teeth by the appliance that was

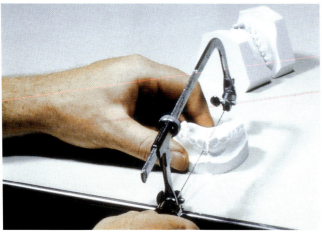

FIG 1-4 Teeth are sawed off the cast with a fine jeweler's saw.

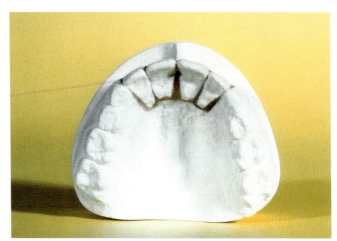

FIG 1-5 Teeth are repositioned on the cast with pink baseplate wax.

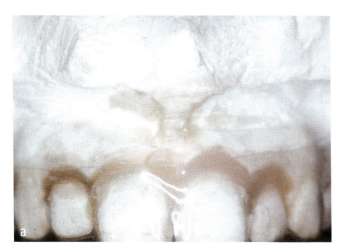

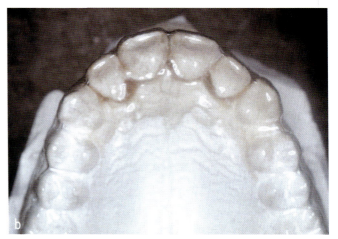

FIG 1-6 (a and b) A clear plastic appliance made on a cast where the maxillary incisors were repositioned and held in place with wax. Note that a thin film of molten wax was spread around the teeth.

made on the corrected model. The appliance is resilient and snaps over the teeth and the mucosa. It exerts pressure until the teeth attain their predetermined positions. This type of appliance is very effective for contraction of a dental arch but not as effective for expansion. A patient treated by the author with this type of appliance had a mandibular incisor that was crowded out of the dental arch and was in crossbite with the maxillary lateral incisor (Figs 1-7a to 1-7e). The incisor was slenderized with a disk on the mesial and distal surfaces so that it could be pushed into the dental arch. Treatment time was 2 months. Note that the appliance extended a convenient distance over the mucosa, past the gingival margin. It was not scalloped.

When the correction is too great to be done in one step, adjustments may be made in increments using two or more appliances. Partial and progressive adjustments are made by moving the teeth gradually and holding them in place with wax. A new vacuum-formed appliance is made for each phase. When the teeth are properly aligned, the final appliance is used as a retainer to maintain the teeth in their corrected positions. Corrections made with this type of appliance are most effective when they are limited to the six anterior teeth.

Contoured orthodontic appliances are made for either one or both dental arches and may be worn at all times. If only one arch is being treated, the patient is able to eat

FIG 1-7 A patient with the mandibular right lateral incisor crowded out of the dental arch and in crossbite (September 1960).

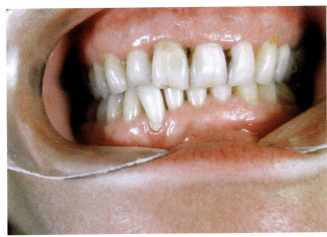

FIG 1-7a The mandibular right lateral incisor has been slenderized. A disk was used on the mesial and distal surfaces.

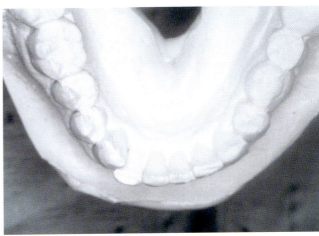

FIG 1-7b Occlusal view of the cast.

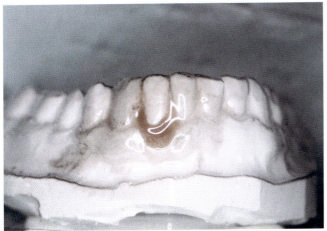

FIG 1-7c The mandibular incisor was repositioned and held with wax. A clear plastic appliance was made on the altered model.

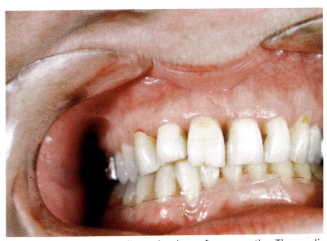

FIG 1-7d View of the appliance in place after 2 months. The appliance is not scalloped.

with the appliance in position. When maxillary and mandibular appliances are used simultaneously, hooks for maxillomandibular elastics can be bonded with acrylic, or another compatible adhesive, in appropriate locations. Unfortunately, stability of the appliances then becomes a problem. When indicated, a maxillary and a mandibular contour appliance can be bonded together for finishing of an orthodontic case (Fig 1-8). Minor intercuspal corrections can be made in this way. Repositioning of the mandible, of course, is questionable.

For en masse movement of teeth with an extraoral appliance, tubes may be bonded to the appliance over the maxillary first molars. An extraoral facebow is inserted into

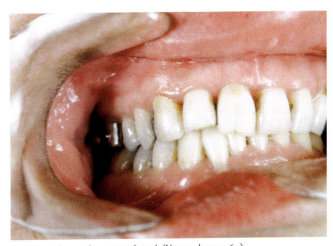

FIG 1-7e Correction completed (November 1960).

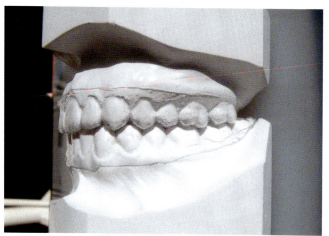

FIG 1-8 Maxillary and mandibular contour appliances bonded together for final finishing.

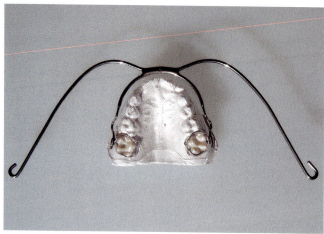

FIG 1-9 A clear plastic appliance made over a model with bands on the maxillary first molars. A facebow, for extraoral force, is inserted into the tubes on the bands through an opening in the plastic.

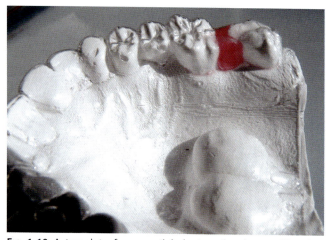

FIG 1-10 A template for a partial denture for the maxillary left quadrant. Note the wax pontic.

Other Uses in Dentistry

The contour appliance is not limited to orthodontic procedures.[5] It has many dental uses.[5] Dental contour appliances can be used as a splint to limit the mobility of loose or periodontally involved teeth. When used as a nightguard to prevent bruxism, the contour appliance is made with a maxillary biteplate or a smooth, rigid mandibular occlusal plane that prevents intercuspation with the opposing dentition. Self-curing, clear acrylic is processed over the appliance into the grooves and over the cusps of the teeth to create a smooth occlusal plane. Acetate is not used for the thermoformed appliance because acrylic does not bond to acetate. Contour appliances may also be used to carry medicaments to the gingival tissues, hold a surgical pack in place, and control hemorrhage following a surgical procedure. They also can transport chemicals, such as fluoride gels, to the teeth.

In restorative dentistry, it is a fast, convenient way to make an esthetic provisional crown or partial denture. An impression is taken and a plaster cast is made. Missing teeth are replaced with artificial teeth and held in place on the cast with baseplate wax. Any teeth that require recontouring are corrected with wax or trimmed with a finishing stone (Fig 1-10). The occlusion is checked, and then a full, clear acetate thermoformed appliance is made. The teeth that require preparation for crowns are ground down in the mouth. The provisional partial denture, splint, or crowns are made by pouring quick, self-curing acrylic of an appropriate shade into the appropriate area of the contour appliance. The appliance is insert-

the tubes and activated with elastics from a head cap or neck strap. An alternative method is to fit and cement molar bands with buccal tubes on the first molars. Impressions are taken with the bands in place, and a model is made for a thermoplastic appliance that fits over the bands. In this case, the vacuum-formed appliance can be used in conjunction with an extraoral facebow that is inserted directly into the tubes on the molar bands through an opening in the plastic (Fig 1-9).

ed in the mouth, and the excess acrylic is removed. The acrylic can be observed through the clear appliance so that color, contour, and voids may be corrected. The occlusion is established by having the patient close his or her mouth onto the appliance. As soon as the acrylic begins to set, it becomes hot (flash setting point). It is possible to feel the warmth through the clear plastic and remove the appliance immediately, thus avoiding trauma to the tissues. The final set takes place out of the mouth. The appliance requires very little trimming of excess acrylic, and there is no need for polishing. The final product is as smooth as glass. Veneers can be made in the same way within a clear plastic appliance. These veneers are useful for photography, performances, speeches, etc. These procedures have been illustrated and described in detail in the dental literature for the past 40 years.[6–8]

Summary

The introduction of pressure forming of calendered thermoplastics to make dental appliances has had a significant impact on the practice of dentistry. This process simplified many existing procedures and facilitated the introduction of new concepts for treating patients. Since these appliances can be made of clear plastic, which is inconspicuous, they are readily accepted by patients. New materials are constantly being introduced, accuracy has improved, and the fabrication processes have become automated. The process keeps evolving.

References

1. Butzko R, Stratton E. Thermoplastic sheet forming. Modern Plastics Encyclopedia 1957;35:736.
2. Butzko R. Plastic Sheet Forming. New York: Reinhold, 1958.
3. Nahoum H. The vacuum formed dental contour appliance. N Y State Dent J 1964;9:385–390.
4. Kesling H. The philosophy of the tooth positioning appliance. Am J Orthod 1945;31:297–304.
5. Nahoum H. What price progress? Am J Orthod Dentofacial Orthop 2002;122:15A–16A.
6. Fiasconaro JE, Sherman H. Vacuum-formed prostheses. I. A temporary fixed bridge or splint. J Am Dent Assoc 1968; 76(1):74–78.
7. Hirshfeld L, Geiger A. Minor tooth movement in general practice, ed 2. St Louis: Mosby, 1966.
8. McNamara J Jr, Brudon W. Orthodontics and Dentofacial Orthopedics. Ann Arbor: Needham Press, 2001.

chapter 2

ESSIX TECHNOLOGY:
TOOTH MOVEMENT AND RETENTION

by
John Sheridan, DDS

The two contemporary systems for moving teeth with plastic appliances are the Invisalign and Essix systems. The Invisalign System is unique in that the clinician must be able to plan the path to optimal results before treatment is initiated so that a series of aligners can be constructed to achieve treatment objectives. The Essix System is based on in-course adjustments of what is essentially a single appliance to achieve the treatment goals.[1-3] This chapter presents the concepts and techniques of the Essix System.

Clear plastic tooth-moving appliances are excellent options for adults or responsible adolescents who might be reluctant to wear fixed appliances, who will follow the clinician's directions, and whose chief complaint centers around mild to moderate alignment problems. But, this discipline requires the essential elements of orthodontic tooth movement, force, space, and time (ie, there must be adequate force to move a tooth without inducing pathology, there must be enough space to accomplish the desired tooth movement, and the appliance must be in place for an appropriate length of time for the force to be effective). The clinician can control two of these essential prerequisites: force and space. As with any dynamic removable appliance, however, the patient must provide the third essential: time. Therefore, the target population that is most eligible for tooth movement with plastic appliances is, primarily, adults. In adult patients, the dentition has been milling itself in for perhaps decades. Although the occlusion may not have ideal dental relationships, the bite has usually adapted to a nonpathologic efficiency that is satisfactory for that particular patient. In the absence of functional distress or the resolution of extant or impending pathology, the focus of treatment with Essix appliances should be directed at the patient's chief complaint, and that is usually the appearance of the anterior teeth. The clinician, of course, is responsible for maintaining the pretreatment symptom-free functional occlusion.

Adolescents are usually not included in the plastic alignment population because strict adherence to clinical instructions is not predictable in that age group. Some clinicians believe that children and adolescent patients are best treated with conventional fixed appliances. The occlusion in the younger population, unlike in adults, has not had the chance to adapt to decades of function. It is hoped that the establishment of accepted occlusal parameters will be of value in adapting the masticatory system to the impending variables of diet, lifestyle, age, and stress.

The Essix Tooth-Moving System

Conventional fixed appliances are constantly modified because of the multiple variables that arise during treatment; so it is with Essix technology. Tooth movement is possible in all planes of space, and the fabrication expense is a fraction of the cost of multiple laboratory-fabricated appliances that must be used sequentially. Because Essix plastic appliances can be fabricated in the office, the cost of fabrication is minimal.

Creating space

There are two types of space that must be evident for tooth movement with Essix appliances: space within the appliance and space within the dentition. Space within the appliance is obtained by blocking out the working cast or cutting a window in the thermoformed appliance. The clinician has the option of using the method that is most efficient for the particular circumstance.

Creating space within the appliance: Blocking out the cast or cutting a window into the plastic

Blocking out the cast to create space into which the target tooth can move is achieved by placing a thickness of time-cured or light-cured composite on the working cast that is proportional to the amount of projected tooth movement (Fig 2-1). The cast must not be blocked out with wax because it will melt during thermoforming. The blockout material forms a bulge in the thermoformed appliance, and if normal overbite and overjet are evident, the bulge in the plastic can cause incisal interference if it is on the lingual of the maxillary incisors or the facial of the mandibular incisors. Additionally, if the blocked-out area is on the facial of the appliance, the bulge in the thermoformed plastic will slightly detract from the esthetic presentation. These conditions seem to be well tolerated by the patient.

The alternative method of creating tooth-moving space within the dental arches is to cut a window into the thermoformed appliance with a plastic trimming bur in a slow-speed handpiece. The bur causes a frayed border to the window that can be smoothed with a scalpel (Fig 2-2). Because tooth movement must be unimpeded, particular attention must be given to the size of the window. It is best to err on the side of a bigger rather than a smaller

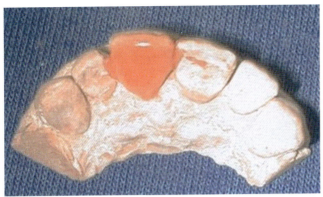

FIG 2-1 Space within the appliance is obtained by blocking out the cast.

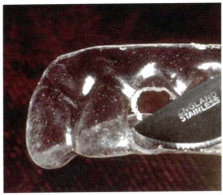

FIG 2-2 A window cut into the thermoformed appliance with a plastic trimming bur and finished with a scalpel creates space into which the tooth can move.

window. A 2.0- to 3.0-mm gingival border of plastic is necessary for adequate strength and resiliency.

Tongue irritation may develop from the presence of a lingual window because patients have a tendency to rub their tongue against the window's border. Patients can be supplied with bracket wax to wipe into the lingual window to alleviate this aggravation.

Creating space within the dental arches with interproximal reduction

Creating space within the dental arches usually involves expansion, extraction, or interdental reduction. Extraction is not a suitable option for gaining space with plastic appliances because it is difficult to upright roots and to efficiently close any remaining extraction space after the crowding is resolved. Expansion with a clear plastic appliance is possible, but arch coordination is difficult during the finishing stage and there is the liability of possibly moving the teeth past the limits of alveolar bone. Additionally, the patient's chief complaint frequently involves the resolution of crowding in a single arch. If, for instance, maxillary incisor crowding were the patient's chief complaint, expanding this arch would necessarily involve the complexity of adapting the mandibular arch to it to establish incisor or canine guidance. Caution is advised when rearranging established occlusal patterns by expansion when the patient's chief complaint is centered on mild to moderate incisor alignment problems and not functional distress.

To avoid the complexities associated with extraction or expansion, the judicious removal of interproximal enamel, if possible, is indicated. There are various techniques to do this. Using hand-pulled abrasive strips is too laborious

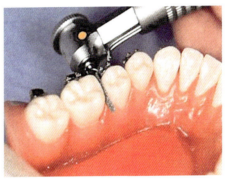

FIG 2-3 Interproximal reduction with the air-rotor stripping technique.

and is minimally effective for other than very modest dimensions because forcing the metal strip between proximal surfaces moves the teeth laterally into the periodontal space and does not create the needed interdental reduction.

Handpiece-mounted reducing disks can be dangerous because of the proximity of the tongue and cheeks to the rotating disk. This risk can be decreased with a disk guard, but this obstructs the clinician's vision of the reduction site. The safest and most efficient system for gaining space within the arch is by interproximal reduction with the disciplined utilization of an air-turbine handpiece. The Invisalign and Essix techniques recommend this method.

Air-rotor stripping (ARS) is a contemporary clinical procedure that involves the use of an air-turbine handpiece to reduce interproximal enamel for the alleviation of mild to moderate crowding (Fig 2-3).[4–5] There is ample evidence that ARS does not induce pathology of the hard or soft tissues.[6–9] Additionally, the space generated by ARS does not have to be estimated; it can be measured in increments of 0.10 mm with commercially available gauges (Fig 2-4).

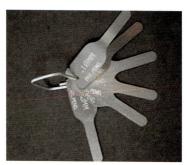

FIG 2-4 Commercially available gauges can be used separately or in tandem to measure the space generated by interproximal reduction.

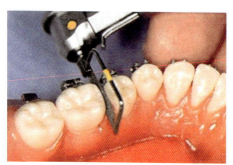

FIG 2-5 The Intensive Ortho-Strip System reduces proximal enamel with appropriate blades in a handpiece that generates a back-and-forth shuttle action.

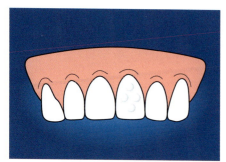

FIG 2-6 Force can be directed on any part of the clinical crown to create the most desired effect.

A conservative guideline would be to remove no more than 0.75 mm of interproximal enamel between the anterior contact points, and no more than 1.0 mm for contact points (0.5 mm for proximal surfaces) in the buccal sections. The suggested guidelines for ARS are as follows:

- Prior to ARS, establish a slight open field with coil springs or separators to improve the visual and mechanical access to the contact area.
- Contour the reduced proximal surfaces to resemble the acceptable morphology.
- Finish the reduced proximal surfaces to acceptable smoothness with fine-grit diamond burs.
- Prescribe a fluoride gel or rinse to supplement the already powerful remineralization potential of the reduced proximal surfaces. Data indicate that when the fully reacted outer layer of enamel is removed, the abraded (stripped) enamel surface is more prone to remineralization. When that occurs, the remineralized enamel surface is more, not less, resistant to caries initiation.[7,8,10]

The Intensive Ortho-Strip System (GAC) is an alternative method of reducing interproximal enamel with a handpiece but without a rotating bur. It involves the use of handpiece-driven abrasive strips with different configurations and abrasive potentials (Fig 2-5). The instrument removes enamel with a 0.8-mm oscillation movement (back-and-forth shuttle action). Metallic strips with different abrasive grain sizes may be used for the initial reduction of proximal surfaces. Also, there are flexible blades to contour and smooth the reduced proximal surface with abrasive grain sizes from 15 to 125 μm (see Fig 2-5).

Inducing Tooth-Moving Force in an Essix System

With Essix tooth-moving mechanics, the clinician has the option of placing force wherever on the crown surface would have the most desirable effect. Unlike an edgewise bracket that confines force application to the bracket slot, an Essix appliance permits force application on any area of the clinical crown. This, in turn, determines the type of tooth movement. For instance, if the force is placed incisally, more tipping is evident on the target tooth. If the force is placed gingivally, more bodily movement occurs. If the force is placed distally, movement about the mesial vertical axis occurs, and if the force is directed medially, movement about the distal vertical axis is evident (Fig 2-6).

There are two primary systems of creating a tooth-moving force with an Essix appliance. The first uses Hilliard thermopliers to alter the appliance by spot-thermoforming it. The second system, called mounding, does not involve altering the appliance to induce force. It involves the sequential placement of small mounds (layers) of bonding composite to the surface of the tooth.[10] These two force-inducing systems will be described separately.

Hilliard thermoforming pliers: Inducing force by altering the appliance

The Hilliard thermoplier technique efficiently induces a tooth-moving force into an Essix plastic appliance usually within a few seconds, and it can be done at chairside. The pliers can spot-thermoform a projection into the appliance that induces force as the resilient plastic returns to its resting state. These projections in the plastic can be mod-

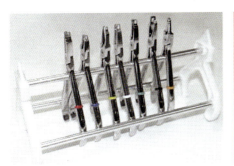

FIG 2-7 Various Hilliard thermopliers can induce a variety of biomechanical effects.

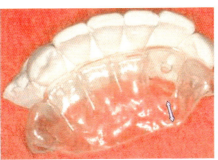

FIG 2-8 The thermoformed tooth-moving bump is always made toward the tooth surface, and an adequate gingival amount of plastic should be apparent on the gingival aspect of the window (*arrow*).

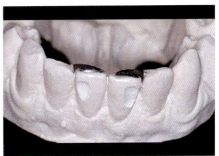

FIG 2-9 A 1.0-mm depression in the working cast allows the plastic to have maximum thickness for future adjustments.

ified to induce additional force on the same appliance as the case progresses. Various pliers are designed to induce force, create space within the appliance, create bite ramps, tighten an Essix appliance for a better fit, and create attachment hooks for Class II or III elastics (Fig 2-7). These pliers are capable of generating forces that can move teeth in all three planes of space and can move teeth that are adjacent to each other in different directions at the same time.

The force-inducing thermoformed projection (bump) created by the pliers is always made toward the tooth surface (Fig 2-8). To spot-thermoform this projection into the Essix plastic, the thermoplier tip is heated to approximately 200°F for Essix C+ plastic. When this temperature is achieved and measured, handles of the thermoplier are gently squeezed together to create a force-inducing projection in the plastic appliance. It must be cautioned, however, that in subsequent adjustments this periodic stretching of the plastic causes the projection to become thinner and decreases its force potential. Creating the first projection, by cutting a 1.0-mm depression in the working cast, allows the material to have a maximum thickness for future adjustments (Fig 2-9).

A heat source that generates temperatures in the 180°F to 215°F range is necessary to heat the thermoplier tip for spot-thermoforming the plastic. Because thermopliers are usually used at chairside, an open flame near the patient is a safety concern. A touch-activated burner is recommended for this reason (Fig 2-10). It has a "dead man's switch" that turns off automatically when the operator's hand is removed from the activation button. Heat sources such as a butane flame or a bead sterilizer may be used in the lab, but caution dictates that they should not be used at chairside.

Measuring the temperature of the thermoplier tip prior to thermoforming is required. If the thermoplier temperature is below the thermoforming range, the plastic will only stretch and tend to revert back to its original sheet form, thereby compromising tooth movement. If the temperature is too hot, the pliers will burn through the plastic. To preclude these difficulties, the exact thermoforming temperature can be recorded with a Hakko digital thermometer that displays on a readout scale the precise temperatures, in Fahrenheit or centigrade (Fig 2-11).

Mounding: Inducing force by placing composite on the tooth surface

Mounding reverses the technique of altering the plastic appliance by placing a force-inducing projection into it. Instead, a small mound of composite is placed on the enamel surface of the tooth to be moved. The resilient plastic presses against the mound and induces tooth movement. Whether there is a thermoformed projection in the plastic appliance or a small mound of composite on the tooth makes little difference because the biomechanical principle is the same; both methods deliver force to the target tooth as a result of the interference of the resilient plastic returning to its resting state (Fig 2-12).

The mound is placed on the enamel surface after the Essix appliance has been thermoformed. The technique is described below.

A conventional acid-etch procedure is done on the enamel surface that is to receive the mounding composite. The etched area should be of sufficient dimension to place a 1.0-mm thick composite mound. It is not necessary, or desirable, to etch the complete enamel surface. A 1.0-mm thick composite mound (any bonding composite is

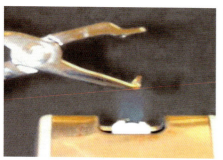

FIG 2-10 The touch-activated burner is a safe method of heating the tips of the thermopliers at chairside.

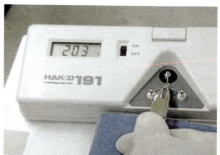

FIG 2-11 The Hakko digital thermometer can accurately record the temperature at the tip of the thermopliers.

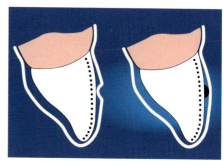

FIG 2-12 A projection in the plastic or a composite mound on the enamel surface delivers equivalent forces on the target tooth as the resilient plastic returns to its resting state.

adequate) is placed on the prepared surface and cured. The height of the mound can be determined with before-and-after readings with a Boley gauge (Figs 2-13a and 2-13b).

The Essix appliance is placed on the teeth. The only modification made to the appliance is to create enough space for the tooth to move into by the methods previously described (ie, cutting a window in the plastic or by blocking out the cast prior to thermoforming the appliance).

At the subsequent visits, additional force can be induced to create additional tooth movement by adding 1.0-mm composite layers to the original mound. If the patient feels force on the target tooth, the force is usually adequate. If the patient feels no force, a slight amount of additional composite should be placed on the established mound. Occasionally, the patient feels no force when the appliance is seated but experiences a proprioceptive feeling of pressure on the target tooth after it has been placed and then removed. If the force is so great that it is difficult to seat the appliance, the height of the composite mound should be decreased with a sandpaper disk or a fluted plastic trimming bur.

Types of Tooth Movement That Can Be Achieved with Essix Mechanics

Labial and lingual movement

Labial and lingual movement is accomplished by placing the force-inducing projection in the plastic or a composite mound on the enamel surface, on the side that the tooth is to tip away from, and by relieving the cast with blockout compound or a window cut into the plastic on the side the tooth is to tip towards. If, for example, an incisor is to tip lingually, a composite mound (or Hilliard thermoplier projection) is placed on the facial enamel surface. Space for the tooth to move into is obtained with blockout relief or a window cut into the plastic. Additionally, adequate proximal space must be evident or obtained with interproximal reduction. If the tooth is tipped too far, the force-inducing composite mound or thermoplier projection can be reduced. This allows the target tooth to rebound to the desired position. The case report described below illustrates this principle.

An adult male had a maxillary left lateral incisor that was conspicuously out of alignment (Fig 2-14). It required proximal lateral incisor stripping and 2.5 mm of maxillary lateral incisor movement to the lingual. The buccal section intercuspation was acceptable. After the Essix appliance was fabricated, a mound of composite was placed on the facial surface of the aberrant lateral incisor. A lingual window was cut out of the plastic to establish the space for the tooth to move into. When the resilient plastic pressed against the composite mound, tooth movement was initiated. Using the same appliance, three separate mounding modifications (two of 1.0 mm and one of 0.5 mm) induced the force necessary for alignment of the lateral incisor.

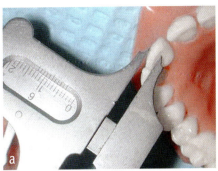
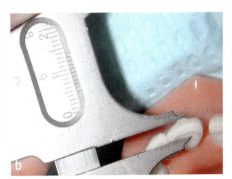
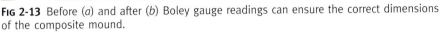
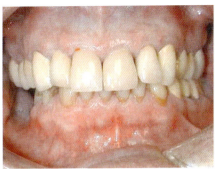

Fig 2-13 Before (*a*) and after (*b*) Boley gauge readings can ensure the correct dimensions of the composite mound.

Fig 2-14 The maxillary left lateral incisor is flared to the facial and requires 2.5 mm of lingual movement.

Treatment time was 3 months. Adjustment appointments were scheduled every 2 to 3 weeks. Chair time was minimal and involved making impressions, bonding the initial mound to the facial enamel, and adding the additional composite layers to the initial mound.

Lateral movement

On the working cast, blockout material—preferably Triad light-cured gel (Dentsply)—is placed on the side of the tooth where the lateral movement is to be accomplished. This creates a channel within the thermoformed plastic for the tooth to move into. For example, if a maxillary central incisor is to move to the mesial, blockout material is placed in the mesial interproximal area on the working cast before fabricating the Essix appliance (Fig 2-15). Space in the arch is obtained with interproximal reduction after the appliance is thermoformed. The blockout relief must be slightly above the incisal edge of the target tooth to prevent the incisal edge from contacting the inside of the Essix appliance and interfering with tooth movement.

Once space is obtained within the appliance and within the arch, the seated appliance induces initial movement. For additional movement, this force can be augmented with composite additions to the original mound or amplification of a thermoplier projection during the patient's sequential visits.

Torque

Torque is routinely established in an edgewise bracket by creating a couple, established with equal and opposite moments, within the bracket-to-wire complex. In effect, the tooth rotates around the bracket slot axis with the root mov-

ing one way and the crown moving in the opposite direction. Because of this, the efficiency of the edgewise moments are constrained because the width of the bracket limits the distance between the torquing moments to 0.022 inch or 0.018 inch (ie, the slot width of commercially available brackets). Essix-induced torque is more efficient because the distance between the opposing moments is only limited by the length of the clinical crown, measured in millimeters, rather than the width of a rectangular bracket slot measured in thousandths of an inch (Fig 2-16).

Essix torque is accomplished by creating a force-inducing projection in the plastic with Hilliard thermopliers or by mounding composite on the enamel surface. This is done in conjunction with a blockout material on the cast to allow tooth movement. For instance, if incisor torque involves moving the incisal edge lingually and the root labially, the working model is prepared by placing a force-inducing projection, or composite mound, on the incisal third of the labial surface of the crown and on the lingual surface on the gingival third of the crown. These forces induce a mechanical couple that will torque the incisor, moving the incisal edge lingually while the gingival section of the crown moves labially.

If incisor torque involves holding the incisal edge of the target tooth stationary and obtaining exclusive root movement, the Essix appliance is constructed to have 2.0 mm of the incisal edge covered with plastic and is, therefore, locked within the appliance. This incisal edge plastic cap holds the incisal edge in place while the root rotates under it due to the induced gingival force (Fig 2-17). The following case report illustrates this principle.

A middle-aged female had a lingually positioned mandibular central incisor that required significant facial tipping and labial root torque (Fig 2-18a). After appropriate

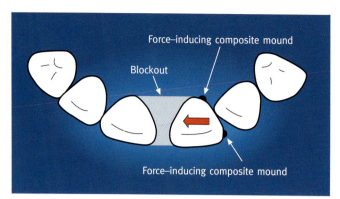

FIG 2-15 A channel for lateral tooth movement is constructed by placing blockout compound on the working cast before thermoforming the appliance.

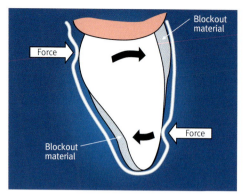

FIG 2-16 An efficient torquing couple, to move the root while slightly rotating the incisal edge, is established with an induced force and appropriate sections of the working cast blocked out.

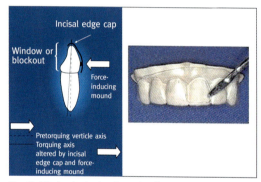

FIG 2-17 An incisal edge plastic cap and a cervically placed mound or thermoplier bump torques the root while holding the position of the incisal edge.

interproximal reduction, a canine-to-canine Essix appliance was constructed, a 1.0-mm mound of composite was bonded to the lingual surface of the out-of-line incisor, and a facial window was cut into the appliance to create space into which the incisor could move. The initial mound was amplified twice with additional 1.0-mm layers of composite. These mechanics tipped the incisor into alignment, but the root still needed to be torqued under the crown. A second appliance was constructed with an incisal cap and a cervically placed lingual mound to induce facial root movement. After the addition of two 1.0-mm composite layers to the original torquing mound, root position was acceptable, as is evidenced by the lingual alignment of the mandibular incisors (Fig 2-18b). An Essix retainer for nighttime wear was constructed to retain the correction.

Rotation

To rotate an incisor about a central axis, it is necessary to induce a rotational force on diagonally opposed tooth surfaces and block out the appropriate space on the working cast. For example, if an incisor is to rotate lingually on one side and labially on the other side, the mounds or force-inducing projections would be distolingual and mesiolabial, and the relief would be distolabial and mesiolingual (Fig 2-19).

Interproximal reduction is usually necessary to create the room for the proximal surfaces to rotate into. It is best to reduce these surfaces incrementally in conjunction with the applied rotational force during subsequent visits. If one does all the reduction at one time, there is a possibility of generating too much space. A more conservative approach would be to reduce a little, then rotate the tooth a little. This sequence can be maintained until the target tooth is aligned. The rotational efficiency of an Essix appliance is apparent in the following case report.

This adult female's chief complaint was "crooked upper front teeth." Resolving this situation required minor interproximal reduction mesial and distal to the maxillary left central incisor to rotate it into arch form, a slight rotation about the distal contact point of the maxillary right lateral incisor and facial movement of the maxillary left lateral incisor (Fig 2-20a).

A rotational plastic appliance was constructed after blockout space was obtained on the working cast to create room for the proximal surfaces to move into. Air-rotor stripping was not done at one time but a little at each sequential appointment (ie, stripped a little, then moved

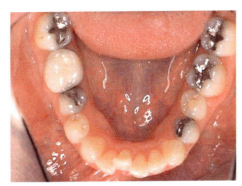

FIG 2-18a The out-of-line incisor needs to be moved labially, and the root needs to be torqued under the crown.

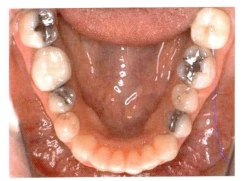

FIG 2-18b The finished case indicates that the tooth was tipped and then torqued into acceptable alignment.

a little). After the rotations were resolved, the minor facial movement of the left lateral incisor was achieved. Satisfactory alignment was achieved (Fig 2-20b).

Additionally, rotation can be induced in an out-of-line proximal surface while maintaining the proximal surface that is acceptable. For example, to rotate the tooth on the mesial while holding an acceptable distal contact point, the distolingual aspect of the tooth is not blocked out while space for movement of the out-of-line mesial contact point is obtained with blockout compound. This absence of relief on the distal of the tooth locks the acceptable contact point in place and the target tooth pivots mesiolingually like a door on a hinge as a result of the force induced by the resilient plastic returning to its resting state. A guideline for the amount of tooth to have held within the appliance is 10% of the acceptable proximal surface. This approach is demonstrated in another case.

The distal contact point of the maxillary right lateral incisor is acceptable (Fig 2-21a). The mesial contact point needs to be rotated about a distal vertical axis to achieve acceptable alignment. Additionally, the right central incisor needs to be slightly tipped facially after appropriate and sequential interproximal reduction.

The progress photograph indicates that the rotation of the right lateral incisor has been partially corrected and that the central incisors are in approximate alignment (Fig 2-21b). Figure 2-21c shows the successful alignment of the rotated lateral incisor about an acceptable distal contact point in conjunction with alignment of the central incisors.

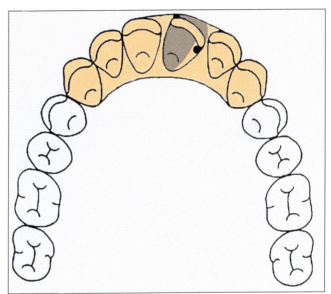

FIG 2-19 Rotation about a central axis requires force induction on diagonally opposed tooth surfaces and blocking out space on the working cast.

Extrusion and intrusion

The Essix appliance can serve as an anchor for elastics to extrude or intrude an anterior or posterior tooth. The suggested appliance for anterior teeth involves cutting a complete window into the thermoformed plastic to create the space for the target tooth to move into and to allow the bonding of a clear plastic button to the facial enamel for attachment of an intrusive or extrusive force-inducing elastic. Elastic attachment tabs are constructed, and light elastics, to be changed every day, are attached from the tabs on the appliance to the button bonded on the facial enamel. A diagram of the extrusion appliance used to intrude anterior teeth is shown in Fig 2-22.

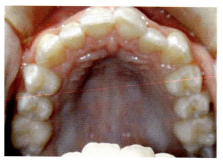

FIG 2-20a The maxillary central incisor needs to be rotated about its center line to be placed in acceptable arch form.

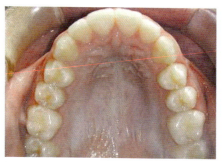

FIG 2-20b The center-line rotation was achieved by periodic interproximal stripping and incremental additions to the initial composite mound.

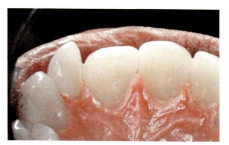

FIG 2-21a The mesial of the lateral incisor is rotated out of arch form. The distal contact point is acceptable.

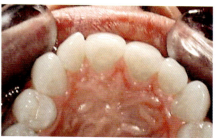

FIG 2-21b The out-of-line contact point is being corrected by periodic stripping while the force on the same Essix appliance is gradually increased.

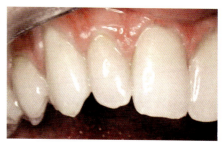

FIG 2-21c The incisor has been rotated about the distal axis and is in acceptable alignment.

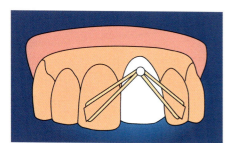

FIG 2-22 Anterior extrusion appliances utilize an elastic force stretched between elastic attachment tabs and strategically placed on a clear plastic button on the clinical crown.

Elastic attachment tabs can be constructed in various ways, such as cutting two horizontal slits, 3 to 4 mm apart, into the appliance with a scalpel and extending them 2 to 3 mm from the center of the facial surface toward the interproximal. A vertical scalpel cut is then made near the interproximal to connect the horizontal slits (Figs 2-23a to 2-23c). To minimize tissue irritation, the vertical edge of the tab should be well into the curvature of the interproximal area, and the corners of the tab should be rounded. The created tab is then flexed away from the body of the plastic, elastics are attached, and the patient is instructed as to their use.

Additionally, Hilliard thermopliers can be used to construct elastic attachment buttons on plastics. Two thermopliers are necessary to construct the elastic attachment button. The first plier thermoforms a cylindrical projection in the appliance when the tip of the pliers is heated and pressed into the plastic. A Hakko digital thermometer is used to determine the appropriate thermoforming temperature. Then, the heated thermoplier is placed at the desired location on the appliance and the handles are gently squeezed to create the initial cylindrical indentation into the plastic (Fig 2-24a). After 15 seconds, the pliers are removed with a rolling motion (rather than being pulled straight out of the plastic).

Next, the second slot-forming plier is heated, the "lipped" edge is placed around the base of the previously formed cylinder, and the plier handles are squeezed together. This indentation on the base of the cylinder forms an undercut to which an elastic can be attached (Fig 2-24b). The elastic will be held in place even when it is oriented up to 30 degrees away from the button (Fig 2-24c).

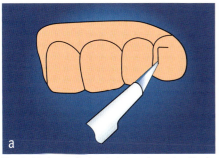
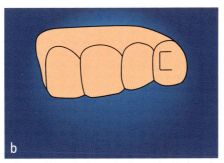
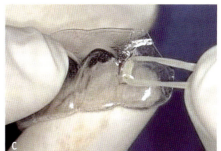

FIG 2-23 (a to c) A tab is cut into the Essix appliance for attachment of an elastic band.

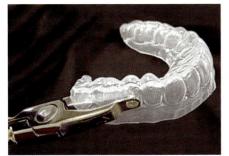
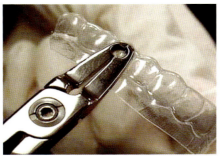
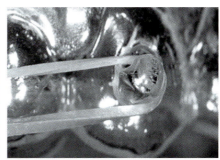

FIG 2-24a The initial heated plier thermoforms a cylinder into the appliance.

FIG 2-24b The second heated plier crimps the base of the cylinder to form an elastic attachment.

FIG 2-24c An elastic can be attached to the thermoformed button.

Intruding posterior teeth

Resolving excessively erupted posterior teeth with fixed appliances is biomechanically frustrating because, all things being equal, the simultaneous extrusion of adjacent teeth will be more evident than intrusion of the targeted teeth. This imbalance inevitably induces orthodontic complexities that can be avoided when intrusion is achieved with minimal, if any, effect on adjacent teeth. When intrusion or extrusion is indicated, an initial stage with an Essix appliance can reduce the complexities that are associated with trying to resolve the condition with fixed appliances.[11] Construction of the posterior intrusion appliance is described below.

The working cast is fabricated from die stone and subsequently trimmed to no more than 2.0 cm in height. Excessive undercuts, such as the three-cornered spaces that are gingival to contact points, are blocked out on the working cast with acrylic or stone.

Essix 1.0-mm C+ plastic is thermoformed over the unaltered cast, and the basic outline of the appliance is obtained by cutting the extraneous plastic away from the cast with a serrated metal disk. The plastic, gingival to the tooth to be intruded, is extended to give a plastic base for the elastic attachments. When the appliance is removed from the cast, the plastic outline is established with a curved Mayo scissors and extends 2 to 3 mm onto the gingival surface. The plastic covering the crown of the tooth to be intruded is then cut away.

A small rubber band (3/8 inches, 4.5 oz) exerting light force is secured to the facial and lingual tabs so that it crosses the crown of the extruded tooth. The rubber band is rotated to form an X. The rubber band, because of this configuration, does not slide into the interproximal area. The effectiveness of this appliance is apparent in Figs 2-25a and 2-25b.

The reciprocal force of the stretched elastic tends to unseat the appliance. Therefore, it is critical for the plastic to be well adapted to all retentive undercuts gingival to contact points. The retention potential of the appliance can be increased further by emphasizing the retentive undercuts gingival to contact points with a Hilliard thermoplier specifically designed for that purpose. Additionally, small composite mounds can be placed on the facial of selected teeth prior to making the impression. When the appliance is seated, it will snap over these composite mounds, and consequently form mechanical locks that will make the appliance resistant to displacement.

21

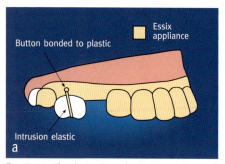
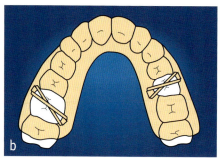

FIG 2-25 The intrusive elastic force is applied directly to the excessively extruded tooth. The effectiveness of the molar intrusion appliance is apparent. (*a*) Mechanics of the intrusion appliance. (*b*) Intrusion elastics in place.

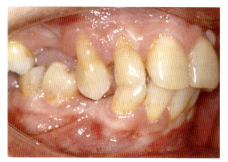
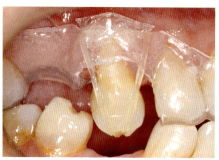
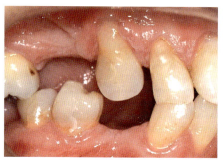

FIG 2-26a The right canine had excessively erupted until it was touching the tissue of the opposing side.

FIG 2-26b The elastic force directed a pure intrusion effect on the canine.

FIG 2-26c The canine was intruded into successful alignment without affecting the occlusal status of the bordering teeth.

The intrusion elastic is attached to the attachment tabs or buttons. Since intrusion requires light force, the elastic should induce no more than 50 to 75 g of force. Also, as the target tooth starts to intrude, any occlusal force on the rubber band is eliminated and the tendency for it to break is reduced.

The following case report illustrates the intrusive capabilities of an Essix appliance. This case involved full-mouth rehabilitation. The right maxillary canine had excessively erupted until it was touching the tissue in the opposing arch (Fig 2-26a). A full-arch Essix intrusion appliance was constructed from a 1.0-mm Essix C+ plastic sheet. An elastic-securing notch could be cut into the tip of the canine because a veneer was to be constructed during the prosthetic phase of the patient's treatment. Alternatively, composite mounds could be bonded on each side of the tip of the canine and would serve to stabilize the intrusive elastic.

To induce an intrusive force, elastic attachment tabs were cut into the periphery of the appliance, and an elastic was placed from these tabs over the notch on the canine (Fig 2-26b).

The appliance was worn for 3.5 months. The canine was intruded 4.5 mm while the occlusion of the remaining teeth was not disturbed (Fig 2-26c). The elastic attachment notches cut into the tip of the canine were reduced with a sandpaper disk to approximate normal morphology. The canine remained vital and the facial periodontal defect did not improve or worsen; however, a tissue graft was planned to resolve the facial periodontal defect.

Class II and Class III elastic applications

The biomechanical effects of Essix appliances are significantly increased when Class II or Class III elastics can be used to adjust arch relationships. A full-arch Essix appliance is required to support these elastics. Interarch elastics, in conjunction with removable plastic appliances, require two essentials: a method of attaching the elastics to the appliance, and a method of stabilizing the Essix appliance to counter the displacement effect of the elastic force.

In addition to the construction of elastic attachment methods previously described, a cemented band, or a bonded bracket can be used. Sokolina and Bloomstein,

FIG 2-27 (*right*) The bonded molar attachment is the base for the Class II elastic. The molar is encapsulated in the Essix appliance and is therefore resistant to displacement.

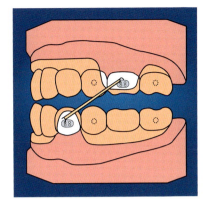
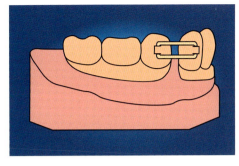

FIG 2-28 (*far right*) A stretched elastic between the sections of the Essix appliance creates the force necessary to close the buccal section space. A stretched elastic between the sections of an anterior Essix appliance induces enough force to close the midline diastema.

combining ARS and Essix anchor technology, first described this method.[12] It involves (1) bonding an attachment (bracket or button) to the facial surface of a tooth that is the base for the elastic vector (a hook on a cemented band would work as well), and (2) constructing the full-arch Essix appliance and cutting a facial window over the area of the bonded attachment (Fig 2-27). The appliance still covers the occlusal and lingual surfaces of the tooth that has the attachment bonded to it and, because of this configuration, the appliance counteracts any extrusive elastic force on the anchor tooth.

Closing spaces: Reopened buccal section extraction and anterior diastema spaces

Clinicians are frequently frustrated when an extraction site, diastema, or idiopathic spacing becomes evident during retention because no one is enthusiastic about another round of fixed appliances to correct the problem. The offending space can be quickly resolved with a modified Essix appliance. The advantages to the patient are that the device is unnoticeable and very thin (< 0.5 mm), it does not interfere with function, and it is not difficult to place.

The biomechanical principle of closing spaces with an Essix appliance is to induce an elastic force across the space to be closed without tipping the teeth into said space. To close a reopened extraction space or, for that matter, any relatively minor buccal section space, 0.040-inch Essix plastic is thermoformed over the full-arch working cast, and the cast is removed from the plastic by cutting around the periphery of the appliance with a serrated disk and prying it out of the plastic with a thin-bladed instrument. The resultant appliance is trimmed 2 to 3 mm above the gingival margin with a curved Mayo scissors, thereby incorporating the retentive undercuts that are gingival to

the interproximal contact points into the appliance. The technique used to close a reopened extraction site is described below.

The appliance is sectioned in the opened extraction space, which converts the Essix appliance into two pieces. (Or, to close reopened bilateral premolar extraction sites, for instance, one anterior and two posterior sections would be created.)

With the appliance placed, thin-walled elastics, approximately 0.25 in, 4.5 oz, are attached to the elastic attachment tabs on each side of the space (Fig 2-28). These relatively thin-walled elastics are stretched tightly and with enough force to move multiple roots bodily through bone.

The patient is instructed to change the elastics at least every 2 days. The appliance is to be cleaned with a toothbrush and water or a commercial retainer cleaner, but not with dentifrice. The abrasive particles in dentifrice dull the surface of the appliance and compromise its esthetic appeal.

Because the teeth are in slightly different positions after the extraction space is closed, it is advisable to equilibrate the occlusal surfaces to coordinate centric relation with centric occlusion.

Appliance construction to close a midline diastema

Midline diastemata are frequently the patient's chief complaint because this unsightly space is evident in the middle of his or her smile. Additionally, when retention instructions have not been followed, diastemata frequently reoccur. The offending space can be closed with a clear Essix appliance.

Presuming that the incisal spacing is not due to forces induced by the occlusion, the previously described procedure for closing extraction spaces with

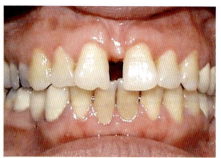
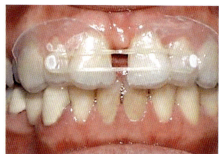
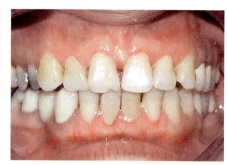

FIG 2-29a The midline diastema was the patient's chief complaint. (Figs 2-29a to 2-29c courtesy of Dr Anacar.)

FIG 2-29b The canine-to-canine plastic appliance was sectioned in the diastema area, and an elastic was stretched across the offending space.

FIG 2-29c The diastema was closed in 3 months; when the incisal edges of the central incisors are esthetically contoured, the esthetic improvement will be evident.

a sectioned Essix appliance and elastics can be applied to close a midline diastema. Following is the technique to be used.

A canine-to-canine Essix appliance, fabricated from 1.0-mm Essix plastic, is sectioned in the diastema space. Half of the appliance is placed on each side of the midline, and each section is extended 2 to 3 mm onto the gingiva. Previously described elastic attachment tabs are placed in the distal of each section. A clear thin-walled rubber band (approximately 0.25 in, 4.5 oz) is attached to the tabs and stretched tightly across the diastema space to create enough force, approximately 150 g, to bodily move the canine and lateral and central incisors on each side of the diastema through bone.

The appliance is worn full-time, with the exception of cleaning and eating, and the elastics are replaced every day. A diastema space of up to 3 mm should be closed within 5 or 6 weeks. At that time, the midline diastema will be closed but half of that space is now distal to the canines, and the teeth can move back into it. This redistributed space should be filled with a small composite thickness on the mesial of the first premolar or distal of the canine. This step may decrease the tendency for relapse. For additional retention, it would be advisable, bite permitting, to bond a lingual wire to the teeth on each side of the closed diastema. A conventional Essix retainer can be fabricated to fit over it to amplify the retention potential. And since the anterior bite will be slightly affected by the diastema closure, the anterior teeth should be equilibrated to assure balanced incisal coupling.

The following case report illustrates the effectiveness of Essix diastema-closing mechanics. This adult patient's chief complaint was the significant midline diastema (Fig

2-29a). A canine-to-canine Essix appliance was fabricated on the working cast, trimmed, and sectioned at the midline. An elastic with moderate force was secured to the elastic attachment tabs that were cut into the appliance (Fig 2-29b). The diastema was closed within 3 months (Fig 2-29c). Additional esthetic contouring of the incisal edges and composite bondings in the midline three-cornered space completed the esthetic treatment goal.

References

1. Sheridan JJ, LeDoux W, McMinn R. Essix retainers: Fabrication and supervision for permanent retention. J Clin Orthod 1993;27:37–45.
2. Sheridan JJ, LeDoux W, Robert MC. Essix appliances: Minor tooth movement with divots and windows. J Clin Orthod 1994;28:659–663.
3. Sheridan JJ, McMinn R, LeDoux W. Essix thermosealed appliances: Various orthodontic uses. J Clin Orthod 1995;29:108–113.
4. Sheridan JJ. Air-rotor stripping. J Clin Orthod 1985;19:43–59.
5. Sheridan JJ. Air-rotor stripping update. J Clin Orthod 1987;21:781–788.
6. Sheridan JJ. The physiologic rationale for air-rotor stripping. J Clin Orthod 1997;31:609–612.
7. el-Mangoury NH, Moussa MM, Mostafa YA, Girgis AS. In-vivo remineralization after air-rotor stripping. J Clin Orthod 1991;25:75–78.
8. Brudevold F, Tehrani A, Bakhos Y. Intraoral mineralization of abraded dental enamel. J Dent Res 1982;61:456–459.
9. Pinheiro ML. Interproximal enamel reduction. World J Orthod 2002;3:223–232.
10. Sheridan JJ, Armbruster P, Nguyen P, Pulitzer S. Tooth movement with Essix mounding. J Clin Orthod 2004;38:435–441.
11. Armbruster P, Sheridan JJ, Nguyen P. An Essix intrusion appliance. J Clin Orthod 2003;37:412–416.
12. Sokolina M, Bloomstein R. Air-rotor stripping technique for treatment of Class III malocclusion: Case report. World J Orthod 2002;3:233–238.

chapter 3

History and Overview of the Invisalign system

by
Trang Duong, DDS

Several major developments have changed the field of orthodontics in the second half of the 20th century. Digital imaging and computers, for example, have improved the diagnostic process. Similarly, the introduction of prescription brackets, bonding, glass-ionomer cements, and nickel titanium and other alloy wires have improved treatment efficiency and efficacy.

The latest technological advance in orthodontics is the Invisalign System, which combines the idea of using overlay appliances and the application of three-dimensional technology to move teeth (Figs 3-1a and 3-1b).

History of Overlay Appliances

Moving teeth with overlay appliances was popularized by Kesling, who in 1945 reported the use of a Vulcanite tooth-positioning appliance[1] (Fig 3-2). As early as 1926, however, Remensnyder had introduced the Flex-O-Tite gum-massaging appliance, with which he reported achieving minor tooth movements.[2] Since then, various types of overlay appliances, such as invisible retainers, have been used.[3–7] Following the approach of Nahoum (see chapter 1), Sheridan popularized the Raintree Essix technique of using clear aligners formed over plaster models[6] (see chapter 2).

History of Align Technology

Align Technology was founded in 1997 to develop the next-generation esthetic appliance. Invisalign takes the principles pioneered by Remensnyder, Kesling, Nahoum, Sheridan, and others and integrates CAD/CAM (computer-aided-design/computer-aided-manufacture) technology. This innovative approach combines orthodontic principles with three-dimensional computer and mass-customization technologies.[1,3–7] Advances and innovations in these technologies have further improved and enhanced the Invisalign System. This chapter tells the story of Invisalign: how it was conceived and how it has evolved.

The Invisalign Concept

Kelsey Wirth and Zia Chishti, two MBA students from Stanford University, founded Align Technology in April 1997. The concept on which the company was founded came from Chishti, who had undergone adult orthodontic treatment, but like many patients was not consistent in wearing his clear retainer. After experiencing recrowding of his mandibular teeth, Chishti returned to wearing his overlay retainer, and this realigned his anterior teeth. Frustrated with the relatively slow and modest progress achieved with his overlay retainer, Chishti came up with the idea of using multiple appliances and computer imaging technology to effect

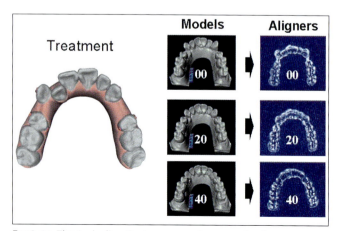

FIG 3-1a The Invisalign System generates gross tooth movements via a series of smaller tooth movements.

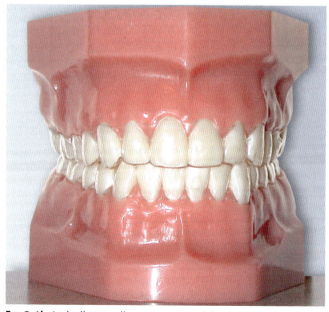

FIG 3-1b Invisalign appliances on a model.

major tooth movements. From this revolutionary concept, Chishti and Wirth, two orthodontists, along with a software engineer, formed Align Technology in a garage in Palo Alto, California. Today, the company is based in Santa Clara, California, employs over 800 employees, and has divisions in Europe, Mexico, and Costa Rica.

The Invisalign Process

The Invisalign process involves several steps. The first step is the acquisition of complete patient records from the treating orthodontist. Once received at Santa Clara, the records go through a series of steps from scanning to case setup and then back to the clinician for a review called ClinCheck (see chapter 11). The process of manipulating virtual tooth movements is completed when the clinician approves the ClinCheck. Once the ClinCheck is approved, the aligners are processed and sent to the clinician. Figure 3-3 shows the Invisalign process and the individual steps within the entire process from beginning to end.

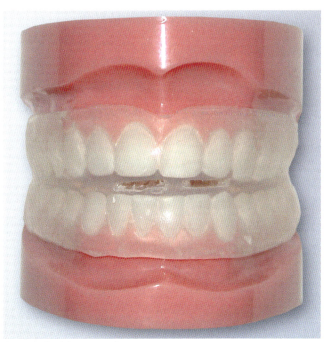

FIG 3-2 Positioner appliance.

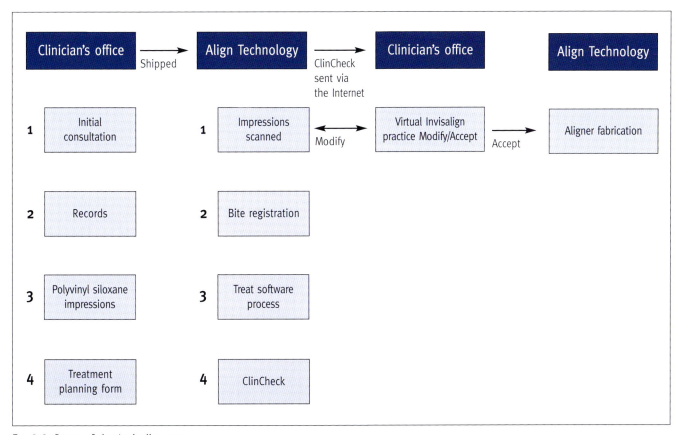

FIG 3-3 Steps of the Invisalign process.

Polyvinyl siloxane impressions

An essential component of the Invisalign process is getting an accurate representation of the teeth. When the Invisalign process was in development, several potential impression materials were tested, including alginate and various polyvinyl siloxane (PVS)–based materials. PVS was chosen because it provided the greatest degree of accuracy and stability. Today, PVS impressions are still required; however, the clinician can use the one- or two-step technique (Fig 3-4). Tests are currently in progress to evaluate an alginate-based material that can provide the accuracy and stability of PVS while allowing easier and more efficient handling.

Scanning

The first Invisalign patient's dental images were initially captured by laser scanning. By the time Invisalign was commercially launched, however, an altogether different

scanning technique was used: the PVS impressions were poured in dental plaster and encased with epoxy and urethane (Figs 3-5a to 3-5c). The models were destructively scanned with rotating blades that made numerous passes over the epoxy-encased models. After each pass, an image of the newly shaved surface was captured. A computer linked to the scanner then assembled the scan data to create a three-dimensional reconstruction of the models. Today, the impressions are scanned directly using a computerized tomography (CT) scanner, thereby bypassing the steps of pouring and encasing the models. This method greatly increased the efficiency of the scanning process. More information on the scanning process can be found in chapter 6.

Bite registration

To accurately capture the occlusion of the two arches together, a bite registration is required. The bite registration is based on centric occlusion because a virtual typodont with a virtual hinge axis is not currently available. The proper occlusal registration of the two arches is created using the bite registration material (Figs 3-6a and 3-6b).

Treat software

After the bite has been established, an Invisalign virtual orthodontic technician uses software to "cut" the virtual models and separate the teeth, thus allowing them to be moved individually. In 1997, because of the limitations of the software tools used to perform the cutting of the teeth, each virtual tooth had to be separated and

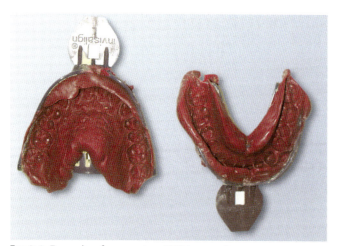

FIG 3-4 Example of a one-step PVS impression.

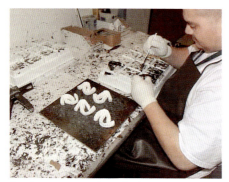

FIG 3-5a Preparation of plaster models for encasing in epoxy in preparation for early method of destructive scanning.

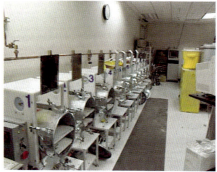

FIG 3-5b Machines used to encase the models.

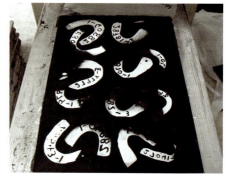

FIG 3-5c Plaster models after they have been encased in epoxy.

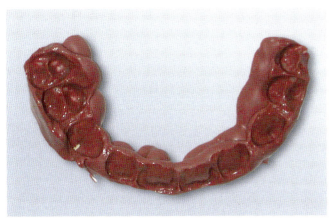

FIG 3-6a Polyvinyl siloxane registration material.

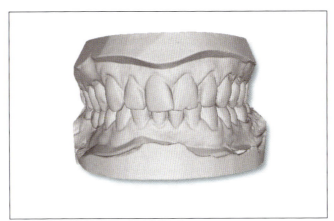

FIG 3-6b Bite registration.

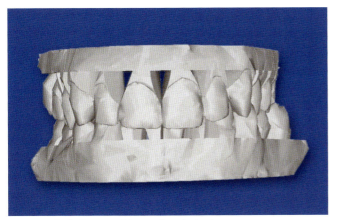

FIG 3-7a Early image with no virtual gingiva.

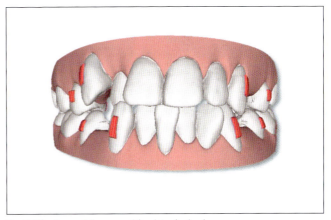

FIG 3-7b Current image with virtual gingiva.

sectioned, which was a time-consuming process. This process took about 48 hours for a single case. The resulting images were grainy and had defects. The file size for one case was about 10 MB. There was no virtual gingiva at this time, so the extension of the cuts was visible (Figs 3-7a and 3-7b). When the Invisalign process was in its earliest stages of development, the clinician was required to fill out not only a treatment planning form but also a staging form on which he or she indicated which teeth were to be moved and in what sequence. The clinician then sent the forms to the company. This approach demanded a great deal of time from the clinician, who was compelled to determine, based on the treatment goals, the best sequences for moving the teeth into the desired alignment. Today, the staging is done by Align Technology based on the clinician's treatment plan.

However, the clinician can still specify changes to the staging via ClinCheck. Once the case is set up and staged based on the clinician's prescription, the virtual data are converted to a ClinCheck file that can be sent electronical-

ly to the clinician's Virtual Invisalign Practice (VIP) website for review (see chapter 15). After reviewing the ClinCheck file, the clinician can either accept it (thus, authorize production and delivery of the aligners) or modify it by providing instructions through the VIP website (Figs 3-8a and 3-8b).

Aligner production

Once the clinician approves the ClinCheck, the three-dimensional computer images are converted to physical models using a process called rapid prototyping. Specifically, stereolithography is the rapid prototyping technology used to create the models (Fig 3-9). These models are still used to fabricate the aligners on a Biostar (Scheu-Dental) pressure-molding machine (Figs 3-10 and 3-11). Previously, the aligners were manually trimmed, laser-etched, disinfected, packaged, and sent to the clinician. Today, the trimming process is performed robotically on a mechanical five-axis milling machine.

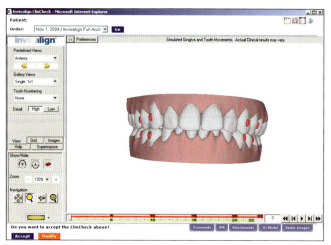

FIG 3-8a ClinCheck virtual image.

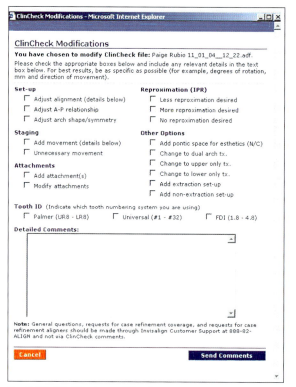

FIG 3-8b ClinCheck modification page.

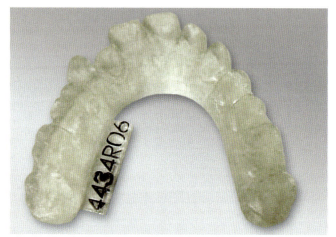

FIG 3-9 Stereolithography model.

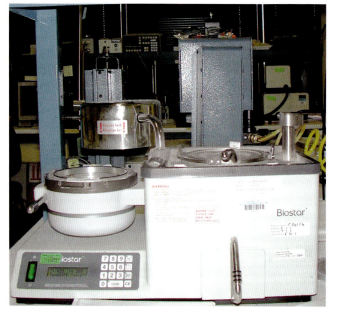

FIG 3-10 Biostar machine used to fabricate the aligners.

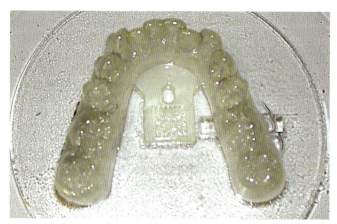

FIG 3-11 Pressure-formed aligner over the stereolithographic model.

Invisalign Patents

Given the unique and innovative nature of the Invisalign System, Align Technology filed patents to protect the Invisalign technology. Align Technology, Inc, holds approximately 60 patents covering a wide range of techniques for scanning teeth and designing and manufacturing removable dental appliances. The patents also cover computer techniques for modeling dental structures and compressing and transmitting the dental data to the orthodontist and general practioner's workstation through ClinCheck. Patents range from defining tooth-moving appliances computationally to methods and systems for incrementally moving teeth.

Invisalign: The Future

The concept of moving teeth with clear overlay appliances has been around since 1926. Align Technology, however, is the first company to incorporate modern technology in a way that makes this concept a feasible, viable, efficient, and effective orthodontic treatment option. Without the innovative computer technology and advanced manufacturing processes, which are the hallmarks of the Invisalign System,

it would be extremely difficult—if not impossible—to produce aligners in such large numbers and with such great accuracy.

The Invisalign process has evolved and improved since 1997, and even today continues to change and adapt to better meet the needs of clinicians and their patients. In the chapters that follow, each step in the Invisalign process will be discussed in detail to provide information on the technology behind this innovative process.

References

1. Kesling HD. The philosophy of the tooth-positioning appliance. J Dent Res 1945;31:297.
2. Remensnyder O. A gum-massaging appliance in the treatment of pyorrhea. Dent Cosmos 1926;28:381–384.
3. Nahoum H. The vacuum-formed dental contour appliance. N Y State Dent J 1964;9:385–390.
4. Pontiz RJ. Invisible retainers. J Dent Res 1971;59:266–271.
5. McNamara JA Jr, Kramer KL, Juenker JP. Invisible retainers. J Clin Orthod 1985;19:570–578.
6. Sheridan J, LeDoux W, McMinn R. Essix retainers: Fabrication and supervision for permanent retention. J Clin Orthod 1993;27:37–45.
7. Rinchuse DJ, Rinchuse DJ. Active tooth movement with Essix-based appliances. J Clin Orthod 1997;31:109–112.

SECTION II

MODELING IN THE INVISALIGN SYSTEM

chapter 4

POLYVINYL SILOXANE IMPRESSION MATERIALS

by
John M. Powers, PhD

Impression materials are used to accurately record the dimensions and spatial relationships of oral tissues.[1] Alginate hydrocolloid impression materials have been used for many years in orthodontics to produce study models. Improvements in alginates have allowed the orthodontist to send alginate impressions to the dental laboratory for fabrication of study models. However, for increased accuracy and durability of full-arch impressions, elastomeric impression materials, such as addition silicone and polyether, are used. Desirable features of elastomeric impression materials include[2]:

- Appropriate consistencies (tray, wash, monophase) for the desired technique
- Ease of use (automix with static or dynamic delivery)
- Lack of taste or odor
- Wetting of the tissues without bubbles
- Quick setting to minimize deformation in the mouth
- Flexibility (easy to remove from the mouth)
- High elastic recovery on removal from the mouth
- Excellent detail reproduction
- Ease of disinfection
- Long-term dimensional stability

Wax bite registrations are traditional but are highly susceptible to distortion on removal from the mouth and during storage.[3] Elastomeric bite-registration materials offer improved accuracy and dimensional stability. Desirable features of elastomeric bite-registration materials include:

- Ease of use (automix cartridge)
- Adequate working time with quick setting in the mouth
- Resistance to deformation
- Long-term dimensional stability[4]

Types, Composition, and Setting

Silicones

Addition silicone (polyvinyl siloxane, PVS) impression materials are most commonly used in the dental office, whereas the older condensation silicones are primarily used in the dental laboratory for duplicating procedures. Examples of commercial addition silicone impression materials and their manufacturers are listed in Table 4-1.

Addition silicones are available as two pastes or putties, one of which is the base and the other the catalyst. Many consistencies are available, including light (syringe, wash), medium (tray), monophase, heavy, and putty. In most instances, the two pastes are mixed from a cartridge using an automix gun with static mixing tips or a benchtop dynamic mixer (MixStar, Zenith/DMG; Pentamix 2, 3M ESPE). Two-putty systems are usually mixed by hand-kneading, but injectable putties are now available. The newest addition silicones contain nonionic surfactants that achieve increased wettability of the dental tissues. Many products are available in regular and rapid-set formulations.

The polymerization reaction of addition silicones occurs between vinyl and hydrogen groups with no by-product being formed, so the addition silicones are dimensionally stable. Latex rubber gloves contain sulfur compounds that adversely affect the setting reaction of addition silicones.[5]

TABLE 4-1 Impression materials by type, product name, and manufacturer	
Product	**Manufacturer**
Addition silicone	
Affinis	Coltène/Whaledent
Aquasil Ultra	Dentsply/Caulk
Correct Plus	Pentron Clinical Technologies
Examix NDS	GC America
Flexitime	Heraeus Kulzer
1st Impression	Den-Mat
Genie	Sultan Chemists
Honigum	Zenith/DMG
Imprint II Penta	3M ESPE
Splash	Discus Dental
Standout	SDS Kerr
Take 1	SDS Kerr
Virtual	Ivoclar Vivadent
Polyethers	
Impregum Penta Soft	3M ESPE
P2	Heraeus Kulzer
Alginate substitute	
Dimension Penta	3M ESPE
Alginates	
Identic	DUX
Jeltrate	Dentsply/Caulk
Kromopan	LASCOD

These compounds can be transferred to the teeth and soft tissues during preparation for the impression. Vinyl gloves should be used to avoid contamination. The teeth and soft tissues can be rinsed with 2% chlorhexidine to remove contaminants if needed.

Polyethers

Polyether impression materials are available in light, medium, and heavy consistencies. Mixing can be done by hand, using an automix gun with a static mixing tip, or by using a benchtop dynamic mixer. There is no volatile by-product during polymerization of the polyether. Contamination with water can cause an expansion of the setting material and should be avoided. Examples of commercial polyether impression materials and their manufacturers are listed in Table 4-1.

Alginates

Alginate impression materials can be mixed by hand or by a mixing machine (Alginator, Cadco). Because alginates are hydrogels, they shrink on storage as a result of syneresis and evaporation. Disinfection can be accomplished by either spray or immersion. Examples of commercial alginate impression materials and their manufacturers are listed in Table 4-1.

Alginate substitute

An alginate substitute (actually an addition silicone) is available from several manufacturers (see Table 4-1). This material is mixed by a bench-top dynamic mixer.

Properties of Elastomeric Impression Materials and Their Clinical Relevance

A number of physical and mechanical properties affect the performance of impression materials (Table 4-2).[3,6]

Working and setting times

Working time is a measure of the maximum time available before the impression should be seated in the mouth. Setting time is a measure of how long the impression must remain in the mouth before removal can occur. The accuracy of an impression may decrease if the impression is removed from the mouth too early. A snap set will minimize distortion while the impression is in the mouth. A slight improvement in accuracy may result from leaving the impression in the mouth for an additional 30 seconds beyond the manufacturer's recommendation.

Detail reproduction and wettability

Detail reproduction is influenced by the viscosity of the impression material and its ability to wet the tooth structure and soft tissues, especially in the presence of moisture. Wettability is best with a hydrophilic impression material that forms a low contact angle (20 to 60 degrees) with tooth structure. Poor wetting results in bubbles and voids, often requiring that the impression be remade. Addition silicones are formulated to be hydrophilic by the addition of surfactants or by modification of

TABLE 4-2 Properties of addition silicone, polyether, and alginate impression materials			
Property	**Addition silicone***	**Polyether**	**Alginate**
Working time (min)	0.5–5.0	2.5–3.3	1.2–4.5
Setting time (min)	2.0–4.0	3.3	1.5–5.0
Wettability of tissues	Good to fair	Good	Good
Shrinkage on setting (%) 24 hours	0.08–0.40	0.07–0.27	0.6–2.7
1 week	0.08–0.40	0.21–0.55	Not recommended
Flexibility during removal (%)	2.0–11.0	2.5–8.5	14.0
Elastic recovery (%)	98.9–99.9	98.2–99.7	95.7–96.4
Detail reproduction	Excellent	Excellent	Good

*Alginate substitute has similar properties to addition silicone.

the polymer structure. Polyether impression materials are naturally hydrophilic. In general, light-bodied impression materials provide better detail reproduction than other consistencies.

Flexibility

Flexibility is a measure of the ease of removal of the impression from the mouth. An impression that is stiff may become locked into undercuts in the oral structure and be difficult to remove.

Elastic recovery

When an impression is removed from the mouth, it is subjected to tensile and compressive forces that could result in distortion. The set impression must be sufficiently elastic that it will return to its original dimensions with minimal distortion (< 2%).

Dimensional stability

Dimensional change (shrinkage) occurs when an impression material sets and may increase during the time the impression is stored. At 24 hours, the shrinkage of addition silicones and polyethers is similar. After 1 week, the shrinkage of addition silicones does not change much, but the shrinkage of polyethers increases. Some addition silicone impressions are sufficiently stable that a second gypsum cast can be made several weeks after the impression is made.

Manipulation of Elastomeric Impression Materials

Several steps must be taken to achieve a quality impression. Troubleshooting the impression after removal from the mouth can save time and money in the event that the impression needs to be remade (Table 4-3). There are a number of strategies dental assistants and clinicians can use to improve impressions (Box 4-1). Figures 4-1a to 4-1d show an example of an unusable impression.

Selection of a tray

Full-arch trays are available in metal or plastic. A tray of proper dimensions and extension should be selected. The tray can be extended with wax if needed. A rigid tray is desirable to minimize distortion during the impression procedure. It is best to use a rigid tray even if the impression material itself is rigid. The Invisalign System provides plastic mandibular and maxillary trays.

Tray adhesive

Both addition silicone and polyether impression materials require a tray adhesive for metal and plastic trays. The adhesives vary with the type of impression material and are not interchangeable. Although some trays have perforations and other retention modes, use of a tray adhesive can minimize distortion when the impression is removed from the mouth. The tray adhesive should be allowed to dry before the impression material is added.

TABLE 4-3 Troubleshooting orthodontic impressions	
Criteria for a good impression	**Troubleshooting tips**
Impression uniformly mixed	Make sure dispensing tips (base and catalyst) of automix cartridge are open.
Impression supported by the tray	Make sure impression material is uniformly distributed in the tray. Extend the tray with wax if necessary.
No visible defects	Make sure there are no voids or tears.
Impression adheres to tray	Make sure the impression has not detached from the tray, or the impression will be distorted.

BOX 4-1 Tips for improving impressions

Tips for dental assistants
- Apply the proper adhesive to the tray and allow it to dry completely.
- Make sure the tips of the automix cartridge are open.
- Minimize bubbles when loading the impression tray.
- Pay attention to working times to achieve desired viscosity and detail.

Tips for clinicians
- Select a tray of adequate size and extension. Ensure that the tray allows space for 2 to 4 mm of impression material. Provide occlusal stops if needed.
- Avoid touching the teeth with latex gloves. Chemicals in the latex can prevent the silicone from setting.
- Seat the impression in a timely fashion. Minimize movement of the tray after seating to minimize distortion.
- Do not remove the tray too early, to minimize distortion.
- Remove the tray with a uniform motion to minimize distortion; do not rock or twist the tray.

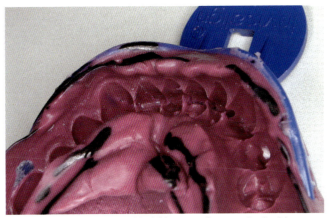

FIG 4-1a Minute voids and bubbles are often overlooked because they might be covered by salivary bubbles.

mixers are cost effective when multiple impressions are made daily.

The tips of the cartridges must be open for the base and catalyst pastes to dispense properly for mixing. Improper mixing of the catalyst and base may result in a poor impression (Figs 4-2a and 4-2b).

Mixing the material

Nearly all addition silicones are available in 50-mL automix cartridges; some products are provided in 75-mL cartridges. Benchtop dynamic mixers utilize large cartridges that contain 360 mL or more of material. The benchtop

Impression techniques

- *One-step technique (monophase)*: The shear thinning property of the monophase consistency allows the impression material to be placed into the tray with minimal slumping.
- *Double-mix technique (tray/wash)*: A wash material is injected around the teeth using a syringe, and the tray filled with a heavy-bodied material is placed.

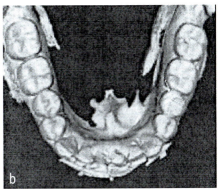
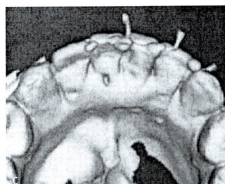
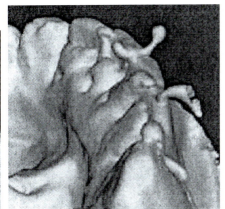

FIG 4-1 (*cont*) (*b*) The scanned image discloses the defects in the impression in the Align return report. As much as Align Technology is reluctant to reject impressions, this impression is not usable. (*c and d*) Closeup views of the scanned image.

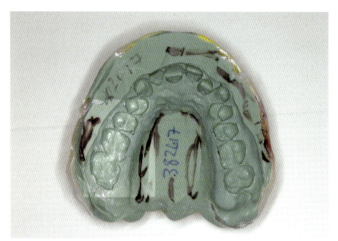

Fig 4-2a At times, the catalyst does not mix in well when the clinician first presses the button on the bench-top automix. It is advised for a modicum of paste to be expelled before the tray is filled. Failure to do so will create nondescript, bubblelike topography.

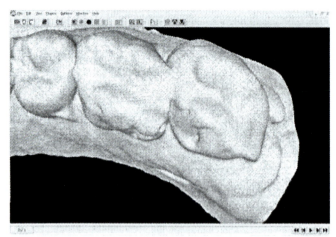

Fig 4-2b The Align return report reveals that the corresponding scanned image lacks detail around these molar teeth. If this impression were to be used, the aligner tray would not fit properly.

• *Two-step technique (tray/wash)*: A preliminary impression is made with the heavy-bodied material (medium consistency or injectable putty) with a cellophane spacer on top. Wash material is added (after removal of the spacer) to the preliminary impression for the final impression. The best accuracy can be achieved by using a tray/wash technique.

Removal and trimming of impressions

Before the impression can be removed, the seal must be broken in the posterior area. The impression can then be removed—a firm, steady motion is best. Unsupported areas of the impression should be trimmed to minimize distortion.

Disinfection of impressions

A variety of disinfectants is available, including neutral glutaraldehyde, acidified glutaraldehyde, neutral phenolated glutaraldehyde, phenol, iodophor, and chlorine dioxide. Addition silicone impressions can be disinfected by immersion per the manufacturer's directions.[7] Polyether impressions can change dimensions on immersion in some disinfectants, so only short times (2 to 3 minutes) in chlorine-type disinfectants are recommended for polyether impressions. Some clinicians prefer to disinfect polyether impressions by a spray-and-wipe technique.

Table 4-4 Addition silicone bite-registration materials by product and manufacturer	
Product	**Manufacturer**
Imprint Bite	3M ESPE
Exabite II NDS	GC America
Genie Bite Registration	Sultan Chemists
Memoreg 2	Heraeus Kulzer
Occlufast Rock	Zhermack
Perfectim Systems 30 Second Blue Velvet	J. Morita
Regisil Rigid	Dentsply/Caulk
Registrado X-tra	Voco

BOX 4-2 Tips for improving bite registrations
Tip for dental assistants
• Make sure the tips of the automix cartridge are open.
Tips for clinicians
• Use trays to improve accuracy.
• Avoid use of excess bite-registration material to minimize rebound.
• Trim carefully since the material is brittle.

Bite registration

Addition silicone bite-registration material is injected using a syringe with a broad tip. Use of a tray improves accuracy. Setting times of addition silicone bite-registration materials vary from 40 to 60 seconds. A number of commercial addition silicone bite-registration materials are available (Table 4-4). Tips for the dental assistant and the clinician for improving bite registrations are listed in Box 4-2.

References

1. Anusavice KJ (ed). Phillip's Science of Dental Materials, ed 11. St Louis: Saunders, 2003.
2. Farah JW, Powers JM (eds). Elastomeric impression materials. Dent Advisor 2003;20(10):2–4.
3. Powers JM, Sakaguchi RL. Craig's Restorative Dental Materials, ed 12. St Louis: Mosby, 2006.
4. Farah JW, Powers JM (eds). Elastomeric bite registration materials. Dent Advisor 2004;21(3):5.
5. Baumann MA. The influence of dental gloves on the setting of impression materials. Br Dent J 1995;179(4):130–135.
6. Lu H, Nguyen B, Powers JM. Mechanical properties of 3 hydrophilic addition silicone and polyether elastomeric impression materials. J Prosthet Dent 2004;92:151–154.
7. Drennon DG, Johnson GH. The effect of immersion disinfection of elastomeric impressions on the surface detail reproduction of improved gypsum casts. J Prosthet Dent 1990;63:233–241.

chapter 5

Align's Standard on Quality Impressions

by
David Chenin, DDS

Making the polyvinyl siloxane (PVS) impression is the most critical stage in the treatment process. A good impression helps to ensure proper identification of tooth anatomy and the manufacture of aligners that fit. After the impression is scanned (see chapter 6), it is inspected by Align technicians. Thus, it is the virtual three-dimensional positive of the impression that is inspected. Technicians are trained and tested in specific protocols and standards. The primary reference used gives technicians who inspect PVS impressions defined visual criteria for the acceptance or rejection of an impression. The clinician's and patient's perspectives are always kept in mind during the inspection process.

The rejection of an impression is taken very seriously. All options and considerations are taken into account and attempted prior to the rejection of an impression. Some of the major areas that are evaluated include the following:

- The impression extends more than 2 mm beyond the free gingival margin (cementoenamel junction if recession is present) on the buccal and lingual surfaces. When high-quality intraoral photographs are provided by the treating clinician, occurrences of small discrepancies along the gingival border can be restored by the technician (Figs 5-1a and 5-1b).

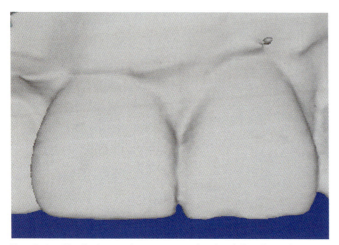

FIG 5-1a Gingival margins are not clearly defined in the scan image.

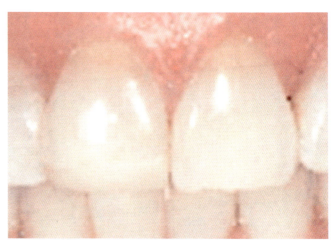

FIG 5-1b Clinical photographs aid the technician in drawing the gingival border.

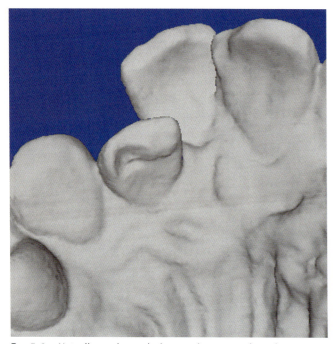

FIG 5-2a Not all poorly made impressions are rejected.

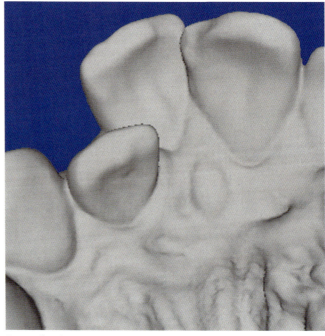

FIG 5-2b The same image after reshaping and smoothing.

- Distortions, bubbles, voids, and wrinkles of teeth are reshaped if they are less than 2 to 3 mm, depending on the location and if the surrounding contours are clearly visible (Figs 5-2a and 5-2b). To properly restore the correct anatomy, high-quality intraoral photographs provided by the treating clinician are critical.
- Incomplete capture of terminal molars may be addressed by trimming away the distal portion of the tooth, which eliminates the part of the tooth where the distortion lies (Figs 5-3a and 5-3b). This may only be possible if the treatment plan outlined on the prescription and diagnosis form allows. For example, the dis-

torted molar may be trimmed if no distalization is requested, no premolar extraction is requested, if the case is for anterior treatment only, if the arch is not being treated, or if the prescription indicates extraction of the distorted tooth.
- More significant distortions may be accepted if the arch is not being treated, since the opposing arch is being used primarily to set the occlusal bite relationship (Fig 5-4).

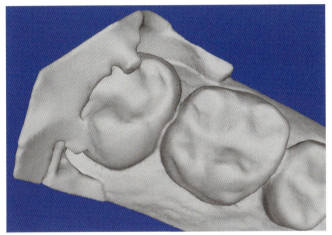

FIG 5-3a The distal side of the second molar is not provided in the impression.

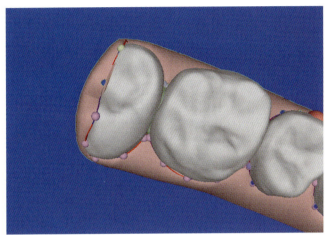

FIG 5-3b The aligner can be created only for the portion of the dentition represented in the image.

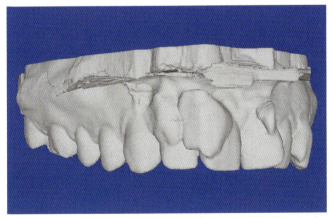

FIG 5-4 This impression is very poor but is usable if only the mandibular arch is being treated. Occlusal surfaces of teeth are adequate to occlude the maxillary and mandibular arches.

chapter 6

Scanning Process and Stereolithography

by
Srinivas Kaza

The term *image acquisition* (or *scanning*) is used to describe the process of converting a physical object into three-dimensional (3-D) electronic data. The scanning process is used in various applications ranging from reverse engineering to nondestructive or destructive testing. Methods and technology of image acquisition have made remarkable progress over the last few years. The Invisalign System uses state-of-the-art scanning technology to accurately capture tooth geometry. This chapter outlines the evolution of scanning technology at Align Technology.

Laser Scanning

Laser scanning was the first scanning technology used by the Invisalign System. In laser scanning, a laser beam is projected on the object being scanned, and the reflection of the beam is recorded. The object being scanned is rotated to several predetermined positions so that multiple views can be recorded. The recordings made from these different views are incorporated together to produce a 3-D electronic image of the object. This scanning technique is one of the most widely used for a variety of applications and is offered by several companies. The scanner used in the Invisalign System was made by Cyberware, located in Monterey, California. During the time laser scanning was used with Invisalign, it posed

certain challenges—for example, acquisition speed and the ability to capture undercuts and small interproximal spaces. In an effort to improve on these aspects, Align Technology turned to the use of destructive scanning technology.

Destructive Scanning

In destructive scanning, cross-sectional information of an object is captured and used to construct a 3-D image. The technique is undertaken as follows (Fig 6-1):

1. Plaster casts are poured for the impressions submitted.
2. The plaster casts are detailed by a lab technician to remove any defects and/or reconstruct partially missing information (see chapter 5).
3. Multiple plaster casts are placed on a plate and encased in a black polymer. The polymer is allowed to solidify, encasing the plaster models in it.
4. The encased block is mounted on a milling machine, and a thin section is sliced off the top.
5. The object is moved to a camera system to capture a two-dimensional view of the top.
6. Additional cross sections are milled and scanned. The process is repeated until the bottom of the object is reached.

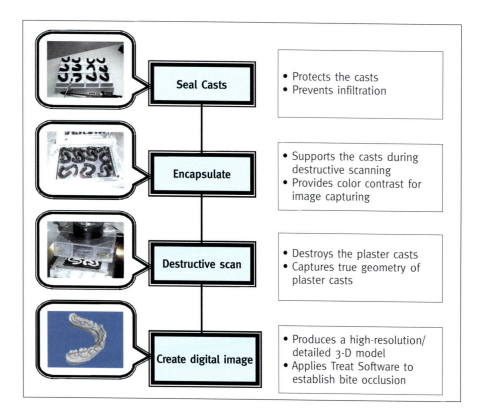

FIG 6-1 Destructive scanning process.

7. Postprocessing software identifies the plaster casts using the contrast between the white plaster casts and the black encasement material. The images of plaster on each layer are then aligned and stacked together to create a 3-D image of the plaster casts being scanned.

Destructive scanning is one of the best methods available to capture intricate geometries, undercuts, and the like. The process of preparing a plaster cast for scanning, however, can be messy, time-consuming, and expensive. For the Invisalign System, the main problems revolved around time, cost, and the fact that the cast is destroyed (necessitating the pouring of two casts, which further increases the cost).

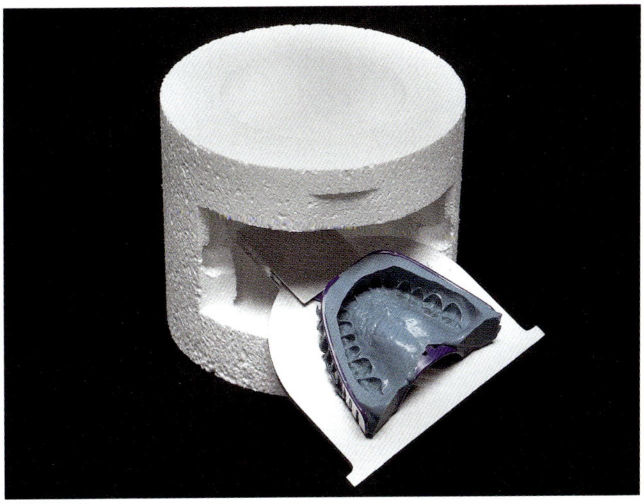

FIG 6-2 Impressions placed in foam fixture.

White-Light Scanning

White-light scanning uses a white-light pattern to capture images of the object being scanned. A pattern of white light (most commonly used is the moiré pattern) is projected on the object, and the reflection is captured by a camera. The captured image is stored, and the process is repeated with the object at a different orientation relative to the camera. Several images are taken at various positions, and the views are then aligned and combined to create a 3-D image of the object.

White-light and laser scanning are the most popular scanning technologies available. For a time, Align Technology utilized white-light scanning in conjunction with destructive-scanning technology. Although this combination of scanning methods offered high accuracy and resolution, the Invisalign System required an imaging technique capable of providing even greater detail to capture deep undercuts and small interproximal gaps. This prompted the move to computerized tomography (CT) technology.

Computerized Tomography

CT uses X-rays to scan an object. A set of impressions is loaded onto a fixture (Fig 6-2) and mounted on a rotary table in the scanner. X-rays are then beamed onto the target. The X-rays pass through the impressions, and the resulting image is captured by a detector positioned behind the impressions. The rotary table is then rotated by a small angle, and another image is captured. Multiple

images are acquired at high speed and stored. Postprocessing software is used to extract information about the teeth, based on the attenuation of the X-ray beams that pass through the impression. CT scanning allows the direct scanning of an impression, thereby eliminating the intermediate step of pouring a plaster cast (Figs 6-3a and 6-3b).

Rapid Manufacturing of Molds

Rapid manufacturing is a term used to describe processes that can fabricate complex geometries in a matter of hours without any tooling. Rapid manufacturing techniques typically involve layered manufacturing processes where objects are produced one layer at a time. The rapid manufacturing process currently used at Align Technology is known as *stereolithography* (SLA) (Figs 6-4 and 6-5). In SLA, a solid object is constructed by curing the part in layers. A 3-D electronic representation (computer-assisted design [CAD] model) of the object to be built is first divided into thin cross sections. The cross-sectional information is then transferred to the SLA machine.

The machine has a vat of liquid photopolymer that cures when exposed to light of a certain wavelength. A laser beam at this wavelength is then used to cure the bottom-most cross section of the object. A layer of liquid photopolymer is then applied on top of the cured layer, and the next layer is cured on top using the laser. The process is repeated until the last layer is cured, resulting in the desired solid object.

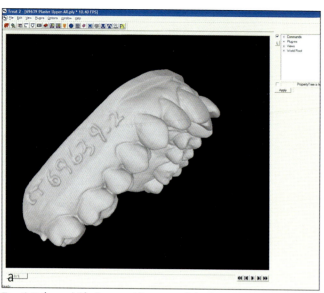
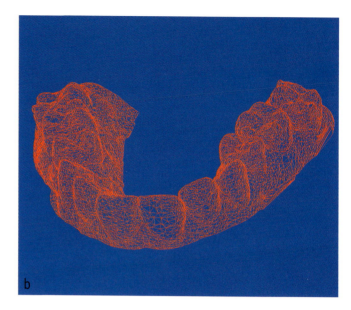

FIG 6-3 (a and b) Scanned images of the impression.

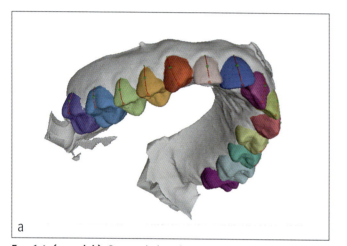
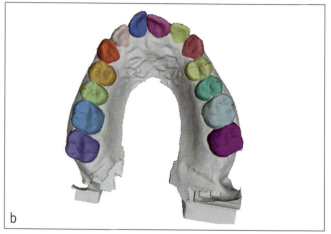

FIG 6-4 (a and b) Scanned data is segmented using the ToothShaper process. (See chapters 7 and 8 for a detailed explanation of ToothShaper.)

SLA Technology and the Invisalign System

The first step in the production of an aligner is the acceptance of the planned treatment by the submitting clinician through ClinCheck (see chapter 11). A clinician's acceptance of the proposed treatment triggers Invisalign's internal information systems. The case information—such as patient information, number of stages in the maxillary and mandibular jaw treatment, tooth movements, attachment designs, and the like—are fed into the custom software designed for the Invisalign SLA system. Subsequently, the treatment files are converted into a triangulated file format. The software then lays out the various cases within the build area of the SLA machines (currently 500 × 500

mm) to optimize space utilization. The electronic data are separated into multiple slices of a specified thickness. The slice data are then transferred to the SLA machine for manufacturing. The SLA molds are built on a platform that is located about one-slice thickness below the resin surface. The first layer from the bottom is then drawn by a laser (Figs 6-6a and 6-6b).

The photosensitive resin cures and turns solid upon contact with the laser beam. Once the first layer is completely traced, the build platform moves down a distance equivalent to the thickness of one layer. The second layer is then traced and cured on top of the previous layer. The process is repeated until the top of the object is reached. At the end of the process, the build platform consists of the molds; the rest of the photopolymer in the vat remains liquid.

Fig 6-5 SLA build process. (Images courtesy of Hong Kong Polytechnic University.)

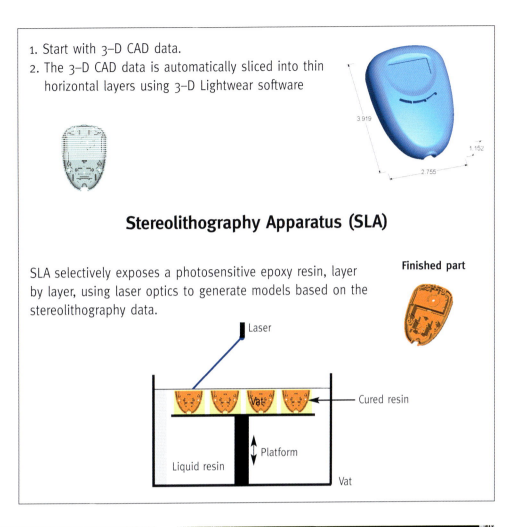

1. Start with 3–D CAD data.
2. The 3–D CAD data is automatically sliced into thin horizontal layers using 3–D Lightwear software

Stereolithography Apparatus (SLA)

SLA selectively exposes a photosensitive epoxy resin, layer by layer, using laser optics to generate models based on the stereolithography data.

Finished part

Laser

Cured resin

Platform

Liquid resin

Vat

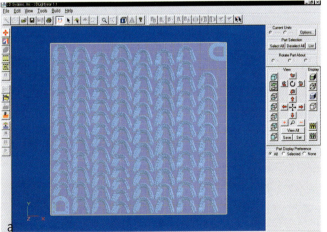

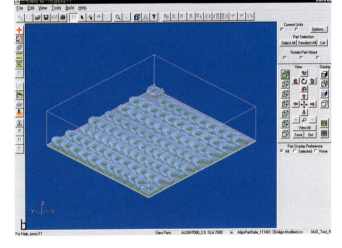

Fig 6-6 (a and b) Patient data layout on an SLA tray.

After the process is complete, the build platform that contains the molds is removed from the machine and transferred to an automated postprocessing line (Fig 6-7). In postprocessing, the platform is first spun at high speeds to remove any excess liquid resin on the molds. Upon completion of the spin, the platform is automatically loaded into a wash system that uses high-pressure water to clean the molds of any remaining uncured resin and debris. The platform is then automatically transferred to an ultraviolet (UV) curing station. The molds are exposed to specific wavelengths of high-intensity UV light that completely cures them. The molds are then automatically transferred to a

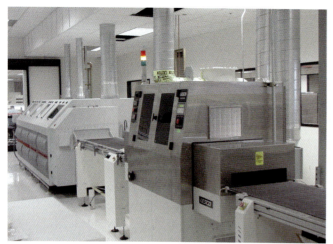

FIG 6-7 Postprocessing system for SLA molds.

mold-and-support-removal machine that removes the molds from the platform and cleans them to ensure that no debris remains on the molds. The molds are then packaged and shipped to the facility in Mexico for the aligner fabrication process (Fig 6-8).

An SLA mold created at Align has some embedded tracking features in it. First, readable text is engraved on the side of the mold to indicate the patient identification and the stage number (Fig 6-9a). Second, each SLA mold has two-dimensional bar code information (commonly known as the data matrix), which contains similar information (Fig 6-9b). The bar code is used by the automation processes to automatically detect the information on the mold and direct the part accordingly.

Aligner Fabrication

Aligner fabrication represents the back end of the process, whereby a sheet of plastic is formed over the SLA molds, trimmed, removed from the mold, polished, and packaged.

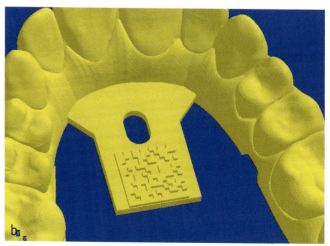

FIG 6-8 Fabricated SLA molds.

The process of creating an aligner starts when the SLA molds are received in the forming area. Upon arrival in the forming area, the molds go through an automated marking machine where the two-dimensional data matrix is hot-stamped with black ink to provide contrast that allows bar code readers to process the information. Next, the molds are sprayed with an organic silicone release agent to help with the aligner removal process after forming (Fig 6-10). Each mold is then read with a bar code reader to ensure that the information can be accurately read and verified.

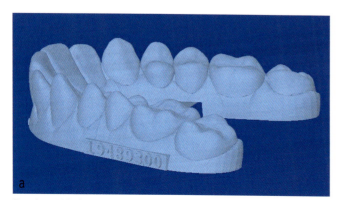

FIG 6-9 Side-lettering identification feature (*a*) and two-dimensional bar code information (*b*).

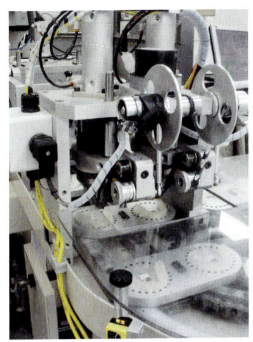

FIG 6-10 SLA molds are loaded onto a machine that reads the bar code information and applies a release agent for forming.

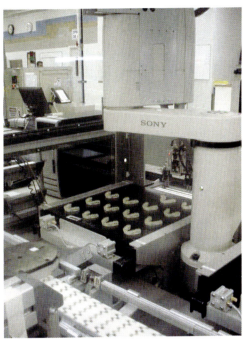

FIG 6-11 SLA molds being processed in an automation line.

The molds are then placed on a 20 5 20–inch pallet and loaded onto a conveyer line. The pallets are routed to an automated forming machine (Figs 6-11 and 6-12). Each SLA mold is picked up from the pallet by a robot. Prior to further processing, the bar code is read by a reader. Once the read is complete, plastic is formed on the SLA mold. This plastic mold then goes under a laser marker, which downloads information from the network as to where to place the aligner information for that particular aligner (for each aligner, the Invisalign software automatically creates and stores a marking box that indicates where the aligner can be marked without compromising its esthetic quality).

After the forming and marking process is complete, the molds are automatically routed to one of several five-axis trimming machines (Fig 6-13). Of course, prior to loading on the trimming machines, the relevant cut information (based on the bar code) is downloaded into the trimming machine. This information indicates where the gingival line is located for that particular stage, thus ensuring that the trimming machine cuts along a line that produces an accurate aligner fit. A robot loads the mold onto the trimming machine, and the cutter trims the aligner along the specified path (Fig 6-14). Upon completion of the trimming process, the aligners are removed from the SLA molds and transferred to a tumbling/deburring machine that removes most of the aligner's

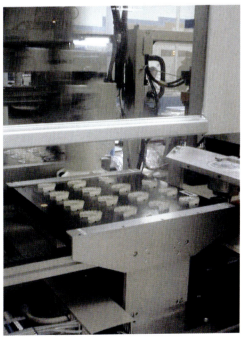

FIG 6-12 SLA molds being loaded onto the forming machine.

sharp edges (Fig 6-15). After the tumbling cycle is complete, each aligner is hand finished and polished to ensure that no sharp edges remain (Fig 6-16). The aligners are then disinfected in an ultrasonic bath to ensure they are safe to

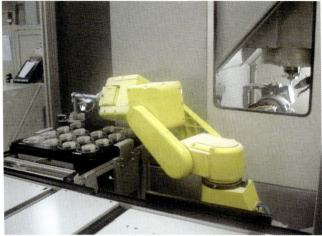

FIG 6-13 After forming, the formed parts are loaded onto a five-axis cutting machine for aligner trimming.

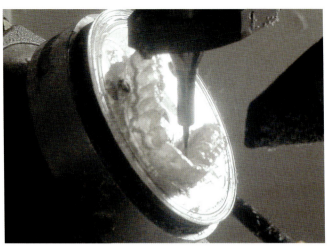

FIG 6-14 Aligner trimming process.

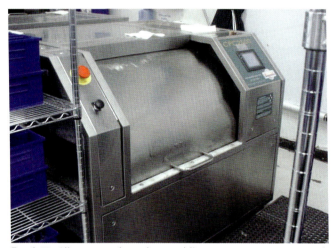

FIG 6-15 Aligners go through a tumbling process to remove rough edges.

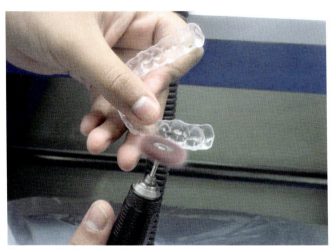

FIG 6-16 Final trim and polish by hand.

wear. This is the final product that is now ready to ship (Fig 6-17). At the end of the disinfection cycle, the aligners are removed and placed and sealed in Invisalign packaging. The packages are then shipped to the prescribing clinician.

Summary

The manufacturing systems described above produce aligners that perform well. Further streamlining of the process, however, has the potential to expedite the process. To this point, clinicians can look forward to self-starting machines, self-diagnosing machines, pallet changer and conveyer systems, automated postprocessing systems, and part tracking and work flow routing.

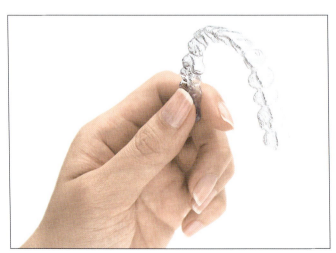

FIG 6-17 Final product.

chapter 7

INVISALIGN SOFTWARE

by
Andrew Beers, PhD

From Invisalign's inception in early 1997, software was envisioned as a key component of the technology of the system. Advances in scanning and rapid prototyping systems allowed physical objects to be scanned, manipulated digitally on a computer system, and re-created as a physical object. Actually, these technologies had been in place for computer-aided design (CAD) applications. For Invisalign, what was needed was CAD software that could be readily applied to orthodontic appliance design. The software would allow a virtual model to replace the standard dental cast used in conventional orthodontic appliance manufacture. The virtual model could ultimately be called upon to be much more than a simple replacement for a dental cast. Analyses difficult to perform on a physical model may be more easily done on a virtual model. For instance, "what if" treatment scenarios could be performed on a computer model with greater ease than on a physical model. At a minimum, sophisticated computer algorithms would facilitate the automation of some aspects of the appliance design process, allowing the company to support a broad customer base.

What other advantages does the virtual model offer? Manual, laboratory-based methods have already been used to create appliances similar to those used in the Invisalign System.[1] In these methods, individual teeth are cut from dental casts, set into wax or a similar substance, and manually repositioned into a new configuration. An appliance is then created from this new configuration using common processes—typically, vacuum-forming or pressure-forming. By repeating the process and generating multiple configurations from the segmented dental cast, appliances can be created for each configuration (see chapters 1 and 2).

Such manufacturing methods present clear limitations. The detailed, manual nature of the process can be tedious and prone to errors. Fundamentally, manually prescribed tooth movements on cut plaster teeth cannot be precisely calibrated for the force systems they will generate. In turn, the envisioned tooth movement may never happen. Finally, creating a series of appliances that put the teeth in good final positions is difficult because the ideal final position could exist only in the mind of the person preparing the models but not be orthodontically feasible. Planning each appliance in the series such that the teeth in each model lie along a sensible path to the final position could be impossibly challenging by manual methods.

Many of these limitations disappear when virtual three-dimensional (3-D) models are used. They are unfettered by the physical constraints that make up the core of the limitations described above. The key is to design software that creates a virtual model that can facilitate the manufacture of a physically attainable device. To meet this requirement, the software behind the Invisalign System had to successfully achieve several challenging tasks:

- Model the hard and soft tissues of the mouth
- Plan a final, treated position for the teeth that takes into account proper occlusion
- Plan and execute how the movement from the initial to the final position will take place
- Produce a virtual model that could be fabricated using rapid prototyping technology, to allow the forming of the individual aligners through conventional processes

The software performs these key modeling functions in the context of a larger manufacturing process that begins with the acquisition of the initial dental model and ends with the creation of the dental models used to make the Invisalign appliance. Between these steps, the teeth are only represented virtually.

The Invisalign manufacturing process, from the perspective of the software technology, was broken into a series of steps: segmentation, final setup, staging, review, and fabrication. The initial dental model is one surface and looks like a virtual dental cast. In segmentation, this virtual cast model is divided into a set of smaller surfaces, one for each tooth. Additionally, a model of the gingiva is created. Software called ToothShaper is used during this step.

In final setup, the individual teeth are placed into a clinically and esthetically acceptable final position. A key requirement at this step is to provide methods to evaluate the final position of the teeth. Software called Treat is used during this step. Once the final position is defined, the path that each tooth will take from its initial position to its final position needs to be defined. These motions are planned during the staging process, which also includes projections of the rate of movement for each tooth as well as the time required. The Treat software is also used here. In the review step, the clinician is shown the virtual treatment model and is given the opportunity to comment and request any changes to the final position, tooth movements, or both. The clinician uses ClinCheck software to view the virtual models (see chapter 11). In fabrication, the virtual model is prepared for production into physical models that can be used to create the final appliances. Software called Fab finishes the preparation of the virtual model for manufacture.

History and Background of 3-D Software

The genesis of the Invisalign software lies in a variety of areas, including two-dimensional (2-D) and 3-D computer geometry and graphics, human-computer interaction, and imaging. Advances achieved in such engineering disciplines as image and surface acquisition further pushed these areas to create ways of processing new kinds of data. In dentistry, these ideas have already been applied in oral surgery and in the treatment of craniofacial deformities.

A software package named Sketchpad is credited with being the earliest known CAD system.[2] Authored in 1963 as part of Ivan Sutherland's PhD thesis,[2] Sketchpad employed a graphical user interface (the first of its kind) to allow a draftsman to easily and interactively create a drawing on a computer system using a light pen. It pioneered the idea that one could create a subdrawing once as a master drawing and reuse it many times. Furthermore, if the master drawing were changed, then all copies of it would change. This is an idea that many systems employ today.

A system from which the Invisalign process drew inspiration is the "3-D fax machine" described by Levoy et al.[3] This system made possible the sending of a 3-D object over a communications system like the Internet, much in the same way that a fax machine allows a document to be sent over telephone lines. At the sender's end, the object is scanned and a 3-D model of its surface is created. This model is then sent over the Internet to a remote site, where it can be fabricated using, for example, a rapid prototyping process such as stereolithography. Of course, prior to fabrication, the model can be manipulated by either the sender or the receiver.

Numerous CAD techniques have been applied in many fields, including dentistry and orthodontics. For example, computer-assisted orthodontic treatment planning systems use the computer as an analytical tool to aid the orthodontist during the treatment planning process. Some other early systems focused on using the computer to ease the analysis of cephalometric tracings.[4] This model was subsequently extended, and it allowed the practitioner to also view changes to the tracing that would result from treatment.[5] The 2-D models of orthodontic treatment proposed by Biggerstaff[6] provided an early visual means of planning and evaluating posttreatment tooth positions with a computer.

Three-dimensional techniques have been applied to research in dentistry and orthodontics, as well. An early system developed by van der Linden et al that enabled recording of 3-D information from a dental cast was the Optocom.[7] In this system, two dimensions were specified by moving a microscope to bring the desired point on the cast in line with a set of crosshairs. The third dimension was captured with a touch probe attached to the mechanism that supported the microscope.

Later systems relied on scanning and imaging techniques to acquire a 3-D surface model of a cast or impression. The points used in an analysis could then be captured using an interactive computer application. One such system, by Laurendeau et al,[8] scanned a dental impression using a technique that could determine the 3-D location of certain points based on how the impression and the medium it was contained in (colored water) absorbed light. A simple boundary was computed between each tooth on the resulting virtual model. The positional relationship between the roughly segmented teeth was then analyzed to provide a simple, automated diagnosis. Kuroda et al developed a similar system to analyze dental casts and to perform virtual setups.[9] Their system involved the use of a slit-ray laser scanner to acquire approximately 90,000 3-D coordinates to create a 3-D model of a dental cast. A computer system can be used to perform measurements and conduct basic treatment planning on the resultant model.

Another area where 3-D geometric techniques have been applied is in the area of craniofacial research and surgery. Currently, there is significant interest in computer-aided surgical treatment planning. Using techniques described above, Motohashi and Kuroda[10] developed a system for planning orthognathic surgery from a scan of a dental cast. The cast is segmented into individual teeth, which are then moved by a user into their postoperative positions, where they can be evaluated using digital tools. Other approaches begin with a 3-D scan to capture the geometry of the patient's head. This scan is usually a computed tomography (CT) or magnetic resonance imaging (MRI) scan to capture the internal structures of the head and mouth. Hassfeld and Mühling[11] surveyed the technology that has been applied in this area. McCance et al[12] used pre- and postoperative CT scans of surgical patients to illustrate the movements achieved in both soft tissue and bone.

Others contemporaneous with Invisalign have attempted to build complete treatment planning systems that could be used in the orthodontic office. These systems incorporated 3-D input to more accurately capture the patient's unique geometry. Alcañiz et al[13] describe work on a product named Magallanes, which is a treatment-planning system based on a scan of a standard dental impression. A laser scanner is used to scan a dental cast to create a 3-D surface representation of the cast. Automated routines segment the model by detecting boundaries of teeth. It should be noted, however, that these routines work well only when the teeth are nearly vertical. The software allows interactive specification of a treatment plan and the simulation of the tooth motions that would be obtained through the use of specified archwires. The latter is accomplished via a simple biomechanical model of how teeth may behave when a simulated archwire applies mechanical forces.

Recent commercial products such as those produced by OrthoCAD, Geodigm, OraMetrix, and others expand on the ideas listed above, bringing together computer graphics technology and modern scanning systems. OrthoCAD and Geodigm both yield digital models that can replace a plaster cast for diagnosis, treatment planning, and long-term storage. SureSmile by OraMetrix goes one step further: it provides a system[14] that allows detailed treatment planning and the fabrication of a device designed to execute the formulated treatment.

A Brief History of Invisalign Software

The development of the software used in the Invisalign System began in early 1997. At the time, the 3-D graphics on Microsoft Windows–based computers was a niche market—specialized computers that ran Windows and had high-end graphics cards were geared toward the entertainment and design industries, but still did not have much of a following. Most 3-D computer graphics at the time were done on computers manufactured by Silicon Graphics.

In early 1997, the software component of the Invisalign process was broken into two parts: modeling the teeth and moving them. Two corresponding software packages were created: Clipper and Aligner. The Clipper package mimicked what happened in a dental laboratory by allowing a user to "cut" a virtual dental model into multiple pieces, each one representing a tooth. The Aligner package took the virtual model created by Clipper and allowed a user to move the teeth into a final position; Aligner also defined how the teeth moved into those positions over time. It was, essentially, a package for animating the movement of tooth models.

Clipper's basic tools were the eraser and the saw. The eraser did exactly what its name promised: it allowed the

operator to eliminate part of the model. This was used, for example, to create a flat base on the bottom of the model, in the same way that a technician might on a plaster cast. The saw allowed the user to create U-shaped cuts. Looking at a tooth from the labial direction, a curve was specified that started above the marginal ridge, descended along the interproximal region and along the gingival line, and finally curved up to the opposite marginal ridge. The same curve was created on the lingual side and connected to the first curve by a flexible surface. This surface would cut the model into two pieces, with the tooth above and the rest of the model below. The saw would be applied to each tooth until all teeth were segmented. The remaining part of the model was left to approximate the gingiva. This model was also represented at two levels of detail: a highly detailed model was used to manufacture the appliances, and a less detailed model was used for quicker interaction with the user of the software. Examples of the two levels of detail are shown in Figs 7-1a and 7-1b.

Aligner was, at its heart, an application that allowed a user to create a key-framed animation[15] of a set of teeth. Put simply, in a key-framed animation, the positions of the teeth are specified by the user at the beginning and the end of the treatment, and potentially at a small number of points during the treatment. These user-specified positions are key frames. The computer fills in the intermediate positions, smoothly interpolating the position and orientation of the teeth between the specified key frames (Fig 7-2).

Over time, the functionality of Clipper and Aligner grew increasingly similar, to the point where they differed in only a few key ways. These programs were eventually merged into a single application called Treat. This new application has the ability to do real-time contact detection,[16] which allows for an analysis of occlusion at the beginning and end of treatment, as well as any time in between.

As Invisalign grew, Align Technology recognized the need to involve the practitioner in the treatment-design process. To accomplish this, a new application called ClinCheck was created to allow the practitioner to view the results of the treatment-design process and provide feedback to the technicians at Align on how it should be improved. This was made possible by advances in personal computers that allowed the display of Invisalign's 3-D models on commercial-grade equipment.

The initial virtual models used by Treat and ClinCheck were very basic. In Treat, the teeth would move during the course of treatment, but the gingiva would not change

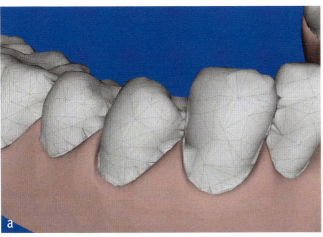
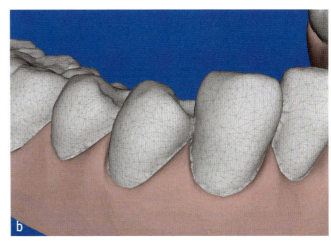

Fig 7-1 Virtual models are represented at two levels of detail: (*a*) low resolution and (*b*) high resolution.

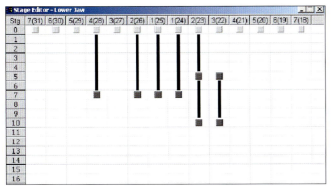

Fig 7-2 Key frame editor. *Gray boxes* indicate when a technician has specified a position for a tooth at a particular stage of treatment. *Black lines* denote periods of time over which a tooth will move between specified tooth positions.

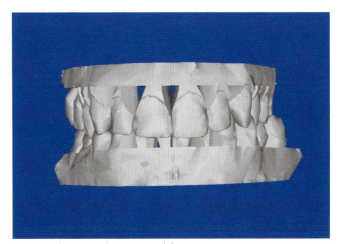

Fig 7-3 The "Stonehenge" model.

shape. The resulting sharp edges and folds in the model were fixed with a virtual wax, which could be stretched and deformed along with the motion of the teeth. The interproximal regions were oddly shaped, and there was a sharp transition at the gingival margin.

Initial ClinCheck models did not have the virtual wax; nevertheless, the virtual models tended to be trimmed more anatomically correctly and smoothly after ClinCheck was in use. The virtual model was, however, still a series of whitish-gray teeth sitting over a horseshoe-shaped whitish-gray approximation of the gingiva (which never changed shape) and was at a much lower level of detail than the model used for manufacturing the aligners. These models quickly earned the name "Stonehenge" for their striking resemblance to the monument (Fig 7-3). To make matters worse, the virtual models ranged in size from 1 to 2 MB. These took a long time to download—between 4 and 10 minutes for the connections typical at the time, at the end of which was a less-than-exciting virtual tooth model.

The next stage in the evolution of the ClinCheck and Treat models happened on two fronts: the models were made smaller, and the virtual gingiva model was added. The models were made smaller by creating a simpler description for teeth (this is described in more detail in the next section), which drastically reduced the size needed to store teeth. It also had the effect of smoothing out the rough, undesirable features of the raw virtual model. Furthermore, this simpler description was based on the highly detailed Treat model, which meant that not only did the models take up less space, but they were also more accurate than the previous ClinCheck models in most cases.

The virtual gingiva was a flexible surface that was attached to each tooth and to a horseshoe-shaped "base." As the teeth moved, the surface deformed to follow the teeth. This behavior, along with its more realistic pinkish color, made the model presentable to a wider audience, including patients. The gingival model is described in more detail in the next section.

59

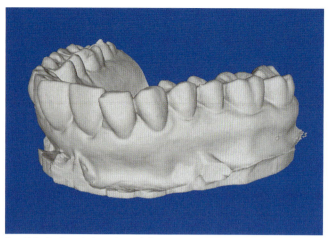

FIG 7-4 A virtual dental model.

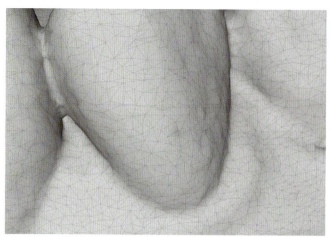

FIG 7-5 The surface is composed of many small triangles.

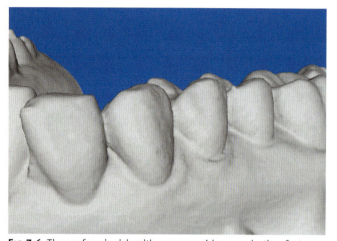

FIG 7-6 The surface is rich with grooves, ridges, and other features.

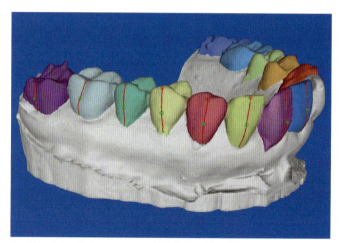

FIG 7-7 Potential crowns are highlighted in different colors.

Modeling

After the impression has been scanned, a 3-D model is created that looks very similar to a dental cast (Fig 7-4). This surface, like many surfaces found in 3-D computer graphics models, is composed of many small triangles (Fig 7-5). These triangles depict the surface of the virtual cast with a high degree of accuracy. The surface is also referred to as watertight, which is to say that the surface is closed and contains no holes. In the modeling step, the model is processed into a form that can be used to create an Invisalign aligner.

A virtual dental model that is appropriate for use in the Invisalign process should satisfy two important criteria. First, the geometry of all tooth surfaces must be captured accurately. Second, the gingiva must be modeled such that it responds to the motion of the teeth in a visually and clinically acceptable way. Accuracy of the crowns is important for

two reasons. First, a tight-fitting appliance can only be made from accurate geometry. Second, any inaccuracy in the shape of the teeth may produce planned motions that are not achievable in the patient's mouth, which can lead to complications during treatment. Root geometry should also be included, since evaluation of root position is standard practice at the end of treatment. The roots can also be used in the analysis of possible motions.

To satisfy the first criterion, the single surface of the scanned data must be segmented into multiple surfaces, one surface per tooth. One way to create separate models of the teeth is to take the approach Kesling did in a dental laboratory: cut a stone dental model into several pieces with a small saw to create independent tooth models.[1] While this approach could be more or less directly implemented using a computer system, more accurate and less labor-intensive approaches for segmenting the virtual model are possible and are necessary to create digital models in any quantity.

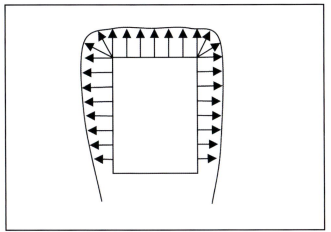

FIG 7-8 A simple tooth model for an incisor. *Arrows* indicate an offset from an underlying basic kernel shape (*solid line*).

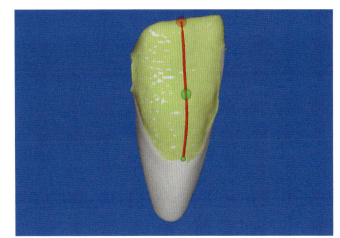

FIG 7-9 A crown and the "best" generated surface. *Red line* denotes user-specified facial axis of the clinical crown.

A more refined approach takes advantage of the rich features of the surface of the virtual model (Fig 7-6), as embodied by Invisalign's ToothShaper software. The surface contains many grooves, ridges, and other features that indicate the boundaries between teeth and also between teeth and the gingival tissue. The approach first looks for high-curvature regions on the surface (ie, regions that are not flat), then connects these regions to form lines of high curvature. For teeth, these lines connect into loops that surround each tooth. The surface contained within each loop is a possible tooth crown, which is displayed to the user in a different color (Fig 7-7).

The crowns identified in this manner are incomplete. They are typically missing geometry in the interproximal regions where adjacent teeth contact each other in the patient's mouth, and no geometry is displayed below the gingival margin. The next step, therefore, is to complete the model of the tooth by creating the missing surfaces. There are two regions in which surfaces need to be added: on the crown region to create interproximal surfaces and below the crown to create a root surface.

While having root geometry would be advantageous, most sources of dental models (ie, impressions and the dental casts created from them) do not have enough data from which to determine the shape of the roots. There are methods of creating approximate root data,[14] but it is the crown data that are most crucial to the Invisalign process. If the model is limited to just crown data, a simple, short surface can be added below the gingival line to complete the model. This short surface is created such that it is parallel to the long axis of the tooth, which helps clarify the overall orientation of the tooth.

To create these missing surfaces, a simple model of tooth geometry is fit to the identified crown (Fig 7-8). The model is a roughly cylindrical surface with its parameters in θ and φ, where φ is the rotation angle around the long tooth axis, and θ represents the parameter along that axis. The function $F(\theta, \varphi)$ represents an offset (the arrows in the picture) from an underlying basic kernel shape (the solid line in the picture). Different incisor shapes are represented by changing the function F (ie, changing the offsets from the basic shape). The shape of this simple model is distorted such that it fits the crown data closely and also satisfies the following set of properties, which describe the "ideal" properties of the missing surfaces:

- The reconstructed surface passes through (or fits to) the border of the scanned part of the crown.
- The horizontal cross section in the root part approximately mirrors the crown cross section and shrinks toward the end of this "approximate root."
- The surface varies smoothly, minimizing the overall curvature.
- The surface is approximately symmetric with respect to the tooth's vertical middle section.

The tooth surface is created by representing the difference of these properties from the simple surface $F(\theta, \varphi)$ as a mathematical "cost" function, and then finding the function $F(\theta, \varphi)$ that minimizes the value of this "cost" function. This surface best matches the original crown data and satisfies these properties most closely (Fig 7-9).

This surface may not be perfect, especially in the interproximal regions. The ToothShaper application therefore provides an interface for shaping these regions. This tool

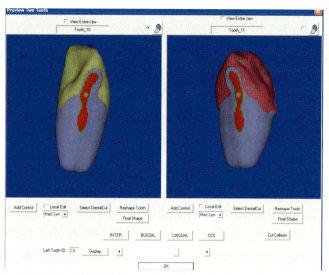

Fig 7-10 A tool in ToothShaper that allows shaping of the interproximal regions and the setup of accurate tooth-to-tooth contacts.

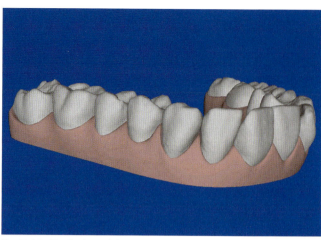

Fig 7-11 Gingival model.

(Fig 7-10) displays regions that are close to neighboring teeth or that contact them and allows a user to accurately shape the teeth in these regions. Photographs are often used as a reference for this operation.

This method of describing tooth geometry does not fully capture all of the details of the tooth surface, but it does come very close. It also has a very small representation on disk that is very similar to those used in early versions of ClinCheck, which were reduced in size so they could be more quickly sent to clinicians.

The final part of the model is the addition of a flexible gingiva model. Align chose a simple flexible surface model for Invisalign. The base data consists of two items: a curve that lies on the tooth and represents the gingival line, and a curve that forms the perimeter of the base of the gingiva. The line on the tooth is derived from the boundary of the segmented crown. It is composed of a lingual half and a buccal half. The line on the base is formed by determining the intersection of the gingival geometry on the scan with a plane that is located below all of the crowns in the model.

To form the gingival surface, the lingual curves are first connected into one continuous curve that forms the overall lingual gingival line. The lingual gingival line is then connected to the lingual part of the base by a surface patch. This process is repeated on the buccal side (Fig 7-11). As the teeth move during the virtual treatment plan, the surfaces of the gingival model change as the line on the tooth changes position with the tooth. This model has a relatively small description, and thus was ideal for quick transfer to the clinician for viewing with ClinCheck.

Display of 3-D Models

The rendering of computer-generated images of 3-D objects as 2-D representations started in 1960 when William Fetter used a plotter to create a series of images of a 3-D model of a human body that he was using to design an aircraft cockpit. A few years later, Ivan Sutherland's Sketchpad system took these images to an early computer screen and made them interactive. In this early system, 3-D models were rendered as a series of lines that represented, very generally, the edges of the original object. Images created in this way were called vector graphics.

In the 1970s, a new technology called the raster display was created and is now in use in virtually all computer systems. In this kind of display, images are represented by a grid of pixels that covers the screen. Pixels can be active (light) or inactive (dark), and in modern systems can take on a variety of colors when active. The process of rendering a 3-D object into a 2-D image thus involves determining which pixels correspond to the various parts of the object and coloring them appropriately.

An image produced in this manner, however, is still 2-D. How do we perceive this image as a 3-D object? The human perceptual system relies on a set of cues to convert a 2-D image into a 3-D conceptualization of the object represented by the image.[17] Binocular vision allows us to integrate two different pictures, each seen with a different eye, to understand 3-D spatial relationships for objects that are relatively close. However, a desktop computer system does not generally have the ability to present a different image to each eye, though specialized systems for doing this do exist.

Certain features of a 2-D image can allow us to imagine a third dimension. Occlusion of one object by another in a 2-D image suggests that one object is in front of the other. As in perspective drawings, the relative size of images that represent objects known to be similar in size suggests that one object is closer than the other. The shading of an image suggests a reflected light source, which can suggest what the object's 3-D shape might be. Perspective views of familiar objects suggest an overall 3-D orientation of that object and its rough shape.

Series of images taken of an object while it is moving make the 3-D relationships clearer. Images taken of an object in motion often show wildly varying occlusal relationships and shading, which makes the shape and relationships between objects in the image very clear. Changes in shading on moving objects can also suggest the 3-D shape of the object. Finally, parts of the object that are farther away appear to move more slowly than parts that are closer, further reinforcing the perception of depth to the object.

Invisalign's software renders images of the 3-D tooth and gingival models by determining the pixels that correspond to each triangle in the model and coloring them appropriately. The base color of a triangle is determined by what the triangle represents—white for teeth and pink for gingiva. This process is further refined by applying a lighting model to the colors. The software defines the position, color, and intensity of a light in relation to the model. The color of each triangle is then modulated by the intensity of the light falling on it.

The intensity of the light that falls on each triangle is computed through a comparison of the direction between the triangle and the light with the direction that the triangle is facing (called the triangle normal direction). When the triangle directly faces the light, the light intensity will be at its brightest. As the angle between the direction to the light and the triangle normal direction increases, the intensity of the light decreases. The intensity of the light can vary across the surface of the triangle. Computing this at each pixel that corresponds to the triangle would be very expensive. Instead, this computation is performed at each vertex of the triangle, and the results are interpolated across the triangle. This technique is called Gouraud shading.[18]

The rendering style used in the Invisalign software has limitations. The teeth have a simple white color. Real teeth have a semitransparent outer layer that is difficult, but not

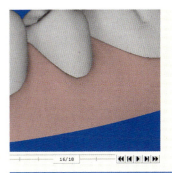

FIG 7-12 Controls along the bottom of the window allow a user to control time.

impossible, to reproduce in real-time rendering. Also, the rendering method does not employ any shadows. The lighting computations are done independent of any objects located between the triangle being rendered and the light source, which would normally cause a shadow. Real-time shadow computations on complex models are difficult to perform. Thus, shadowing cues (similar to the shading cues discussed above) in the mouth that would provide depth and dimension to an image are not captured in the rendering of the virtual teeth.

Final Setup and Staging

After the virtual model is created, the movements of the separated teeth need to be specified throughout the treatment. Invisalign's Treat software performs this function. The process of specifying tooth movements is broken into two steps: specifying the final position of the teeth and then specifying the paths that each tooth will take between its initial and final positions.

The Treat software is similar to the ToothShaper software, but adds a new dimension to the model: time. Time is expressed in units called stages, where one stage corresponds exactly to one Invisalign appliance, and thus represents approximately 2 weeks of elapsed time based on wear times recommended by the company. On the Treat software display screen, time is expressed along the bottom of the window as a slider bar with a set of VCR-like controls that allow time to be played forward and backward (Fig 7-12).

A technician uses the Treat software to arrange the teeth in their final position by moving each tooth individually to a new location. To do this, the technician clicks on a tooth to display a "widget" that allows the tooth to be moved (Fig 7-13). Clicking and dragging on any of the three axes (red, green, or blue) moves the tooth along the indicated

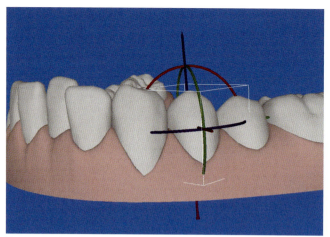

FIG 7-13 The interaction widget allows a user to move a tooth along or around any axis.

Once a good final position is established, the technician goes through a process called staging to determine all of the intermediate positions of the teeth. The Stage Editor tool in Treat, which allows the technician to specify when each tooth in the jaw is moving, aids in this process. Stage numbers are listed vertically down the left side of the Stage Editor, and tooth numbers are listed horizontally across the top, forming a grid of cells (Fig 7-15).

A box in a cell in Stage Editor means that a tooth position has been specified by the technician (in this case, the initial and final positions for that tooth) for that particular stage. The line connecting the boxes signifies that the tooth will move between those two positions over the specified time period. Between those two positions, the tooth will move linearly (ie, it will move in a straight line, at a constant rate). The tooth's orientation will also change at a constant rate.

Stage Editor also allows the technician to analyze the movements created during the staging process. Tabs on the Stage Editor screen display movement distance per stage, plus the degree of space or "overlap" between teeth during each stage (Figs 7-16a to 16-d). The amount of movement per stage is a key component of the treatment, as it directly relates to the amount of force placed on the teeth by the aligner. If the tooth is moved too quickly, high forces on the tooth will result, which is undesirable.

axis. Clicking and dragging on any of the three circles (red, green, or blue) rotates the tooth around the intersection of the axes. Alternatively, an input device such as a SpaceBall allows for more direct control of the position and orientation of the selected tooth. The SpaceBall is essentially a computer mouse that responds to movements and rotations in three dimensions.

To help accurately set teeth into their final positions, Treat computes regions that are in "collision" or contact. Areas involved in the collision are shown in red (Fig 7-14a). This visualization can help ensure that the contact between neighboring teeth in the same jaw is appropriate. Additionally, by not displaying one of the jaws, collisions on the occlusal surface can be observed to check for good occlusal contacts in the final position or any intermediate position (Fig 7-14b).

Two other functions of note are handled by the Treat software. The first is the placement of "attachments." Attachments are extra geometry added to the tooth model that is used clinically to increase the retention of the aligner on the tooth on which the attachment is placed. Treat allows a variety of attachment shapes to be

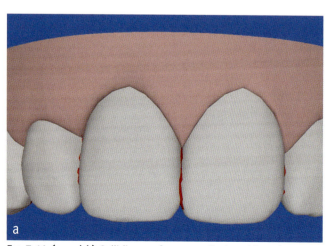

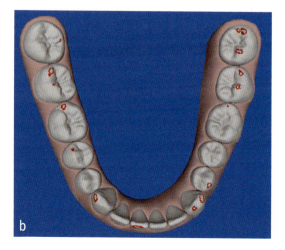

FIG 7-14 (a and b) Colliding surfaces are displayed in red.

placed. (See chapters 9 and 10 for more information on attachments.) Not all (experimental) attachment types are commercially available, however.

Another function of Treat is the modeling of interproximal enamel reduction (IPR). IPR is modeled in Treat by allowing teeth to overlap in the final stage of treatment. Clinically, it is the clinician who will alter the shape of the tooth to achieve a good contact in the mouth. Stage Editor allows the technician to estimate the amount of IPR in real time while planning the treatment.

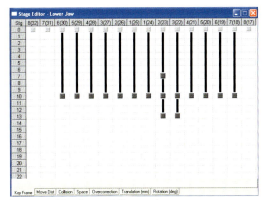

Fig 7-15 The Stage Editor tool.

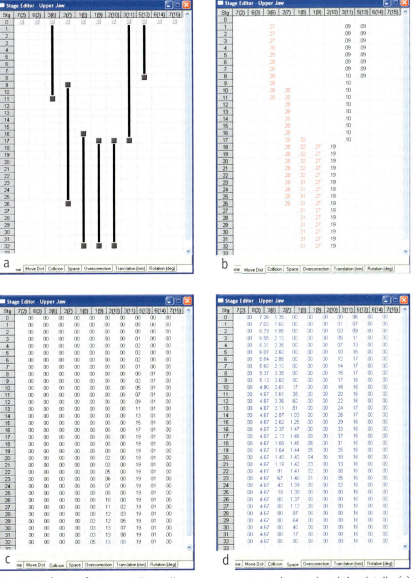

Fig 7-16 (a to d) Stage Editor allows movements to be analyzed in detail. (*a*) Technician-supplied tooth positions and movements. (*b*) Movement of each tooth. (*c*) Contact between adjacent teeth. (*d*) Space between adjacent teeth.

References

1. Kesling H. Coordinating the predetermined pattern and tooth positioner with conventional treatment. Am J Orthod Oral Surg 1946; 32:285–293.

2. Sutherland I. Sketchpad: A Man-Machine Graphical Communication System [technical report 296]. Cambridge, MA: Massachusetts Institute of Technology, Lincoln Laboratory, 1963.

3. Levoy M, Curless B, Goldman D, et al. Project to build a 3D fax machine. Available at: http://www-graphics.stanford.edu/projects/faxing/. Accessed January 8, 2006.

4. Ricketts R. The evolution of diagnosis to computerized cephalometrics. J Dent Res 1969;55:795–803.

5. Faber RD, Burstone CJ, Solonche DJ. Computerized interactive orthodontic treatment planning. J Dent Res 1978;73:36–46.

6. Biggerstaff RH. Computerized diagnostic setups and simulations. Angle Orthod 1970;40:28–36.

7. van der Linden FP, Boersma H, Zelders T, Peters KA, Raaben JH. Three-dimensional analysis of dental casts by means of the optocom. J Dent Res 1972;51:1100.

8. Laurendeau D, Guimond L, Poussdart D. A computer-vision technique for the acquisition and processing of 3-D profiles of dental imprints: An application in orthodontics. IEEE Transactions on Medical Imaging 1991;10:453–461.

9. Kuroda T, Motohashi N, Tominaga R, Iwata K. Three-dimensional dental cast analyzing system using laser scanning. Am J Orthod Dentofacial Orthop 1996;110:365–369.

10. Motohashi N, Kuroda T. A 3D computer-aided design system applied to diagnosis and treatment planning in orthodontics and orthognathic surgery. Eur J Orthod 1999;21:263–274.

11. Hassfeld S, Mühling J. Computer-assisted oral and maxillofacial surgery—A review and an assessment of technology. Int J Oral Maxillofac Surg 2001;30:2–13.

12. McCance AM, Moss JP, Fright WR, et al. Three-dimensional analysis techniques—Part 4: Three-dimensional analysis of bone and soft tissue to bone ratio of movements in 24 cleft palate patients following Le Fort I osteotomy: A preliminary report. Cleft Palate Craniofac J 1997;34:58–62.

13. Alcañiz M, Montserrat C, Grau V, Chinesta F, Ramon A, Albalat S. An advanced system for the simulation and planning of orthodontic treatment. Med Image Anal 1998;2:61–77.

14. Mah J, Sachdeva R. Computer-assisted orthodontic treatment: The SureSmile process. Am J Orthod Dentofacial Orthop 2001;120: 85–87.

15. Burtnyk N, Wein M. Computer-generated key-frame animation. J Soc Motion Picture Television Engineers 1971;8:149–153.

16. Lin M, Manocha D, Cohen J, Gottschalk S. Collision detection: Algorithms and applications. In: Laumond J-P, Overmars M (eds). Algorithms for Robotics Motion and Manipulation. Wellesley, MA: AK Peters, 1996:129–142.

17. Osterloh K, Redmer B, Ewert U. On human perception of 3D images. NDT [serial onine] 2004; 9(5). Available at: http://www.ndt.net/article/ct2003/v26/v26.htm. Accessed February 15, 2006.

18. Foley J, van Dam A, Feiner S, Hughes J. Computer Graphics: Principles and Practice, ed 2. Boston: Addison-Wesley, 1992.

chapter 8

VIRTUAL DIAGNOSTIC SETUP

by
David Chenin, DDS and Kent Verdis

Watercolor painting is a combination of intricately placed strokes and a synthesis of complementary colors. As the artist begins to paint with the end in mind, his or her mental image of the living world is transferred onto blank canvas. Like painting, although much more complex, orthodontic treatment requires one to develop an understanding of an in-depth mental image before any of the initial strokes of paint are applied. Comprehensive visualization and expression of one's objectives, therefore, is a critical step in the creation of the perfect occlusion.

To that end, Invisalign treatment is based on the patient records acquired by the clinician. Five different records are necessary to create a "virtual patient": impressions of the maxillary and mandibular dental arches, bite registration, intraoral and extraoral photographs, panoramic or full-mouth series radiograph, and the prescription and diagnosis form. It is the clinician's responsibility to obtain high-quality impressions and bite registration, along with comprehensive photographs and radiographs, and to devise a clear treatment plan for each patient.

Align Technology converts these patient records into electronic data that can be used to create a three-dimensional (3-D) virtual treatment. To facilitate such conversion of patient records into clinically relevant electronic 3-D data, a series of software-driven steps is incorporated into the manufacturing process. These steps include scanning paper records, generating computed tomography (CT) images of the impressions, and preparing CT-scanned impressions. Once all the records have been digitized, they are sent to a dental technician, who performs additional steps—such as automated tooth segmentation, digital detailing, virtual gingiva creation, and automated occlusion—to prepare the 3-D models for tooth movements, as part of the virtual 3-D treatment plan known as ClinCheck.

Impressions

The polyvinyl siloxane (PVS) impression is the basis of the 3-D representation of a patient's dentition. In the clinical setting, the doctor takes an impression using PVS material with a plastic tray provided by Align Technology (Fig 8-1). PVS is the material of choice because of its extreme accuracy, high dimensional stability, and widespread use in dentistry.[1] The PVS impression is one of the most valuable of the records required for Invisalign treatment (Fig 8-2). The main reason for its importance is because the accuracy of the PVS impression directly correlates to how

well the aligners fit. Impressions of the teeth are the raw data used to fabricate ClinCheck and aligners. Once Align Technology receives the PVS impressions, they are directly scanned by computerized tomography (CT) scanning machines (see chapter 6). Although the dental arches are rendered as separate 3-D units, they are saved as a single electronic file without the teeth in an articulated relationship. The 3-D data file is compressed and stored with the other virtual patient records for later use.

Bite Registration

Capture of accurate occlusal relationships is paramount in 3-D dental software applications. An inaccurate starting point of treatment ensures an inaccurate result. If the occlusion at the start of treatment is correct, all of the movements performed to the final alignment will be accurate. Along with the PVS impression, the treating clinician must also supply Align Technology with a PVS bite registration (Fig 8-3a). The Invisalign virtual diagnostic setup does not employ the use of a virtual articulator at this time; hence, centric relation (CR) records are not used. Centric relation–centric occlusion (CO) shifts should be addressed prior to starting Invisalign treatment. The bite registration recorded by the treating clinician in CO, otherwise known as maximum intercuspation, is a full-arch, complete bite-through record (Fig 8-3b). Digitization of the CO bite registration takes place via the same technology used to acquire the impressions digitally (ie, CT scanning).

Although the nature of how the patient's teeth fit together is stored in the bite registration, we will discuss how the actual anatomy of the patient's teeth is reliably used to re-create the CO bite relationship in most patients. In the Invisalign manufacturing process, the bite registration is used only if additional anatomic information is needed.

The primary method by which the CO is created is based on the geometry and shape of the occlusal surfaces of the teeth. An automated software tool (AutoBite) maximizes tooth-to-tooth interarch contacts through algorithms by matching corresponding tooth-surface contacts of the opposite arch (such as contact points and wear facets) into a maximum intercuspated position. As a result, the original nonoccluded maxillary and mandibular 3-D dental arches are moved virtually into an articulated CO relationship.

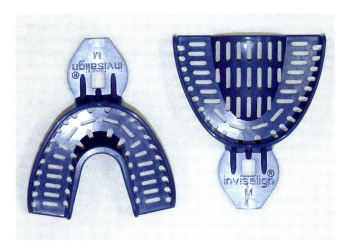

FIG 8-1 Align Technology freely provides impression trays in various sizes for use by the clinician. These trays are robust enough to prevent distortion of the impression material. Perforations provide adequate retention.

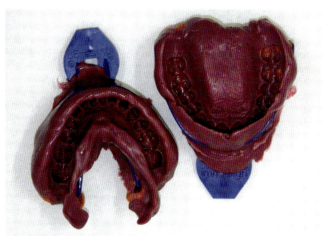

FIG 8-2 Detailed impressions of teeth are critical to Invisalign treatment.

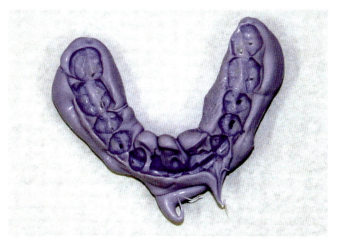

FIG 8-3a Full-coverage PVS bite registration must accompany the impressions.

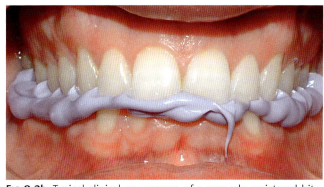

FIG 8-3b Typical clinical appearance of a properly registered bite.

Because of the high level of success achieved with the AutoBite software, bite registration to create CO is required for very few patients. In a small percentage of patients, AutoBite cannot find enough matching tooth surfaces where the teeth uniformly interdigitate in a consistent manner (such as a full cusp molar and canine Class III relationships). Because it is difficult to predict which cases will require PVS bite registration data, treating clinicians must supply it for all of their patients. However, CO is usually created by executing AutoBite based on the shape of the teeth themselves to occlude the models in 3-D space. This process yields highly accurate, consistent, and repeatable CO relationships.[2]

Photographs

Clinical photography supplied by the treating clinician is used for many steps in the manufacturing process. Photographs that are not supplied digitally in jpeg (file interchange format) are scanned by Align Technology via conventional document scanning devices and stored electronically. The eight photographs represented in Fig 8-4 are required for Invisalign treatment.

These images are important for obtaining such additional diagnostic information as a patient's symmetry, facial shape and balance, smile line, restorations, and condition of the dentition and surrounding structures. Such diagnostic information should be interpreted and expressed through the clinician's treatment objectives.

In addition to the diagnostic value for the treating clinician, photographs are used by Align Technology in sever-

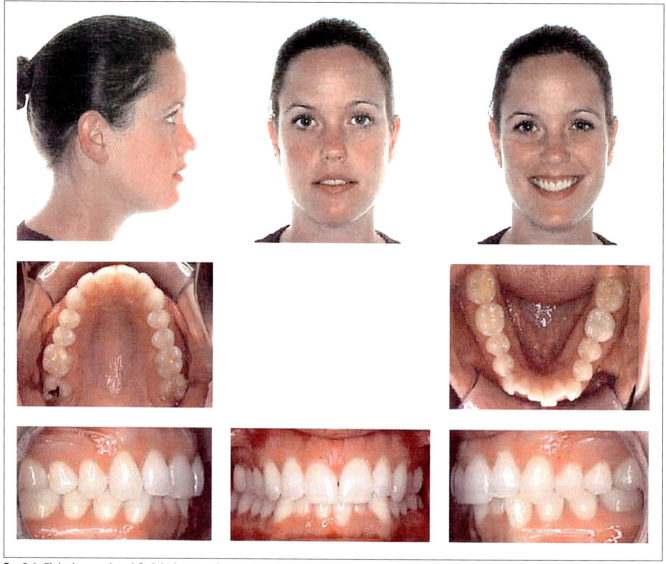

FIG 8-4 Eight intraoral and facial photographs required for Invisalign treatment. All imaging programs offer this template.

al ways. Verification that the dentition shown in the photographs matches that of the 3-D dental models is a quality check performed repeatedly throughout the manufacturing process. Additionally, intraoral photographs can be used for assistance in fixing voids or bubbles in the dental model that may have developed as a result of inconsistencies in the original impression. This ultimately helps to ensure better fit of the aligners. Also, the photographs, particularly the buccal and anterior views, are used in verification of the CO relationship. Photographs are also important in identifying or verifying restorations, tooth movements, and attachments.

Radiographs

Either a panoramic radiograph or a full-mouth series of radiographs may be supplied by the treating clinician (Figs 8-5a and 8-5b) to fulfill the radiograph requirement. Since both types of radiograph are used for the same reasons, there is no advantage or disadvantage in using one type over the other. Radiographs that are not supplied digitally by the treating clinician in jpeg are immediately scanned and stored electronically.

These radiographs are important for the clinician to obtain additional diagnostic information regarding the patient's restorations, caries, skeletal formation, and the condition of the dentition and surrounding bone structures. In addition to their value in quality control (see

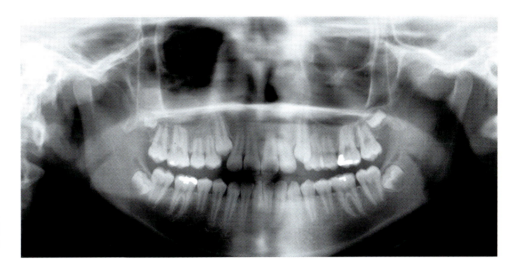

FIG 8-5a The submitted panoramic radiograph should have good definition, especially around the deep periodontal structures.

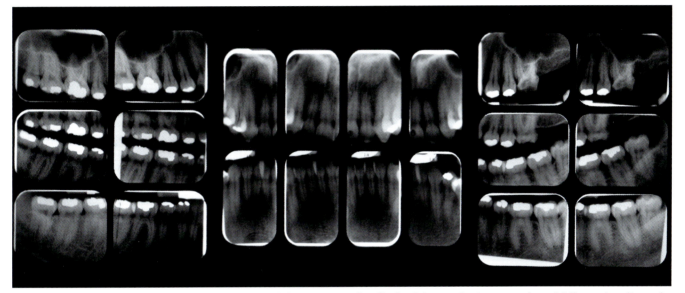

FIG 8-5b Full-mouth periapical series offers more detail, but to set up the ClinCheck images both panoramic and full-mouth radiographs serve equally well.

above), radiographs can reveal the presence of crowns, partial dentures, and implant restorations that may not show on photographs. Therefore, radiographs are also important in identifying or verifying attachments and proper tooth movements.

Additional radiographs taken by the treating clinician for diagnostic purposes do not need to be submitted to Align Technology, as their diagnostic information should be incorporated into the treatment goal information.

Prescription and Diagnosis Form

The treating clinician can provide either an anterior treatment or a full-arch treatment form (Figs 8-6) to Align

Technology. Prescription and diagnosis forms submitted in paper format are scanned and stored for later use. Forms that have been completed digitally by the doctor in VIP (Virtual Invisalign Practice, on the invisalign.com website) are downloaded and stored by Align once the case is received. Each of the clinician's concerns, goals, and treatment objectives must be clearly incorporated and expressed on the prescription and diagnosis form. This form is also used to provide shipping and billing instructions, to indicate the type of case (anterior or full treatment), and to record patient background information.

The prescription and diagnosis form represents an important part of the communication between the treating clinician and Align Technology's technicians. Specific information provided on the prescription and diagnosis form

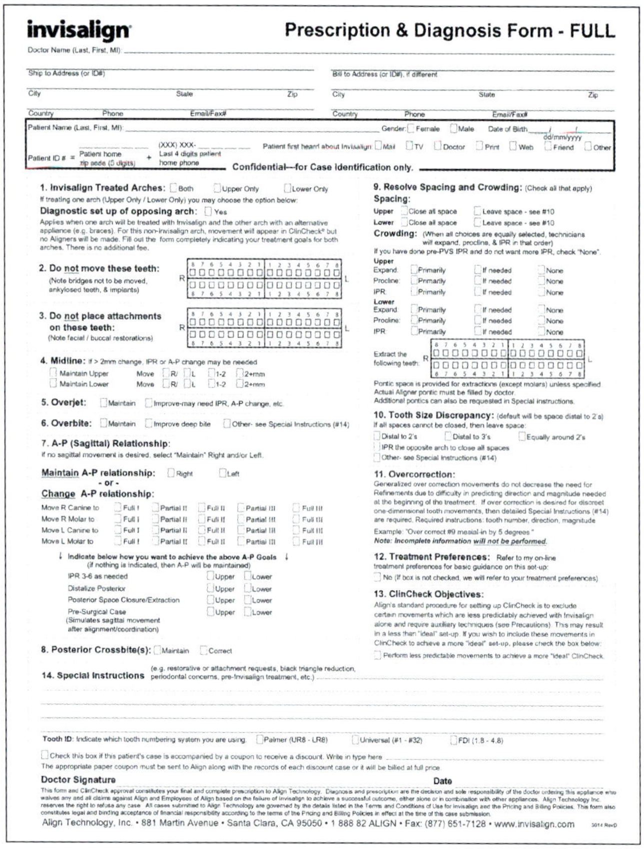
invisalign — Prescription & Diagnosis Form - FULL

Doctor Name (Last, First, MI)

Ship to Address (or ID#) — Bill to Address (or ID#), if different

City — State — Zip — City — State — Zip

Country — Phone — Email/Fax# — Country — Phone — Email/Fax#

Patient Name (Last, First, MI) — Gender: Female / Male — Date of Birth (dd/mm/yyyy)

Patient ID # = Patient home zip code (5 digits) + (XXX) XXX- Last 4 digits patient home phone — Patient first heard about Invisalign: Mail / TV / Doctor / Print / Web / Friend / Other

Confidential—for Case Identification only.

1. Invisalign Treated Arches: Both / Upper Only / Lower Only

Diagnostic set up of opposing arch: Yes

2. Do not move these teeth: (Note bridges not to be moved, ankylosed teeth, & implants)

3. Do not place attachments on these teeth: (Note facial / buccal restorations)

4. Midline: Maintain Upper / Maintain Lower — Move R / L, 1-2 / 2+mm

5. Overjet: Maintain / Improve-may need IPR, A-P change, etc.

6. Overbite: Maintain / Improve deep bite / Other- see Special Instructions (#14)

7. A-P (Sagittal) Relationship:

Maintain A-P relationship: Right / Left

- or -

Change A-P relationship: Move R Canine to / Move R Molar to / Move L Canine to / Move L Molar to — Full I / Partial II / Full II / Partial III / Full III

IPR 3-6 as needed / Distalize Posterior / Posterior Space Closure/Extraction / Pre-Surgical Case — Upper / Lower

8. Posterior Crossbite(s): Maintain / Correct

9. Resolve Spacing and Crowding:

Spacing: Upper / Lower — Close all space / Leave space - see #10

Crowding: Upper / Lower — Expand / Procline / IPR — Primarily / If needed / None

Extract the following teeth:

10. Tooth Size Discrepancy: Distal to 2's / Distal to 3's / Equally around 2's / IPR the opposite arch to close all spaces / Other- see Special Instructions (#14)

11. Overcorrection:

12. Treatment Preferences:

13. ClinCheck Objectives:

14. Special Instructions

Tooth ID: Palmer (UR8 - LR8) / Universal (#1 - #32) / FDI (1.8 - 4.8)

Doctor Signature — Date

Align Technology, Inc. • 881 Martin Avenue • Santa Clara, CA 95050 • 1 888 82 ALIGN • Fax: (877) 651-7128 • www.invisalign.com

Fig 8-6 Prescription form used to submit cases to Align Technology. It may be submitted on paper (shown) or online.

includes the following: arch(es) treated, diagnostic setup, teeth not to be moved, teeth not to have attachments, overbite and overjet goals, sagittal goals and instructions, posterior crossbite correction, information on correction of crowding or spacing, handling of tooth size discrepancies, and other general preferences and special instructions of the virtual setup. Clinicians use this form, which is also available in electronic html format in VIP, to indicate their goals and objectives. An in-depth discussion of how elements of the prescription and diagnosis form are utilized by Align Technology's technicians can be found in chapters 11 and 15.

ToothShaper

ToothShaper is the proprietary name given to the software used to prepare the impression, section the teeth, and remove all virtual gingiva. This software was developed from a rudimentary cutting technique that used a flat "plane"-style cutting tool (Fig 8-7) and has evolved into an almost fully automated cutting and detailing tool. After the PVS impression is scanned, the electronic files are sent to an offshore facility that will send the virtual setup to the prescribing clinician.

The first step undertaken at the offshore (Costa Rica) facility is to inspect all records that are received for each patient. This includes maxillary and mandibular impressions, treatment planning form, patient photos, radiographs (if provided), and bite registration. For each patient, the ToothShaper technician verifies that the information is complete and consistent, and that the quality of the records is acceptable to proceed with treatment.

If all the records pass the initial inspection, the technician begins to cut the teeth—evaluating once again the quality of the impressions. If the impression is of poor quality, the technician captures images of the area(s) that are unacceptable and calls the customer to request another impression. The old impression and the images of the unacceptable area are returned to the clinician so he or she can learn from whatever problems led to the poor quality of the initial impression. Some of the most common reasons for unacceptable impressions are distorted anatomy, bubbles and voids, and incomplete capture of crowns of all teeth.

If the impressions are acceptable, the technician segments the teeth using the ToothShaper software. This process uses many of the same techniques that are used in the traditional dental laboratory; however, it is all done with digital tools in the software. This allows the technicians to get the same or even better quality in significantly less time and with lower scrap rates. There are two basic steps to performing the ToothShaper process: identifying the teeth by marking the facial axis of the clinical crown (FACC), and detailing imperfections in the impression.

The first step is to quickly identify the FACC of each tooth using a point on the incisal edge and a point on the cementoenamel junction (Fig 8-8). The FACCs must be identified first; at the time of this publication, the software cannot fully detect tooth geometry. Identifying the FACC gives the software a starting point from which to run its algorithm. The FACCs are used by the software to estimate the shape and angulation of the crown. When each tooth crown has been identified by the software, the technician fixes any parts that have been missed by the software. This is called "painting" the teeth (Fig 8-9). Once all teeth have been properly identified, the technician simply clicks a button to segment the teeth (Fig 8-10).

The next step is to detail any imperfections in the impression (ie, fill voids, remove excess material, correct

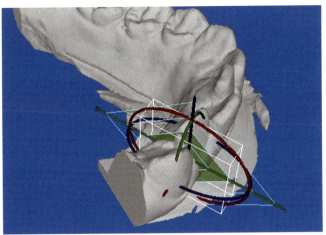

FIG 8-7 ToothShaper cutting tool. In the past, cutting was done manually, but now the cutting and detailing tasks are automated.

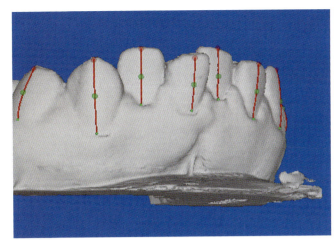

FIG 8-8 The facial axis of the clinical crown for each tooth is identified using a three-point registration.

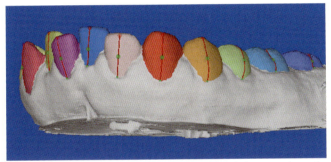

FIG 8-9 The teeth are painted as an aid to discriminate each tooth.

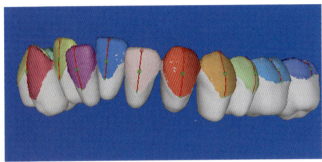

FIG 8-10 The teeth are segmented at the click of a button.

deficiencies in the scan) (Fig 8-11). Mastery of dental anatomy and tooth morphology is a critical component of Align Technology's internal training program. Align's standard on quality impressions is covered in chapter 5.

When all the teeth have been segmented and cleaned up, the technician prepares the models for the setup process. This begins by setting the axis of each tooth. Again, at the time of this publication, this process is performed manually; however, with each passing software release, gains in both cycle time and quality are achieved. The axes are set in the X, Y, and Z directions, which enables the technician to easily move the teeth in the desired position when performing the virtual setup.

When the segmenting of the teeth, detailing of the model, and setting of the axes have been completed, the bite is set in centric occlusion using an automated tool in the software. The AutoBite tool in ToothShaper has been perfected so that all Class I and Class II, and most Class III, bites are nearly all automated. As discussed above under "Bite Registration," the software tool occludes the virtual models based on the anatomy of the teeth and

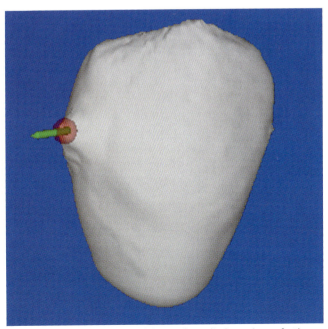

FIG 8-11 The smoothing tool is used to eliminate imperfections.

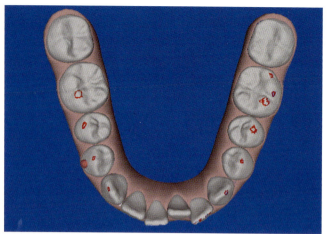

FIG 8-12a Red marks indicate maximum occlusal contact points. These are used to register the occlusion of maxillary and mandibular teeth.

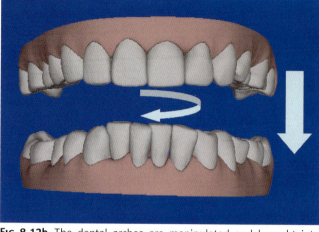

FIG 8-12b The dental arches are manipulated and brought into occlusion.

their maximized occlusion (Figs 8-12a and 8-12b). The technician runs the AutoBite tool and confirms the results with the photos. For cases that feature Class III and open bite conditions, there is sometimes the need to make manual adjustments using the PVS bite registration. The technicians virtually lay the bite registration over one arch and then move the opposing arch to be interdigitated into the bite registrations (Figs 8-13a and 8-13b). AutoBite is the preferred approach to this task because manual adjustments made from the bite registration are difficult, labor intensive, and time consuming. A proper bite set is a key element in a successful Invisalign treatment.

The next and last step for the ToothShaper technician is to adjust the virtual gingiva to replicate the patient's actual gingival tissue. This too is a semimanual step at the time of this publication, but software to automate this step is soon to be released. The virtual gingiva is adjusted with five nodes on the buccal and five nodes on the lingual; the technician moves the nodes to match the gingiva in the original, pre-segmented model (Figs 8-14a to 8-14c). Proper gingiva adjustment is required for a good fitting, comfortable aligner. The file is saved to the patient database and will be submitted to a quality check that is performed by highly trained technicians who again review the pretreated data for records, proper detailing, bite set, and gingiva adjustments. When the ToothShaper process is completed, the case moves onto the setup and stage process, which is explained in chapters 7 and 12.

Summary of Process

Overall, the process of creating the ClinCheck can be summarized in this way: Patient records are scanned into a digital format (unless supplied in digital format by the treating clinician) and stored electronically. Once all records are acquired electronically, a technician uses them to create the virtual patient. The technician locates the facial axis of the clinical crown on all of the teeth, and then the ToothShaper software identifies the shape of all of the teeth. The technician manually adjusts the painting on the teeth so that all of the teeth have only the crowns completely painted. Segmentation occurs automatically. After the segmentation is complete, the technician uses the AutoBite tool to occlude the models into an articulated CO relationship. Finally, the technician manually adjusts the virtual gingiva around each tooth, and the virtual model is complete.

Future Trends

Complete automation is the ultimate goal of almost any manufacturing process. Automation is advantageous because it reduces variability to acceptable levels within controlled ranges. More complex manufacturing processes have variable starting points, contain more steps, and have multiple inputs, which increases the procedure's complexity and variability. As a result of the complexity, incremental improvements are much more achievable and can be implemented in a controlled fashion to ensure reduced variability.

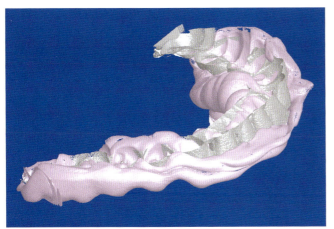

FIG 8-13a Registration of occlusion.

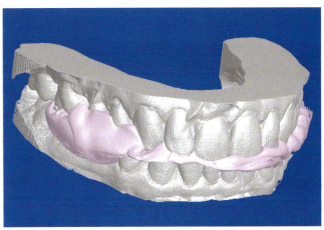

FIG 8-13b Arches registered in occlusion with the aid of occlusal contact points and the bite registration impression.

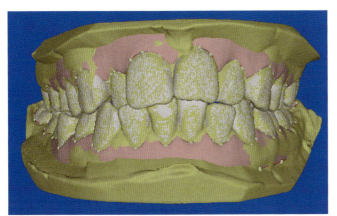

FIG 8-14a Registration of gingival line on the pre-segmented model.

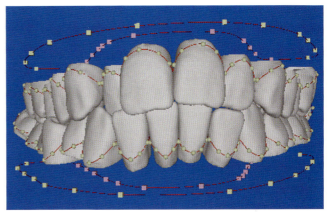

FIG 8-14b Gingival boundaries on the segmented models.

The following timeline of past and expected improvements is presented to better understand the nature of improvements that are in use:

- 1999: Manual cutting with flexible plane-style cutter. Each tooth is manually cut one at a time, with each tooth requiring between 20 and 40 individual slices. Initial detailing was performed on the physical model, which was poured in a dental laboratory.
- 2000: New cutting tool reduces the number of slices to between three and eight per tooth, but is still undertaken one tooth at a time. Initial detailing is still done on the physical model; however, this newer tool and process reduce cutting time by approximately 75%.
- 2002: ToothShaper software was developed, which automates the majority of the cutting and reduces processing time by another 50%. Digital detailing was invented, resulting in the removal of more than 80% of the work done on physically poured models.

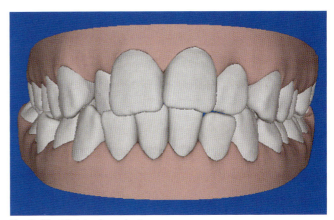

FIG 8-14c Finished product.

- 2003: AutoBite tool was developed, which increases bite set accuracy to 99% for most cases and reduces time by 80%.
- 2005: Automation of gingiva process reduces labor time by 30%.

• 2006: Final automation of ToothShaper steps enables full automation of segmentation and significant amount of detailing, which is expected to reduce labor time to 1/500 of original time from 1999.

References

1. Donovan T, Chee W. A review of contemporary impression materials and techniques. Dent Clin North Am 2004;48:vi–vii, 445–470.
2. Chenin D, Turley A. Analysis of an automated bite creation tool for 3D dental software. 144th Annual ADA Scientific Session Table Clinic, October 2003. Available at: http://www.cheninortho.com/images/Forms-articles/ADA_TableClinic_Handout.pdf. Accessed February 15, 2006

chapter 9

ATTACHMENTS

by
Peter Knopp and Mitra Derakhshan, DDS

Traditional orthodontic appliance systems are designed around components that transmit forces (ie, wires) and elements that apply these forces (ie, brackets) to the teeth. The Invisalign System also follows this design: it directs force application to the teeth through intermediary components—aligners and attachments. Where aligners are analogous to wires, attachments are equivalent to brackets.

The discussion that follows presumes a general understanding of the mechanics of tooth movements. The emphasis is on the concepts underlying, and the uses of, the attachments used in Align Technology's Invisalign System.

Basis of Need

Teeth generally do not have operative purchase points on which any appliance system can act effectively. In conventional appliance systems, this is remedied through the bonding of standardized brackets to the teeth. For the Invisalign System, the necessary purchase points are created through the formation and application of predetermined shapes, which are grouped under the appellation *attachment*.

As with brackets, attachments are necessitated by dental morphologies and mechanics. Further, both brackets and attachments afford an experienced practitioner myriad possible clinical benefits. It should therefore be clear that the informed use of attachments is crucial to achieving effective treatments with the Invisalign System.

Terminology

It is important for users to familiarize themselves with the vernacular of their profession and its related processes. To that end, the following words have particular meanings in the context of an Invisalign System treatment:

- *Attachment*: An object added to the computer representation of a tooth's geometry that may or may not also be added to the real tooth. An attachment is readily identified in a ClinCheck presentation as a red geometric body that lies on one or more tooth surfaces. Figs 9-1a to 9-1c show examples of attachments placed on a computer representation of dentition. There are three types of attachment:
  - *Real*: The physical manifestation of any attachment or the computer representation that becomes reality. This is the shape that is formed (in composite or another material) and bonded to a tooth.
  - *Virtual*: The computer representation of an attachment or a shape that is formed in an aligner but not subsequently reproduced as a physical entity bonded on a tooth.
  - *Window*: An attachment formed partially or wholly around a tooth to create space for it to move into or to isolate it from the movements of other teeth. This is a specialized incarnation of a virtual attachment. The shapes are usually created by scaling the associated tooth by more than 100% and then, as needed, removing buccal and lingual portions to reveal tooth surfaces or bonded attachments on which the aligner can act. Window attachments are always shown in a translucent color so the underlying tooth can also be seen.
- *Base*: The portion of an attachment that penetrates the tooth in the computer representation of a treatment. It is the translucent purple geometry that produces a continuous profile between the tooth and the attachment. In the absence of a base, a gap could exist between an attachment and its underlying tooth. Such a gap would lead to an inexact and, likely, difficult bonding of the attachment to the tooth.
- *Cavity*: The shape formed in the aligner by a real or virtual attachment that is present and visible in the computer representation. In an attachment template aligner, this is the mold to form a real attachment and bond it to a tooth. It is also the shape that most directly contacts a bonded attachment.
- *Channel*: A conduit that runs (generally apically) from the gingival aspect of an attachment or its cavity to the gingival edge of an aligner. It is formed in the aligner by placing one or more virtual attachments gingival to the real attachment (see Figs 9-1b and 9-1c). Alternately, it can be created through the use of an attachment that has sufficient length to extend beyond the gingival margin (Fig 9-2). A channel is created to ease appliance seating and removal, or to benefit the interaction of the cavity and attachment. When a separate attachment is used to form the channel, it may be at a prominence different from that of the real attachment. The shape may also differ from the associated real attachment to control the extent and manner of interactions at the gingival aspect.
- *Dynamic attachment*: A concept wherein the virtual attachment and, consequently, its cavity differ in a predetermined way from the real, bonded attachment. The intentional misfit created between appliance and associ-

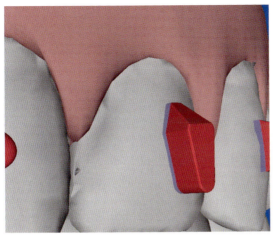

FIG 9-1a Attachment without channel.

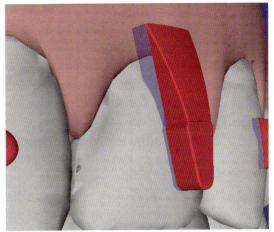

FIG 9-1b Attachment with channel at full.

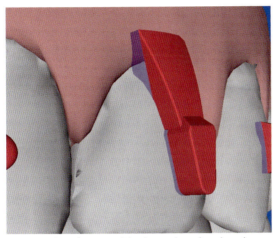

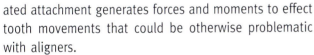

FIG 9-1c Attachment with channel and reduced prominences.

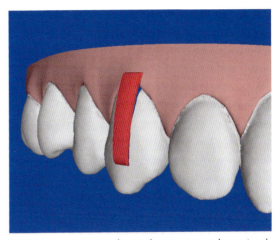

FIG 9-2 A 9-mm curved root tipper on a canine extending past the gingival margin.

ated attachment generates forces and moments to effect tooth movements that could be otherwise problematic with aligners.

- *Engagement*: The degree of attachment and cavity congruence or mating. This is typically more a qualitative than quantitative assessment of how well the two geometries track or join together.

- *Footprint*: The area of contact between a tooth and the attachment bonded to it. The actual footprint of a given attachment varies somewhat among placements because of the wide variations in tooth morphologies.

- *Orientation*: The alignment of an attachment's axes relative to those of another object—usually the underlying tooth. An attachment's default orientation is set at design time. Nevertheless, a practitioner may prescribe any other particular orientation so long as it will not conflict with the footprint and prominence considerations. Figure 9-3 shows two ellipsoid attachments with different orientations.

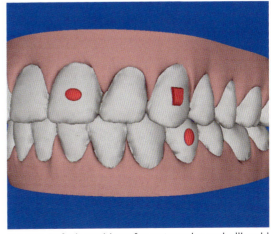

FIG 9-3 Default positions for rectangular and ellipsoid attachments. Note that the orientation has been changed from vertical to horizontal on the maxillary left central incisor.

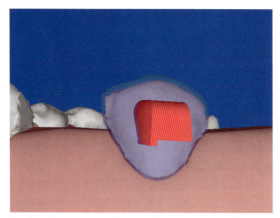

FIG 9-6 The red body is the virtual attachment designed to cause the desired misfit between the aligner and the bonded attachment for both rotation and resistance to intrusion. A scaled-tooth space (translucent purple) is placed around the tooth to eliminate collisions between the tooth and aligner that could impede rotation. (Neighboring teeth were removed for clarity.)

Retention Attachments

Because of factors such as short clinical crowns, insufficient undercuts, missing or extracted teeth, and pronounced tooth-size discrepancies, there are times when appliance retention must be enhanced to ensure that forces of the desired magnitude, direction, and point(s) of application are realized.

This augmented retention is readily accomplished through the inclusion of attachments in the treatment. Since there are no programmed positional changes between the bonded attachment and its cavity in the aligner, attachments placed for retention are always of the congruent type.

The other significant use of retention attachments is for a localized increase in the appliance's resistance to being dislodged on teeth that neighbor a tooth targeted for intrusion. The typical setup is to place one attachment on the buccal surface of each tooth immediately mesial and distal to the tooth that is to be intruded. These bonded attachments provide the leverage points against which the aligner works while the middle tooth's intrusion progresses.

Whether for general or local appliance retention, the current standard is to apply congruent attachments with no greater than 0.75-mm nominal prominence. Nevertheless, it is not unusual for retention attachments of higher prominence to be requested. The obvious risk is that these will be too retentive and the patient will have difficulty removing the aligners. Both in vitro testing and in vivo experience have shown that this does indeed happen. It is therefore advisable to use highly prominent attachments sparingly.

Additionally, the patient should be informed of the possible difficulties and receive instruction in proper aligner-removal methods.

When the need for higher-prominence retention attachments is indicated, the use of channel attachments or attachments that extend beyond the gingival margin may be advisable. The placement of these can mitigate excessive removal forces directed approximately along the occlusogingival axes while still providing mesiodistal retention (see Fig 9-2).

Auxiliary Attachments

Attachments have numerous applications as auxiliary treatment elements. These demonstrate the flexibility and potential of the seemingly simple idea of including additional geometric shapes in the computer representation of teeth. Their functions are the same, of course—the creation of orthodontic forces of the desired magnitude and direction—but how they can be generated and employed may not be so readily apparent. Several of the applications that either have been put into practice or are being developed are described below. In each of the following embodiments, the attachments employed are virtual—their shapes are not applied to the teeth as physical entities.

Force augmentation

It is self-evident that all forces generated by an aligner are due to deformations that alter its unloaded shape. The complexity of the deformation does not necessarily allow for a straightforward determination of the resultant forces. Nevertheless, there are areas of the appliance that are clearly of inadequate strength for the tooth movements they are expected to cause. These areas are predominantly found along the aligner's gingival edge and where there are large spaces between adjacent teeth.

Rather than simply allowing the teeth and their programmed motions to determine the shape and, thus, the strength of the appliance, virtual attachments may be added to the treatment to change the aligner's geometry and the consequent forces it applies to the teeth. These attachments will not be bonded to the underlying teeth, so the chief considerations in the selection of their shape, size, and placement are patient comfort and esthetics.

As an example, consider the appliance morphology that surrounds the maxillary central incisors. This region is typ-

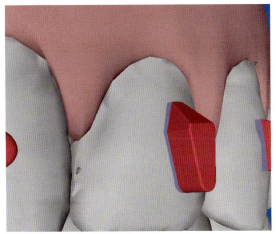

FIG 9-1a Attachment without channel.

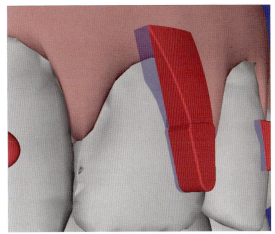

FIG 9-1b Attachment with channel at full.

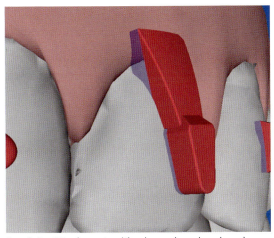

FIG 9-1c Attachment with channel and reduced prominences.

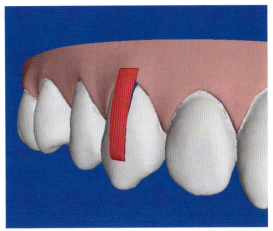

FIG 9-2 A 9-mm curved root tipper on a canine extending past the gingival margin.

ated attachment generates forces and moments to effect tooth movements that could be otherwise problematic with aligners.

- *Engagement*: The degree of attachment and cavity congruence or mating. This is typically more a qualitative than quantitative assessment of how well the two geometries track or join together.
- *Footprint*: The area of contact between a tooth and the attachment bonded to it. The actual footprint of a given attachment varies somewhat among placements because of the wide variations in tooth morphologies.
- *Orientation*: The alignment of an attachment's axes relative to those of another object—usually the underlying tooth. An attachment's default orientation is set at design time. Nevertheless, a practitioner may prescribe any other particular orientation so long as it will not conflict with the footprint and prominence considerations. Figure 9-3 shows two ellipsoid attachments with different orientations.

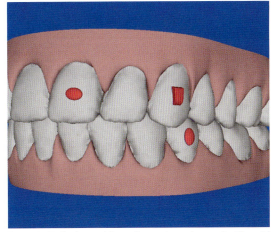

FIG 9-3 Default positions for rectangular and ellipsoid attachments. Note that the orientation has been changed from vertical to horizontal on the maxillary left central incisor.

- *Position*: Self-explanatory, although it should be noted that it is described relative to the underlying tooth or teeth.
- *Prominence*: The projected distance between an attachment's most labial geometry and the nearest point on the tooth on which it is placed. This value is set in every attachment design; however, it must be kept in mind that this is a nominal value. There are several factors that contribute to the alteration of the true prominence of a bonded attachment. First, the achievable placement accuracy of the virtual attachment varies from tooth to tooth. Second, the production of the physical attachment from a template on a tooth can introduce dimensional differences. And third, the attachment composite wears down over the course of treatment due to brushing and chewing, as well as aligner placement and removal.
- *Staging*: The timing of an event during an Invisalign treatment. As used in the context of attachments, it is when an attachment is present or visible in a treatment. Although they are typically placed by default on the teeth in the initial occlusion (stage 0), attachments can be prescribed by the practitioner at any stage. Further, their presence or visibility can be varied over the course of a treatment.
- *Visibility*: Whether or not an attachment that is present can be seen in the computer representation. As noted above, visibility can be changed stage to stage over the course of treatment. An attachment must be present and visible for its shape to be produced in an aligner.

Classifications

There are three fundamental categories of attachments: those that assist movements, those that augment appliance retention, and those that provide or support auxiliary functions. All three act as force transmitters; however, they do so in different ways.

The movement attachments are intended specifically to induce or aid the repositioning of the teeth to which they are bonded. The retention designs typically promote movements in teeth other than the one to which the attachment is affixed; retention attachments serve as relatively fixed points against which the aligner can act. The auxiliary attachments may be placed to act on the teeth they are attached to, on other teeth in the arch, or—in conjunction with other components (eg, elastics)—on teeth in the opposing arch.

Movement Attachments

As noted earlier, sites on which applied forces can act on the teeth are required to effect the intended tooth movements. The principal motions are, of course, extrusion, rotation, and translation. Within the category of movement attachments there are two basic manners of interaction between an aligner and an attachment.

The first is where the virtual and real attachments are identical (ie, the bonded attachment and its cavity in the aligner are produced from the same shape and are hence congruent). The successful application of this concept is predicated on the expectation that successive, small differential displacements between the bonded attachment and its cavity (as caused by the staging of the tooth's movements) engender the necessary deformation in the aligner cavity for it to stretch over the bonded attachment as the aligner is pressed onto the teeth. The cavity's recovery of the induced strain is transferred through the attachment as the intended displacement of the tooth.

This method has had limited success in both clinical study and commercial treatments. The reasons for this are evident. First, the size of the differential displacements is crucial to effective execution. If the displacements are too large, the cavity cannot locally distend sufficiently to fit the attachment, but will "ride up" on the attachment as the aligner bows outward to accommodate the interference. The broad range of factors that determine aligner geometry make it practically impossible to set the differential displacement at a standard magnitude and direction across all treatments or to vary it as a function of the geometry present. These factors include the target tooth's morphology, mesiodistal and occlusogingival dimensions, accessible facial surface, and its programmed path of movement, as well as these same parameters for the surrounding teeth.

Second, any cavity distention would necessarily need to be isotropic with respect to the attachment for the cavity to be able to regain congruency. However, the morphologic and dimensional conditions cited above, as well as the varying thickness of the aligner material, yield anisotropic distention. That is, a uniform force applied to a geometrically inhomogeneous body will cause differing amounts of deflection in that body. There is no means available to impart the varied forces (or, alternately, deflections) to the aligner to cause the cavity to distend in the manner required. Even if the means were created, there would still be the uncertainty in the determination

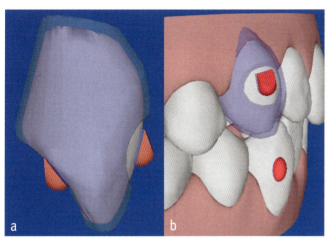

FIG 9-4 (a and b) Window attachments surround the tooth, but allow the aligner access to attachments.

of the appropriate magnitudes of forces (or deflections) discussed previously.

Typically, the attachment and cavity track over several stages; ultimately, however, there is the onset of incongruence that worsens over time. This is reported anecdotally and is also evident in the results from the University of Florida attachment study.[1]

The second manner of attachment/aligner interaction is where the virtual and real attachments are calculatedly different in shape. This causes an interaction that can be thought of as a cam (the real, bonded attachment) and follower (the shape formed in the aligner). This interaction allows for the generation of forces from bowing the aligner outward from the teeth. This deformation is more predictable and quantifiable for a given treatment and, within a determinable range, across treatments. Further, the force caused by the deflection can readily be altered through the addition or removal of geometric effects in the surrounding region. This is discussed in the "Auxiliary" section below.

This interaction has another advantage over congruent interactions in that it has the propensity to be self-correcting. This property led to the appellation of *dynamic attachment*. If the tooth does not track with its movement programmed into the aligner, the followers in the aligner will interfere even more with the underlying cam (bonded) attachments. This causes greater outward deflection in the aligner, which yields more force applied to the tooth through the attachments. The increased force tends to compel the tooth back into accord with the programmed movement.

A dynamic attachment setup follows the following progression: Real attachments are applied to the buccal and lingual tooth surfaces at one stage prior to the onset of the desired movement; these are replaced in the next stage with the attachments' virtual versions, and a window attachment appears at this same stage. The translucent purple bodies seen in Figs 9-4 to 9-6 are window attachments. These are typically removed from the treatment at three stages after the programmed movement has ceased. This is done to allow the tooth movement to be fully expressed.

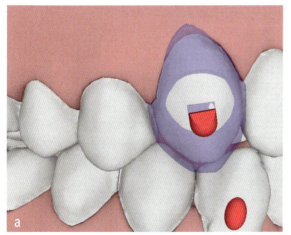

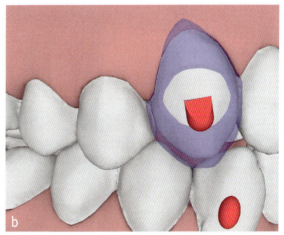

FIG 9-5 (a and b) The purple volume will become a space surrounding the tooth in the aligners. (*a*) The attachments on the canine (the identical lingual one is not shown) slope away from the tooth surface in the occlusal/incisal direction. (*b*) The gingival portion of the attachment has been removed. Starting at stage 01, this will form a step in the aligners that will interfere with the actual bonded attachment. The space around the tooth permits it to move if there are not interproximal contacts with the lateral incisor or first premolar (a judicious amount of interproximal reduction could help).

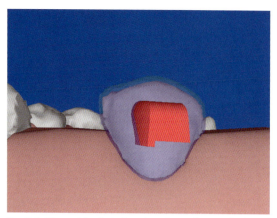

FIG 9-6 The red body is the virtual attachment designed to cause the desired misfit between the aligner and the bonded attachment for both rotation and resistance to intrusion. A scaled-tooth space (translucent purple) is placed around the tooth to eliminate collisions between the tooth and aligner that could impede rotation. (Neighboring teeth were removed for clarity.)

Retention Attachments

Because of factors such as short clinical crowns, insufficient undercuts, missing or extracted teeth, and pronounced tooth-size discrepancies, there are times when appliance retention must be enhanced to ensure that forces of the desired magnitude, direction, and point(s) of application are realized.

This augmented retention is readily accomplished through the inclusion of attachments in the treatment. Since there are no programmed positional changes between the bonded attachment and its cavity in the aligner, attachments placed for retention are always of the congruent type.

The other significant use of retention attachments is for a localized increase in the appliance's resistance to being dislodged on teeth that neighbor a tooth targeted for intrusion. The typical setup is to place one attachment on the buccal surface of each tooth immediately mesial and distal to the tooth that is to be intruded. These bonded attachments provide the leverage points against which the aligner works while the middle tooth's intrusion progresses.

Whether for general or local appliance retention, the current standard is to apply congruent attachments with no greater than 0.75-mm nominal prominence. Nevertheless, it is not unusual for retention attachments of higher prominence to be requested. The obvious risk is that these will be too retentive and the patient will have difficulty removing the aligners. Both in vitro testing and in vivo experience have shown that this does indeed happen. It is therefore advisable to use highly prominent attachments sparingly.

Additionally, the patient should be informed of the possible difficulties and receive instruction in proper aligner-removal methods.

When the need for higher-prominence retention attachments is indicated, the use of channel attachments or attachments that extend beyond the gingival margin may be advisable. The placement of these can mitigate excessive removal forces directed approximately along the occlusogingival axes while still providing mesiodistal retention (see Fig 9-2).

Auxiliary Attachments

Attachments have numerous applications as auxiliary treatment elements. These demonstrate the flexibility and potential of the seemingly simple idea of including additional geometric shapes in the computer representation of teeth. Their functions are the same, of course—the creation of orthodontic forces of the desired magnitude and direction—but how they can be generated and employed may not be so readily apparent. Several of the applications that either have been put into practice or are being developed are described below. In each of the following embodiments, the attachments employed are virtual—their shapes are not applied to the teeth as physical entities.

Force augmentation

It is self-evident that all forces generated by an aligner are due to deformations that alter its unloaded shape. The complexity of the deformation does not necessarily allow for a straightforward determination of the resultant forces. Nevertheless, there are areas of the appliance that are clearly of inadequate strength for the tooth movements they are expected to cause. These areas are predominantly found along the aligner's gingival edge and where there are large spaces between adjacent teeth.

Rather than simply allowing the teeth and their programmed motions to determine the shape and, thus, the strength of the appliance, virtual attachments may be added to the treatment to change the aligner's geometry and the consequent forces it applies to the teeth. These attachments will not be bonded to the underlying teeth, so the chief considerations in the selection of their shape, size, and placement are patient comfort and esthetics.

As an example, consider the appliance morphology that surrounds the maxillary central incisors. This region is typ-

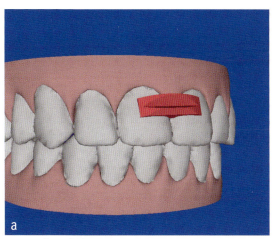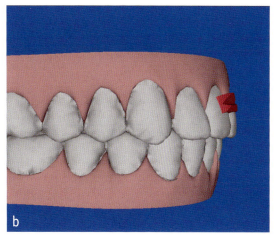

FIG 9-7 (a and b) An attachment placed across the interproximal region of the maxillary central incisors for rigidity.

ically among the weakest points in the aligner for obvious reasons: the teeth are located at what amounts to the keystone of the arch—a distinct inflection point—and they are tall and broad, and have a relatively planar profile. Thus, during appliance formation the plastic thins here more than in any other region. Also, there are no naturally occurring features to add rigidity to the span such as are found with molars. Thickening the plastic over the centrals would tend to make the region stronger; unfortunately, selective thickening of the appliance is not achievable within the constraints of current production methods. Another means of strengthening the region is to cause rigidifying elements to be produced in the aligner. This is easily accomplished through the addition of virtual attachments. Figures 9-7a and 9-7b show a sample ridged attachment placed across the interproximal region of the maxillary central incisors that will form corrugations in the aligner. These will yield more force for a given deformation.

In a similar manner, virtual attachments may be added to other areas to increase an aligner's resistance to shape modification. Their impact on comfort, appliance retention, and esthetics must be kept in mind. It should also be understood that the magnitudes and directions of the resultant forces will be unique to each patient and for each stage of that patient's treatment. So far, no empirical data exist to derive the functional relationship between the attachment's shape and prominence and the ensuing force change.

Fixation points

The production of an attachment that would form a hook or button in an aligner has been a frequent request from practitioners. This is not possible, however, given the means by which both the arch molds and aligners are fabricated. Consult chapter 6 for an explanation of the molding process. Nevertheless, attachments can be utilized to facilitate the use of buttons, hooks, or other linkage components.

Several attachments were created explicitly for the purpose of forming surfaces on which to affix hooks and buttons either through adhesive bonds or mechanical interaction. An attachment on the maxillary arch will create a smooth plateau onto which a linkage component (eg, commercially available button or hook) can be bonded. The body on the mandibular arch will then create a surface with a discernible depression in its center. The diameter and depth of this depression can be altered to serve different purposes (eg, as a more precise locater for component placement on the surface or as a guide to produce a hole for a component that passes through the aligner surface.)

Another particular implementation of virtual attachments as fixation points is created when aligners are used as surgical splints (Figs 9-8a and 9-8b). The attachments form shapes in the aligners that are sufficiently large and rigid to support tying the jaws together through them during postoperative healing. Real attachments may also be placed to augment retention of the appliances.

In a manner similar to perforating the attachments' cavities to use them as fixation points for surgical splints, they may also be slit. The notch that is formed can be used as a hook for elastics. When cutting the slit, care must be taken to ensure that the notch will not propagate into an unwanted tear in the aligner. A way to avoid this is to utilize a rotary tool rather than a fixed blade. The former tends to create a smooth-bottomed crevice whose dimensions are easier to control.

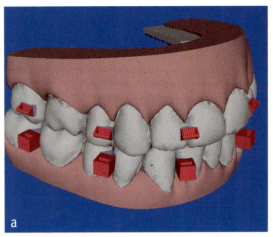
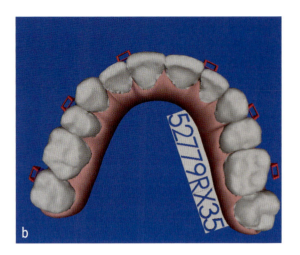

Fig 9-8 (a and b) Surgical splint fixation points.

A fixation point on the exterior surface of an aligner can be viewed as a receptacle on the interior. This concept suggests that additional orthodontic ancillaries may be used in attachments' cavities to place or affix various components. The components could be active (eg, springs) or passive (eg, wedges) and could be changed or adjusted as the treatment progresses.

The advantages of forming fixation points in the aligner are apparent:

• The geometry maintains its position relative to the underlying tooth or teeth over the course of treatment.
• Components can be bonded in the same locations easily and at any stage.
• The geometry can be controlled to be present in the aligner at only those stages it is needed.
• The attachment adds local rigidity to the aligner to reduce unwanted appliance deformation.
• The attachment can be spanned across one or more teeth to cause force systems not otherwise attainable.
• Multiple attachments can be placed adjacently to create a range of fixation points.

Interarch mechanics

Distalization

A novel means of implementing Class II elastics treatment using aligners was proposed by Dr Warren Wakerlin (personal communication, 2002). To this end, an attachment was designed for placement on the maxillary canines. There is a hole through the attachment that runs parallel to the tooth's long axis (Figs 9-9a and 9-9b). This hole is set a distance (prominence) from the tooth surface comparable to that found in canine brackets with hooks. This

hole resolves as depressions in the upper and lower surfaces of the attachment when the aligner is formed. These features act as guides to punch holes into which wire hooks are inserted. The use of a high-speed bur or heated wire to form the hole has produced no problems (ie, tearing) with the aligner even after numerous insertions and removals over a 2-week period.

In some cases, attachments may need to be added on teeth distal to the canine to enhance aligner retention. Figure 9-10 shows the mandibular arch setup with brackets as anchors for the elastics. Very much the same result can be achieved through use of an aligner and retention attachments. Irrespective of the choice of a mandibular-anchorage method, from this point the case proceeds as a typical Class II treatment with traditional appliances, but with the hygiene, comfort, and esthetic benefits of an Invisalign System treatment.

Bite props

As with other treatment methods, some Invisalign System cases require that the bite be propped open to allow for tooth repositioning (eg, correction of an anterior crossbite). With conventional appliances, this is frequently done by bonding composite or a component to teeth to form a wedge. Such a prop can be produced in aligners by using a virtual attachment. As is true for any attachment, props can be present, or not, at any stage prescribed by the treating clinician.

Clinical evidence suggests that aligners correct crossbites more efficiently than do conventional orthodontics. This, coupled with the functional, cosmetic, convenience, and chair-time benefits of an aligner-based bite prop, makes a compelling case for the use of Invisalign in preference to fixed appliances to effect crossbite corrections.

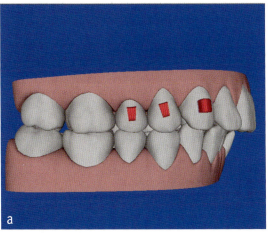 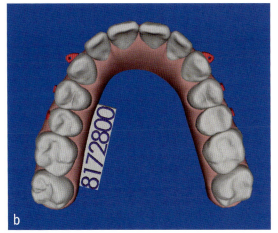

Fig 9-9 (a and b) The holes on the canine attachments are used for distalization.

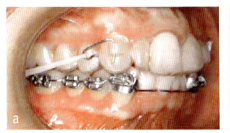 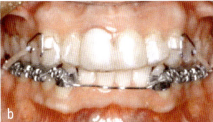 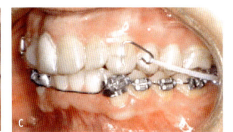

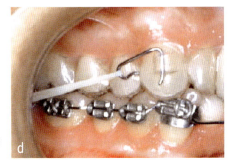 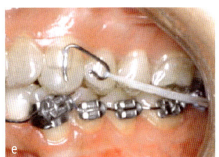

Fig 9-10 (a to e) Clinical use of attachments shown in Fig 9-9b.

Mandibular repositioning devices

Various incarnations of mandibular repositioning devices are available commercially either as laboratory setups or for the practitioner to install. Among them, the mandibular anterior repositioning appliance (MARA) has seen significantly increased usage in recent years—in particular, as an alternative to a Herbst positioner. This has led to MARA design modifications that enhance patient comfort and simplify the installation procedure. Nonetheless, placement of the device remains fairly time-consuming and can require extensive adjustments.

Proponents of a MARA as a mandibular repositioning device cite numerous benefits to both patient and practitioner. Among these are an immediate improvement in profile appearance, more efficient treatment of Class II malocclusions, rapid movement of the maxillary first molars while also causing mesial to buccal rotation, ease of fit, retentive crown coverage, and the ability for simultaneous use with other orthodontic appliances.

The idea of using the Invisalign System to generate a patient-specific, aligner-based device that is very much the same as the MARA was proposed by Dr Robert Fry (personal communication, 2003). Fry is the principal investigator for a clinical study Align has undertaken to evaluate this modified aligner's efficacy. It is expected that this construction will have distinct benefits relative to the existing designs. These include enhanced patient comfort due to the exact custom fit possible with Align's production processes, more precise diagnoses based on the three-dimensional presentation in ClinCheck, greater accuracy and flexibility in setting and adjusting the interarch mechanics by controlling component positioning before committing to device production, and generally

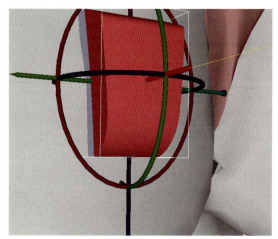

FIG 9-11 Default position of attachments.

improved oral health since the entire appliance is removable and bonding is minimized or eliminated.

Reservoirs

Attachment function need not be confined solely to use as auxiliary components intended to move teeth. The cavity created in an aligner by an attachment can also be exploited as a dispersal point for substances or a receptacle for devices. The former could include drugs to promote an orthodontic treatment (or for a purpose unrelated to orthodontia that has broader health benefits, such as analgesics, antibiotics, etc). The range of devices that could be incorporated into an aligner is fairly extensive, from a wear indicator to modules to monitor a patient's biometrics.

Design Factors

The aspects that drive attachment designs are similar to those that lead to bracket designs—functionality, comfort, and esthetics. As with many other products, interactions and dependencies among these aspects may constrain or guide choices. The following sections provide insight into the attachment development process.

Functionality

The intended output or result is the foremost consideration at the outset of any design. An attachment has several aspects that can be included under the functional designation. For Align's production processes, these aspects include object properties, file size, software compatibility, and appliance fabrication. Only the first and last of these aspects will be discussed here. For the clinician

and patient, the functional aspects include performance, which can be defined as the attachment's role to augment and facilitate the aligner's programmed tooth movement. The performance aspect was discussed earlier in this chapter. Ease, accuracy, and precision of transferral are also covered in chapter 10. Therefore, only the design considerations that affect an attachment's durability will be discussed in this section.

From a practical standpoint, a user need not be concerned with the properties of an attachment. The clinician's awareness of a few fundamentals, however, may provide perspectives on the Invisalign System processes that could lead to improved treatment results.

Every attachment is designed to have the same spatial coordinate system so that consistent, predictable placements are attained when they are applied to teeth. The origin of the coordinates is always positioned at the interface of the attachment proper, and its base is typically placed in the geometric center of the attachment's footprint. The default orientation varies among attachments according to their design intents. As can be seen in Fig 9-11, the coordinate system defines the positional and rotational controls that are used to set an attachment in a particular spatial relationship with respect to the underlying tooth. These controls are not currently accessible from ClinCheck, but are reserved for Align's technicians during case setups.

With some exceptions, an attachment's facial profile defines its footprint. One of the attachment design goals is to minimize this area to produce as unobtrusive a body as possible. There is a countervailing design goal, however, in that the attachment and tooth must have sufficient surface contact area to resist shear or other failure modes when the attachment is loaded to move the associated tooth. It has been determined experimentally that an attachment with a prominence of 0.75 mm must have a footprint of no less than about 5 mm^2 when it is formed in composite and bonded to a tooth. The practical limitations on attachment prominence were discussed previously. There is an additional consideration related to prominence: the footprint typically needs to become larger as an attachment's buccolingual dimension increases.

The physical characteristics of spatial location, contact area, and shape largely define the intended attachment morphology. The thermoforming process used to fabricate aligners determines the geometry's actual representation. There are two main factors that create the differences between the intended and the actual attachment cavity.

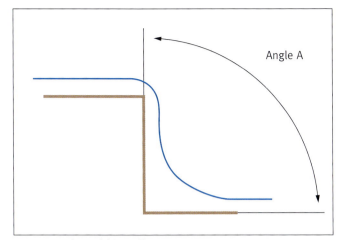

FIG 9-12a The webbing effect.

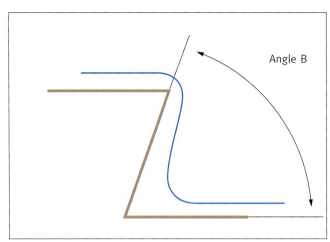

FIG 9-12b An undercut is created to mitigate the webbing effect.

The first is the webbing effect that occurs around the attachment body during aligner thermoforming. Webbing occurs when a material spans a geometric transition rather than conforming to its surfaces (Fig 9-12a). A means of mitigating this effect is shown in Fig 9-12b. It should be clear that if the attachment's profile and consequent cavity are as shown in Fig 9-12a, the aligner will more easily slide over or off the underlying attachment, which diminishes the attachment's effectiveness. To improve the interaction between aligner and bonded attachment, the latter's profile is given an inward bevel. This tends to cause the aligner to form more nearly perpendicular or even inwardly angled surfaces. The slight bevel also helps to reduce the unwanted relative motion between aligner and attachment.

The second main factor that creates differences between the intended and the actual attachment cavity is the bridging effect that results from other local geometries. This is essentially the same phenomenon as seen around the attachment body, but it is caused instead by the proximity of other bodies to the attachment. This is part of the reason for the default placement of an attachment in the locus of the tooth's facial axis point—it is thus removed from the transitions between teeth at the incisal/occlusal edges and between teeth and the gingiva. Webbing and bridging are predominantly beneficial to the comfort and fit of the aligner, but are detrimental to the formation and application of attachments.

The durability of an attachment is a function of three principal components: shape, material, and environment. It had been presupposed and has been effectively demonstrated in actual usage that distinct or sharp edges were not advisable for composite attachments, because they tend to degrade over time more substantially and more quickly than when the attachment's shape flows more smoothly. Where allowable, attachments have limited sharp edges.

The recommended material for attachments has been resin composites, since these are intended for uses not dissimilar to how Invisalign System attachments are employed. Also, the composites' wear resistance is generally well documented and understood. Complete information is provided in chapter 10.

The environment is the unknown and uncontrollable factor in attachment durability. Perhaps the best that can be achieved is to inform patients of some of the caveats given with brackets: avoid hard foods such as nuts and ice and resist over-brushing.

Esthetics

Stating the obvious, the appearance of any geometry bonded to a tooth is determined to a large extent by its size and shape. This is somewhat offset by the fact that the composites used to form attachments can be color-matched to a patient's teeth. The presence of the aligners also mitigates the visual obtrusiveness of the attachments.

Comfort

A patient's comfort is always going to be compromised by bonding anything to the teeth. Efforts are made to minimize the discomfiture by keeping footprints small, prominences low, and shapes free of sharp edges. The edge characteristics are almost exclusively a concern for the short durations when patients are not wearing their aligners. When in place, the appliances create smooth continuous surfaces that minimize discomfort.

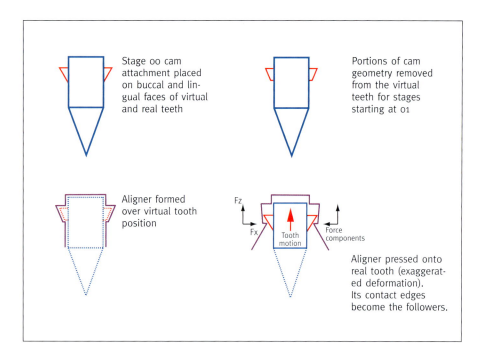

Stage oo cam attachment placed on buccal and lingual faces of virtual and real teeth

Portions of cam geometry removed from the virtual teeth for stages starting at 01

Aligner formed over virtual tooth position

Fz

Fx

Tooth motion

Force components

Aligner pressed onto real tooth (exaggerated deformation). Its contact edges become the followers.

FIG 9-13a Principle behind the dynamic attachment, shown here for extruding a tooth (under development). If the tooth's extrusion begins lagging behind the aligner, the force generated by the deformation will increase, tending to cause the tooth to move more. At a cam angle of 35 degrees, 82% of the force goes to extrusion. Sufficient "head and shoulder" room must be available for the tooth to move into and to avoid binding. This is a simple two-dimensional representation. The complex real geometries of teeth and aligner render actual results less certain.

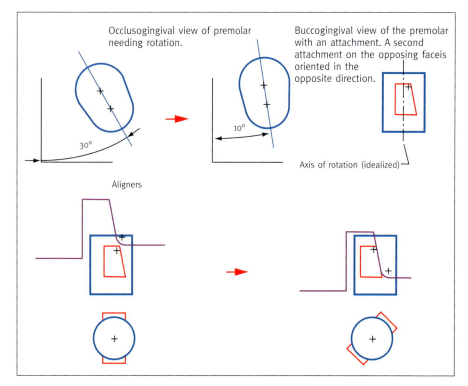

Occlusogingival view of premolar needing rotation.

Buccogingival view of the premolar with an attachment. A second attachment on the opposing face is oriented in the opposite direction.

30°

10°

Axis of rotation (idealized)

Aligners

FIG 9-13b Principle behind the dynamic attachment, shown here for rotating a tooth (under development). The vertical motion of the aligner is converted to rotation of the tooth. There is some intrusive force on the tooth, but this can be counteracted or overcome with, for example, an upward sloping ramp as is used for extrusion.

Imminent Developments

Dynamic attachments

The development of this attachment concept began with the determination of the angles needed to impart the maximum force in the intended direction while minimizing the opposing or otherwise detrimentally directed forces (Figs 9-13a and 9-13b). This was followed by the calculation of a footprint large enough to support more than the expected shear forces. The combination of these factors yielded the attachment prominences, which are substantially greater than those of congruent attachments. Because the interaction is distinctly different, however, no significant increase in difficulty of appliance removal in either in vitro or in vivo evaluations has been realized.

Numerous test cases were set up with the attachments and the respective programmed movements. These cases were produced as models that were mounted on dynamometers to measure the magnitudes and directions of forces. Repeated controlled evaluations demonstrated that the attachments performed as intended and did not pose any additional hazards to the patient.

In August 2003, a study was initiated in several private practices to evaluate two attachment designs—one for rotation and one for extrusion—based on the "dynamic" concept (unpublished data, 2003–2006). The primary objectives of this study were to achieve at least 70% efficacy of movement in more than 70% of the attempts to rotate canines and premolars and attempts to extrude incisors, canines, and premolars. The secondary objective was to obtain and assess clinician and patient reactions to the application and wear of the attachments and appliances.

Subjects were selected from candidates submitted by the participating clinicians for treatment with the Invisalign System. To be enrolled, a patient's treatment had to require 1 mm or more of extrusion for at least one incisor, canine, or premolar or 20 degrees or more rotation for at least one canine or premolar. If an accepted patient evidenced more than one tooth that qualified and the teeth were in the same arch, the teeth were treated consecutively. Teeth in different arches were treated simultaneously when they were not also in opposition, consecutively when they opposed each other. With the exceptions of premolar extraction and orthognathic surgery cases, any type of malocclusion was accepted. It was required that all patients were in adult dentition, had stopped growing, and, if they presented with periodontal disease or active caries, had a clinician or periodontist of record.

Each enrolled patient's treatment was set up using standard Invisalign parameters and methods, but with the following differences: several aligner stages were used to create space around the target teeth, the rotations and extrusions were staged as early as possible in the treatment, the programmed movements were discrete (ie, the teeth were moved along [extrusion] or around [rotation] only one axis), the movement speeds were set based on attachment dimensions, and, of course, the dynamic (buccal and lingual) and window attachments were placed and staged in concert with the timing of the programmed movements.

For each case, attachment usage progressed as follows: All real attachments were bonded at stage 0, the real attachments (in the computer treatment models) were replaced with their virtual counterparts at the first stage of their underlying tooth's programmed movement, the associated window attachments were made visible at this same time, the window attachments were made invisible three stages after the programmed movement ended, and the dynamic attachments remained unchanged for the balance of the treatment.

Though not without some disappointing outcomes, the preliminary results of both motions show great promise. Efficacies are currently distributed over a broad range, but they are generally improving, the range is narrowing, and the contributing elements have been identified. Clinician and patient feedback do not so far suggest complications or negative reactions to the heightened prominence, lingual attachment presence, space-creating window attachment, or outward aligner deflection.

Preformed attachments

Composite attachments can wear noticeably over the course of treatment as a result of repeated removal and replacement of aligners, as well as from speaking, chewing, and brushing. This erosion of their shape may lead to compromised effectiveness.

A possible means of mitigating the wear is being evaluated. This involves preforming attachments and bonding them to teeth in much the same way brackets are. Besides reduced wear, other benefits may arise from the use of preformed shapes. Among these are that the attachment bonding process could become less problematic (eg, reduced flash) and faster, the bonded attachments will have more distinct shapes that could assist efficacy—this is of particular interest for dynamic attachments—and the preformed attachments will likely be even less obtrusive than ones that are currently in use because of the material choices available.

In July 2003, a small investigation was begun, and is still ongoing, to assess the performance and acceptability of preformed shapes. The commercial stalwart attachments curved root tipper (CRT) and ellipsoid were selected as the test vehicles. These were produced in rigid polyurethane. The formation of their attachment template aligner cavities remains unchanged. The preformed attachments are then tacked into the cavities with sticky wax.

The patient selection criteria for this investigation were not particularly restrictive due to the effect in study. The four requirements for inclusion were Class I malocclusion, fully erupted second molars, and no need for premolar extractions. Patients received both preformed and composite attachments. Each arch had only one or the other, and this was assigned randomly. Impressions were made at set time points over the course of treatment. Comparisons of the attachments' geometries at different instances will reveal how well the preformed versions have fared relative to the same shape in composite.

Summary

Attachment use is essential to successful Invisalign treatments. The designs currently available for commercial use are of some assistance but are clearly not up to the task of completely reaching the goal of full expression of tooth movements. Several developments on the near horizon in both processes and product, however, hold promise for dramatically improved outcomes.

Reference

1. Wheeler T. Evaluation of different attachments used in Invisalign treatment. Presented at the 105th Annual Session of the American Association of Orthodontists, San Francisco, 23 May 2005.

chapter 10

INVISALIGN ATTACHMENTS: MATERIALS

by
Eric Kuo, DDS and Trang Duong, DDS

The term *composite material* refers to a three-dimensional (3-D) combination of at least two chemically different materials with a distinct interface that separates the components.[1] The combination of materials provides properties that could not be achieved with one component alone. Therefore, a dental composite material is one in which an inorganic filler is added to a resin matrix to improve the properties of the matrix. Most of the composite restorative materials use the dimethacrylate monomer (bisphenol glycidyl methacrylate, or bis-GMA) molecule.

Resin-based composites have been used since the 1970s for dental restorations. It is well known that when composite is light cured, stresses develop as polymerization and shrinkage occur.[2] Characteristic properties of composites are dependent on the filler content. In resin-based composites, the filler content is directly related to the mechanical and wear-resistance properties.[3,4] The higher filler content also reduces the shrinkage of the composite during polymerization.[5] Because of its effect on both the elastic modulus and shrinkage, the amount of filler content plays an important role on the material properties of the composite.

Low-Viscosity Versus Nonflowable Composites

Low-viscosity flowable composites contain 20% to 25% less filler than do nonflowable materials.[6] Studies have shown considerable differences between elastic modulus and shrinkage properties in flowable and conventional hybrid composite materials.[7,8] Flowable composites can be hybrids or microfilled. Studies have shown that microfilled composites contain lower filler levels than do hybrids.[4,7] According to Hooke's law, stress is determined by the stiffness of the material when subjected to a given strain. The higher the elastic modulus and polymerization shrinkage, the higher the contraction stress.

Composite in Dental Restorations Versus Invisalign Attachments

In a setting such as a Class I or II preparation, extensive polymerization shrinkage can lead to internal stress and exceed the strength of the bond with the surrounding cavity wall and thus lead to failure of the interface.[9] This marginal gap can lead to tooth sensitivity and may provide a site for recurrent caries to develop. In a setting such as bonding brackets or attachments onto the enamel surface of the teeth, this shrinkage does not pose any significant problems. With attachments, however, treatment can extend several months and even a couple of years, so the wear properties and the strength of the bond to the enamel are important properties for selecting a suitable material. Because attachments serve as bonded extensions of the teeth to help achieve specific tooth movements and add retention, they are an important part of the Invisalign System.

Bonding Attachments

With the introduction of bonding composites, the use of orthodontic bands on anterior teeth slowly became obsolete and bonding became popular in the 1980s.[10] Bonding is based on the mechanical locking of an adhesive to irregularities in the enamel surface of the tooth and to mechanical locks formed in the base of the bracket. Orthodontists have used various light-cured and self-cured flowable composites to bond brackets onto teeth. A successful bonding material must meet a set of criteria: it must be dimensionally stable, fluid, able to penetrate the enamel surface, have excellent strength, and be easy to use clinically. Today, filled acrylic (bis-GMA) resins are the preferred bonding materials. These are available in a variety of formulations that differ in the composition and amount of fillers and also in how they are cured (chemical or light).

Attachments

Attachments are composite geometries that are bonded to the facial or lingual surfaces of the teeth for the purpose of increasing aligner retention to the teeth. Because the aligners work by repositioning the teeth according to the new position defined by the next aligner in sequence, the tendency is for the aligner to be slightly displaced at the onset until the teeth respond and conform to the position(s) defined by the new aligner. Once the teeth have moved, the maximum adaptation to the aligner is reached and the cycle repeats with each successive aligner until the final aligner is reached. The attachments are used to create undercuts to help facilitate maximum adaptation of each aligner to the teeth and help avoid aligner displace-

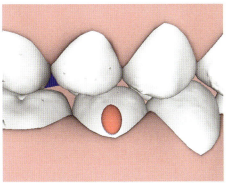

FIG 10-1 Attachments too close to the gingiva may be difficult to bond and maintain.

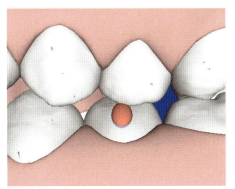

FIG 10-2 Attachments positioned too occlusally or incisally may interfere with the opposing arch.

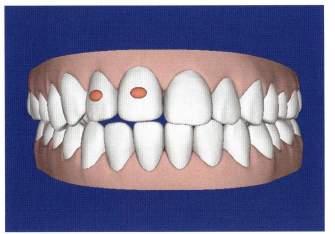

FIG 10-3 Anterior attachments may pose an esthetic concern for some patients.

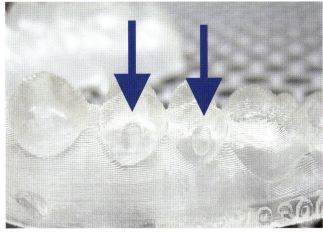

FIG 10-4 Premolar ellipsoid attachments (*arrows*) built into each resin model.

ment, so that the movements programmed into each aligner can be fully expressed. Supplemental retention can also be required in cases where the clinical crowns of the teeth are short or the amount of undercut present is minimal, such as in patients with moderate to severe attrition or gingival hyperplasia. Patients should not be able to remove the aligners with their tongue. Patients with upright teeth or cone-shaped teeth may also experience suboptimal aligner fit without additional appliance anchorage. For these patients, the temporary addition of supplemental undercuts through the use of attachments can significantly enhance aligner retention.

The shape and position of the attachment is determined at the time of the ClinCheck setup. The technician is able to create a virtual attachment on the 3-D model in the Treat software environment that stays on the same position of the tooth at each stage, regardless of the movement programmed for each tooth. The virtual attachment can be positioned anywhere on any tooth, in accor-

dance with the clinician's wishes. Clinical considerations when selecting attachment shape, location, and position should include proximity to the gingiva, proximity to the opposing dental arch, bondability to the tooth surface (metal, porcelain, and dental composite typically require special surface treatment to achieve an adequate bond strength), and esthetics (Figs 10-1 to 10-3).

The attachments placed in the virtual setup are built into the resin models for each aligner stage (Fig 10-4). An attachment template (thin-material aligner) is created to transfer the exact shape and position of the attachment from the 3-D model to the actual tooth. The clinician fills each attachment reservoir in the template with restorative dental composite, etches each tooth to be bonded, seats the filled attachment template on the teeth, cures the composite, and removes the template, leaving the attachments bonded to the teeth in the desired position (Fig 10-5).

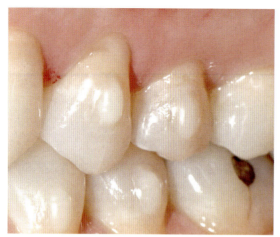

Fig 10-5 Bonded composite ellipsoid attachments on premolars.

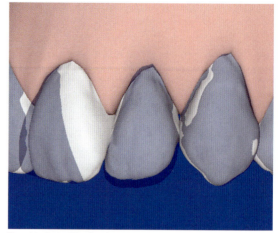

Fig 10-6 A ClinCheck treatment plan superimposition showing the vertical change around the lateral incisor between the initial position and the goal. Mesial-out rotation is planned for the central incisor, mesial-in for the canine.

Biomechanical Considerations

The primary purpose of the Invisalign attachment is to prevent appliance displacement so that the active regions of the aligner can remain in close contact with the teeth until the teeth conform to the desired position within the aligner.[11] This differs from traditional orthodontics, in which the teeth being moved must be included as part of the wire and bracket assembly. With aligner treatment, the teeth being moved do not necessarily have to have an attachment bonded to them. In other words, so long as the aligner material is in close contact with the teeth being moved, the appliance-anchoring attachments may be located on other teeth in the arch and not necessarily on the teeth being moved. This is an important consideration in terms of overall appliance esthetics, since bonding attachments to the facial surfaces of the anterior teeth is esthetically less desirable than bonding attachments to the buccal surfaces of posterior teeth.

Extrusion

The magnitude and direction of tooth movement programmed into each aligner affects the aligner's ability to adapt to the teeth. Tooth movements in the vertical dimension in particular are prone to separating the contact between the aligner and the teeth. With extrusive movements, the aligner by design must pull away from the teeth (Figs 10-6 and 10-7). Since most teeth do not have substantial undercuts along the vertical axis, these movements are least predictable with aligners in the absence of auxiliary treatment with vertical elastics. Composite attachments can

help create an artificial undercut to enable the aligner to better grab the tooth; however, because the aligner material is not sufficiently elastic in the vertical dimension, a mismatch can often develop between the aligner and the attachment. If an interference is created on the facial surface, the tooth may be displaced lingually in response to the force generated from the aligner flex (Figs 10-8 and 10-9).

Intrusion

When dental intrusion is programmed into the aligners, an occlusal interference is naturally created that unseats the aligner from the posterior teeth unless attachments are placed on the posterior teeth to help anchor the aligner (Figs 10-10 and 10-11). Once attachments are placed to prevent the separation of the aligner from the posterior teeth (Fig 10-12), the aligner is able to deliver a vertical force to intrude the incisors. An important point to remember is that the attachments for intrusion are not placed on the incisors themselves, since the aligner displacement forces occur on the posterior section of the aligner and not the incisor section of the aligner.

Intrusion of the posterior teeth poses a greater biomechanical challenge than intrusion of the anterior teeth. This is because, for posterior intrusion, the aligner can only be stabilized by a unilateral anchor to resist the reciprocal vertical forces. The result is a cantilever arm design, which is less stable than the bilateral anchor design typically used to intrude incisors (Figs 10-13 to 10-15). When attempting to intrude posterior teeth, it is important that the interproximal surfaces of the intruding tooth be clear from the adjacent tooth surfaces to avoid tooth-to-tooth

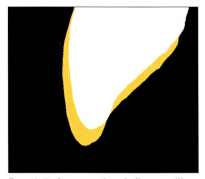

FIG 10-7 Cross-sectional diagram illustrating how extrusion built into the aligner (*yellow*) can lead to separation from the teeth (*white*) because of lack of undercut and insufficient elasticity in the aligner to pull the tooth into the new vertical position.

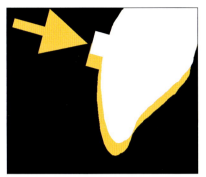

FIG 10-8 Addition of attachment for creation of undercut requires material to be elastic at the point indicated by the arrow to engage the undercut.

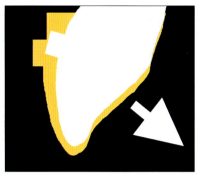

FIG 10-9 The interference created from the aligner-attachment mismatch displaces the tooth lingually (*arrow*) in response to the force generated as the aligner material flexes around the attachment area.

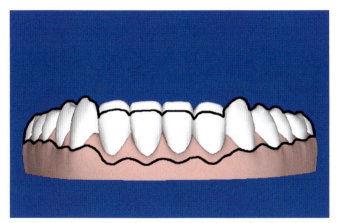

FIG 10-10 The outline of an aligner designed for dental intrusion of the mandibular incisors (*black outline*, movements exaggerated).

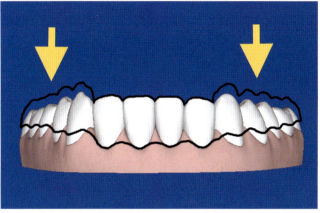

FIG 10-11 How the aligner in Fig 10-10 would sit on the teeth. The point of first contact would be at the incisors, and the posterior section would not seat without additional aligner anchors in the areas indicated by the *arrows*.

binding. Supraerupted molars often present with a coronal tooth width that is greater than the arch length dimension as a result of mesial migration.

Rotation

The derotation of cylindrical teeth also presents biomechanical challenges because of the minimal interproximal surface and undercuts available along the horizontal occlusal plane to the aligner (Fig 10-16). The aligner is prone to slipping along the facial and lingual surfaces as it tries to rotate the tooth. Placement of buccal and lingual attachments is designed to create aligner purchase points for improved tracking during tooth movement (Fig 10-17). Also critical during the derotation of premolars is the absence of friction between the rotated tooth and adjacent teeth, as is the case with the derotation of teeth using conventional fixed appliances.

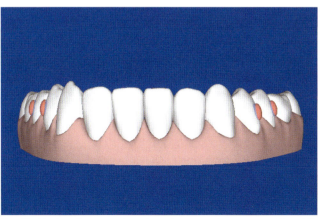

FIG 10-12 Attachments placed on the premolars to provide additional anchorage to counteract the tendency for the aligner to displace from the posterior teeth during incisor intrusion.

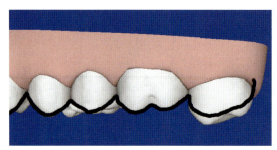

Fig 10-13 Supraerupted second molar with outline of aligner programmed to intrude the second molar.

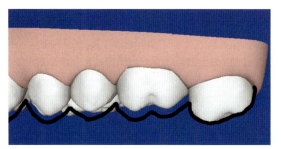

Fig 10-14 Aligner adaptation likely to occur following poor anchoring of the aligner to premolars as a result of inadequate gingival undercuts.

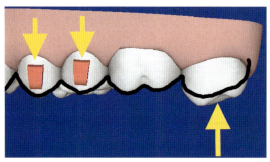

Fig 10-15 Addition of anchoring attachments on the premolars and the resulting cantilever spring designed to deliver intrusion force (*right arrow*) to the second molar in response to the resulting aligner material flex distal to the anchor points. *Left arrows* indicate undercut retention required to deliver intrusion force.

Translation

Improving root translation is a third clinical application for composite attachments. To achieve root translation and avoid tooth tipping, orthodontic force must be generated near the gingival area of the tooth (Fig 10-18). For many teeth, the interproximal surface is suboptimal and must be augmented with additional surface area. Rectangular attachments can be used in this circumstance because the sides of the attachment create additional surface contact with the aligner near the gingival third of the tooth (Fig 10-19).

Attachment Design

A promising development in attachment design is the use of preformed composite attachments. The use of template-formed attachments has three potential areas of improvement. The first is in shape detail and definition. When the template is thermoformed on the stereolithographic (SLA) resin model, some of the attachment edge definition may be lost during the template formation (Fig 10-20). The second area is in the material wear characteristics. Depending on the type of dental composite used for the attachments and the frequency of aligner removal, some attachments may wear or break over time. The third area for improvement is the amount of composite flash formed during the bonding process.

A solution to these problems may be the use of preformed composite attachments. Made from a composite material durable enough to withstand fracture and wear, the preformed attachment can be bonded to the teeth using the attachment template as a guide. The amount of

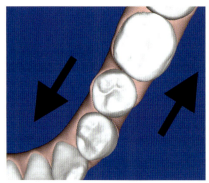

Fig 10-16 Rotation (*arrows*) of a second premolar is needed.

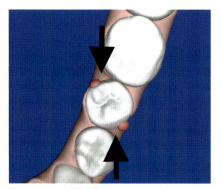

Fig 10-17 Addition of attachments to enhance the undercuts along the horizontal plane to enable better adaptation of the aligner to the tooth during rotational movements. *Arrows* indicate purchase points to facilitate rotation.

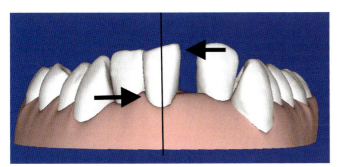

FIG 10-18 The force couple (*arrows*) needed to create root translation.

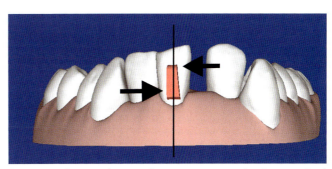

FIG 10-19 Rectangular attachments augment the interproximal surface area near the gingival line to improve the quality of the force couple (*arrows*) needed for root translation.

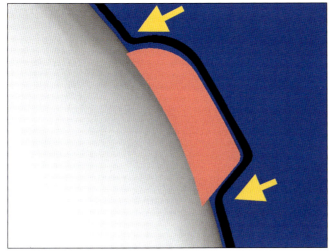

FIG 10-20 Attachment template adaptation can be improved in the areas indicated by the *arrows*.

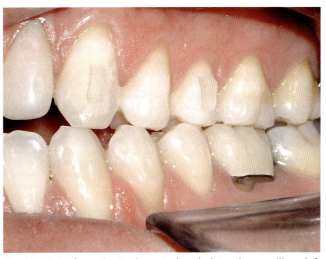

FIG 10-21 Preformed attachments bonded to the maxillary left canine and second premolar. Note the minimal flash formation and detail preserved in the edges of the attachment.

adhesive flash formed can be minimized, and the attachments can be manufactured with great accuracy to preserve the optimum amount of detail in the shape (Fig 10-21).

References

1. Broutman L, Krock R. Modern Composite Materials. Reading, MA: Addison-Wesley, 1967.
2. Chung KH, Greener EH. Correlation between degree of conversion, filler concentration and mechanical properties of posterior composite resins. J Oral Rehabil 1990;17:487–494.
3. Condon JR, Ferracane JL. In vitro wear of composite with varied cure, filler level, and filler treatment. J Dent Res 1997;76:1405–1411.
4. Braga RR, Hilton TJ, Ferracane JL. Contraction stress of flowable composite materials and their efficacy as stress-relieving layers. J Am Dent Assoc 2003;134:721–728.
5. Munksgaard EC, Hansen EK, Kato H. Wall-to-wall polymerization contraction of composite resins versus filler content. Scand J Dent Res 1987;95:526–531.
6. Bayne SC, Thompson JY, Swift EJ Jr, Stamatiades P, Wilkerson M. A characterization of first-generation flowable composites. J Am Dent Assoc 1998;129:567–577.
7. Labella R, Lambrechts P, van Meerbeek B, Vanherle G. Polymerization shrinkage and elasticity of flowable composites and filled adhesives. Dent Mater 1999;15:128–137.
8. Price RB, Rizkalla AS, Hall GC. Effect of stepped light exposure on the volumetric polymerization shrinkage and bulk modulus of dental composites and an unfilled resin. Am J Dent 2000;13: 176–180.
9. Davidson CL, de Gee AJ, Feilzer A. The competition between the composite-dentin bond strength and the polymerization contraction stress. J Dent Res 1984;63:1396–1399.
10. Powers JM, Kim HB, Turner DS. Orthodontic adhesives and bond strength testing. Semin Orthod 1997;3:147–156.
11. Kuo E, Hordt C. Attachments in der Invisalign-Therapie. Kieferorthopädie 2001(special issue):25–28.

chapter 11

ClinCheck:
Overview and Preparation

by
Craig Crawford, DDS

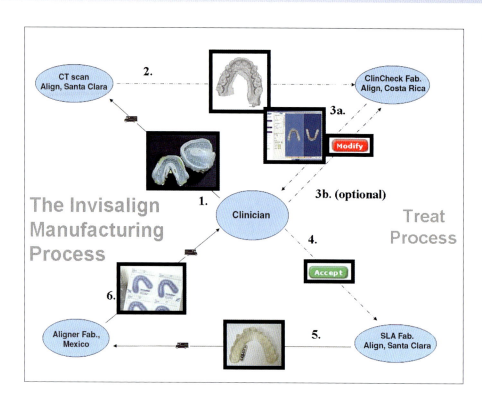

FIG 11-1 Overview of Invisalign process.

A clinician's diagnosis and treatment plan are the two fundamental elements of a successful outcome for any orthodontic treatment. Traditionally, the treatment plan, mechanics, their sequence, and the desired treatment outcome are noted in the patient's chart. These notes trigger visual images in the mind of the operator along the course of the treatment—indeed, the imaginary ideal, or optimal, outcome is always present in the mind of the clinician. In the Invisalign System, however, concrete images replace the mental images.

Once a diagnosis is made (tentative or definitive), the mechanics of treatment are done through a software system called ClinCheck. The ClinCheck file is a three-dimensional (3-D) virtual representation of a clinician's prescribed treatment plan. It reflects the stages of treatment from which aligners are manufactured. ClinCheck software provides viewing and navigation tools that greatly facilitate treatment planning, and ultimately allows for better clinical decisions. The ability of ClinCheck to allow diagnostic setups, treatment planning, and evaluations makes it an invaluable tool for the clinician. Treatment planning should be divided into both a treatment goal (what will be done?) and treatment plan (how will it be done?); ClinCheck enables the clinician to visualize both.

The ClinCheck is made up of two main components: (1) a series of computerized graphic images of the patient's teeth through several stages of movement, from initial to final position; and (2) pressure-formed clear plastic appliances made from stereolithographic (SLA) models of the images in the first component.

The ClinChecks are created by trained technicians using Align Technology's in-house proprietary software along with the supplied patient records (impressions, bite registration, photographs, and radiograph series or panoramic radiograph) and the clinician's treatment form. The ClinCheck is sent via the Internet to the clinician for review, and the clinician can communicate back to the Align technician to accept the ClinCheck or request any changes.

As soon as the clinician accepts the ClinCheck, production of the SLA models begins. Resin models are created for each stage of treatment. These models are sent to Juarez, Mexico, for final manufacture of the aligners. Once completed, the aligners are sent directly to the treating clinician's office (Fig 11-1).

Treat Software

The workforce at the Treat facility consists of specially trained technicians, engineers, clinicians, and managers. The treating technicians and the clinicians undergo rigorous and thorough training in orthodontic principles and the use of Invisalign and the Align software. The Treat

FIG 11-2 Screen shot of Bite Zero, which shows the patient's original occlusion in rough images.

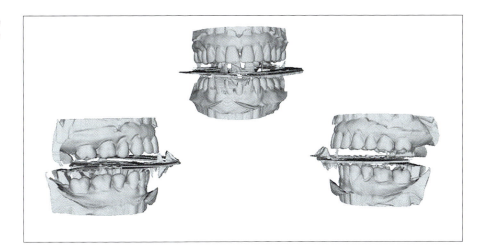

FIG 11-3 Trimming and cutting tools used by the technician to manipulate the teeth.

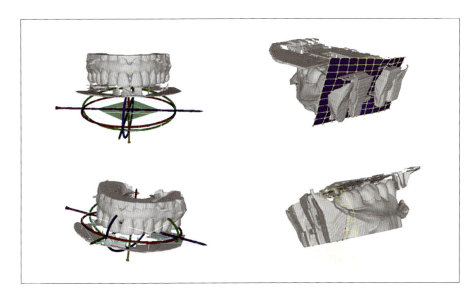

facility uses two different software programs to create ClinCheck files: ToothShaper is the program that allows for the preparation of the models (cleaning, detailing, sectioning of the teeth, and setting of the bite), and Treat is the program used for positioning the teeth, staging the movements of the teeth, placing attachments, and placing the final simulated gingiva. These programs and their use are described thoroughly in chapters 7 and 8.

The process entails four main steps: detail with a digital detailing tool (DDT), cut and detail, setup and stage, and final gingiva. The first three steps are described here; addition of final gingiva to the images is described in chapter 8.

Digital Detailing Tool

Inspection of the scanned data is the first step undertaken by the Treat facility's technicians. The scanned models are inspected for gross impression defects and for inaccuracies in the scan (Fig 11-2) and are cleaned of any extra artifacts from the impression and scan process (Fig 11-3). The "cleaned bite" models are then inspected for impression accuracy (Fig 11-4); patient records are used to help confirm usability of the impression and to ensure patient match. Finally, the scanned models are digitally detailed using the ToothShaper software (Fig 11-5).

Cut and Detail

The facial axes of the clinical crowns (FACCs) are placed on each clinical crown (Fig 11-6). These help identify the individual teeth. Paint Crowns is an application that gives each tooth's clinical crown a different color (Fig 11-7). The teeth are sectioned by the software to produce separate units for each tooth.

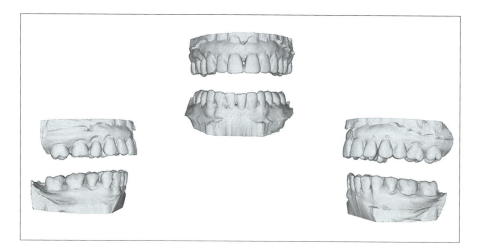

FIG 11-4 Cleaned bite.

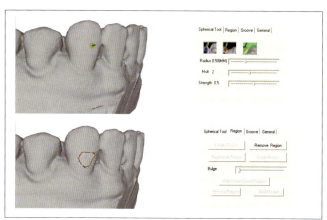

FIG 11-5 Detailing tools.

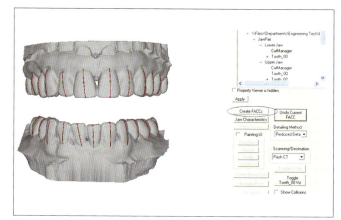

FIG 11-6 Placement of fixed axes of clinical crowns.

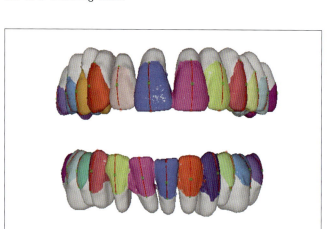

FIG 11-7 Painted crowns.

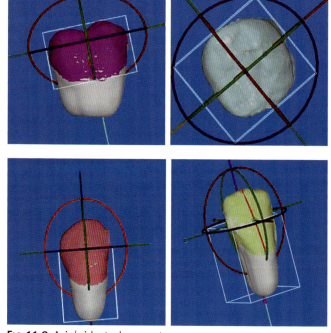

FIG 11-8 Axis/widget placement.

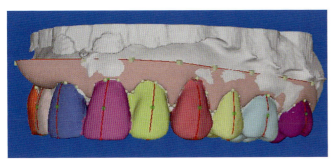

FIG 11-9 Initial gingiva placement.

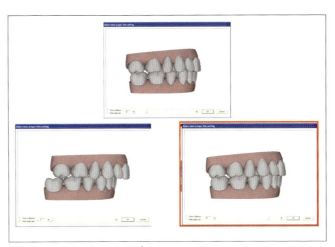

FIG 11-10 AutoBite set tool.

Widgets, used to move the teeth later in the process, are positioned in each tooth (Fig 11-8). Next, the simulated initial gingiva is placed (Fig 11-9).

The majority of bite sets are completed using a software application known as AutoBite. This software takes the opposing models and performs a best fit with the models to achieve at least a tripodization of occlusal contacts (Fig 11-10). The bite set is in centric occlusion or maximum intercuspation. Setting of the bite in centric relation has not been automated and is difficult to do manually with accuracy.

If the software has more than one option to set the bite, the technician is alerted, and a manual bite set is performed using the photos and—in difficult cases—the PVS bite registration.

After the bite is set, the records are reviewed, and the bite set is inspected for accuracy. Photographs and the goals and special instructions of the treatment plan are important for this inspection. If the bite does not appear correct, it will be reset or a comment indicating that there was difficulty setting the bite will be sent to the treating clinician via the ClinCheck.

Setup and Stage

At this point in the process, the scanned models have gone through inspection, detailing, sectioning, bite set, and gingiva placement. The next step, setup and stage, is when the teeth are placed in the final or goal position, reproximation is calculated, staging (the sequence of tooth movements from the initial position to the final position) is performed (see chapter 12), attachments are added, and comments to the treating clinician are placed.

All of this is completed using Treat software. The technicians responsible for this portion of the process rely on the complete and accurate records submitted by the treating clinician to aid in the completion of the case.

To create the treated file, the technicians rely on the completed treatment planning form, the clinician's treatment preferences, and their extensive training in orthodontics and on the Treat software.

The treatment planning form is of great value and is the most important piece of information that the treating clinician provides the setup and stage technician. This is where the clinician provides in written form the mental picture he or she has for the treatment and that he or she expects to see in ClinCheck. The treatment forms can be completed either as a written form that is mailed or as an electronic form that is sent via e-mail.

The clinician's treatment preferences are completed on the clinician's Virtual Invisalign Practice (VIP) page, which consists of a number of questions about general setup for the case. It also allows for free text of special instructions to be applied to most of the clinician's cases. These preferences and instructions are valuable for reducing the time the treating clinician spends on the completion of the treatment forms for each case in the event the clinician wants similar values in different case setups. The clinician can opt out of using the treatment preferences by marking a designated check box on the treatment form (see Fig 8-6).

The file that the technician creates is called a Treat file, which is converted into ClinCheck to facilitate transfer of the file to the clinician via the Internet. The ClinCheck sent to the clinician is the technician's or Align Technology's interpretation of the treatment form.

chapter 12

STAGING

by
Rene Sterental, DDS

Staging is the collection of steps and procedures used to arrive—in sound clinical and biologic fashion—at the final desired position of the teeth using Treat software.

After receiving the final cut model from the ToothShaper technician, the setup and stage technician reads the prescription form and reviews the clinical records that were submitted with the case to determine how the clinician wants to treat the case. The technician also reviews the clinician's preferences for accomplishing the treatment goals, as well as any other details of which the clinician wants the technician to be aware.

The setup and stage technician opens the file in Treat software to begin the ClinCheck setup. The technician aligns and positions the teeth in the Treat file to their final position as determined by the clinician's treatment prescription and preferences. After the correct final position is achieved on both arches, and after the occlusion has been adjusted, two additional stages remain in the setup: stage 0 (the initial position of the teeth before any movements have been applied) and stage 1 (the final position of the teeth).

The technician proceeds to "stage" the setup—that is, set up all the intermediate steps required to guide the teeth from the initial position to the final position, taking into consideration the biologic requirements of tooth movement, the biomechanical requirements of moving teeth with aligners, and any other details that allow the technician to set up the case efficiently and effectively. After the case is staged, the virtual setup contains information on how many stages or steps are required, the velocity at which the teeth are moving (both linear and angular), the timing of the movements for each particular tooth, the amount and timing of interproximal collisions and spaces during the treatment, and the pattern of anchorage that is being used. All this information is presented in the Stage Editor window in Treat, displayed under several tabbed windows to facilitate easy access for the technician.

Stage Editor

The Stage Editor window is used to visualize and quantify how the teeth are moving and comprises seven tabbed windows that display different information. These windows are Key Frame Editor, Move Distance, Collision, Space, Overcorrection, Translation (mm), and Rotation (deg) (Fig 12-1).

Key Frame Editor

The Key Frame Editor is used to set and display, using a graphical format, the staging pattern for the selected case. Lines and key frames are used to show at what stage a particular tooth starts to move, during how many stages it moves, and at what stage it finishes moving. Any intermediate steps are also shown. The pattern used to stage the case can easily be seen and modified; any change to the number of total or individual stages for a particular movement is performed using the Key Frame Editor (Fig 12-2).

Move Distance

The Move Distance window is used to determine the speed at which the crowns of the teeth are moving. Based on the number of stages needed to complete the movement for each tooth, the speed for each movement varies. The maximum speed that a tooth is allowed to move is 0.25 mm/stage. Speeds faster than 0.25 mm/stage are highlighted in red to alert the technician that the speed is too fast and that a larger number of stages is needed for that particular movement (Fig 12-3).

Collision

The Collision window is used to visualize numerically the amount of overlap between adjacent teeth throughout the sequence of stages. The amount of overlap detected and measured by the software is used to determine when adjacent teeth collide while they are being moved. This also determines when the overlap is increased past certain predetermined values, and finally the amount of interproximal reproximation (IPR) needed to create the space that will allow those movements to be performed clinically. These collisions are usually referred to as *microcollisions* and are the reason that contacts have to be monitored clinically with unwaxed dental floss to ensure that they do not become too tight and prevent the teeth from sliding freely against each other.

Per the current Invisalign collision protocol, normal contacts are considered to be those between 0.00 and 0.05 mm; in Treat, they are displayed in black in the Collision window. IPR below 0.2 mm per contact is not allowed, so collisions between 0.06 and 0.14 are highlighted in blue to alert the technician that they need to be removed (Fig 12-4a). A maximum of 0.5 mm of IPR is allowed, unless the clinician specifically overrides it and requests more. Any

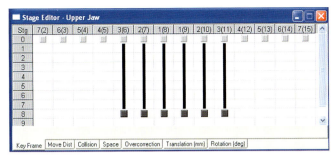

FIG 12-1 Stage Editor window.

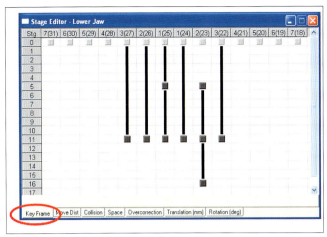

FIG 12-2 Key Frame Editor window.

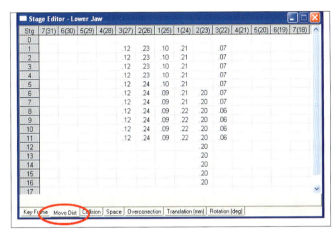

FIG 12-3 Move Distance window (velocity). Excessive velocity is highlighted in red.

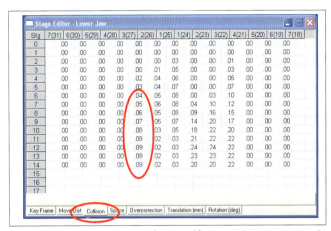

FIG 12-4a Collision window (intra-arch). Normal contacts are in black; high final collision is in blue (IPR < 0.2 mm would result).

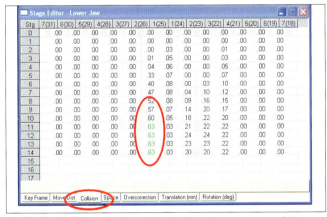

FIG 12-4b Collision window. High final collision in green (IPR > 0.5 mm would result).

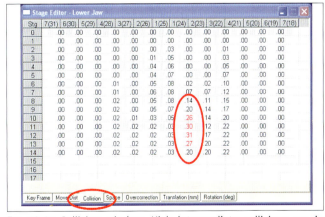

FIG 12-4c Collision window. High intermediate collisions are in red (requires intermediate key frames).

final overlap larger that 0.6 mm is highlighted in green so it is not inadvertently left unchanged by the technician (Fig 12-4b). To prevent intermediate collisions from being larger than the final overlap (which would either prevent the teeth from moving or, if IPR is performed, leave an open contact between the teeth at the end of the treat-

ment), any overlap that is measured at 0.05 mm above the final one is highlighted in red to signal that it requires the technician's immediate attention (Fig 12-4c). Unless the clinician specifically requests that an IPR higher than 0.5 mm/contact be performed, all numbers should be black when the staging of the treatment is complete.

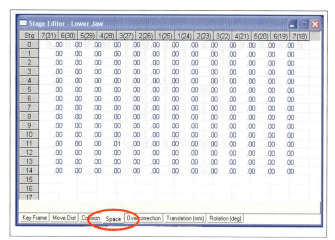

FIG 12-5 Space window.

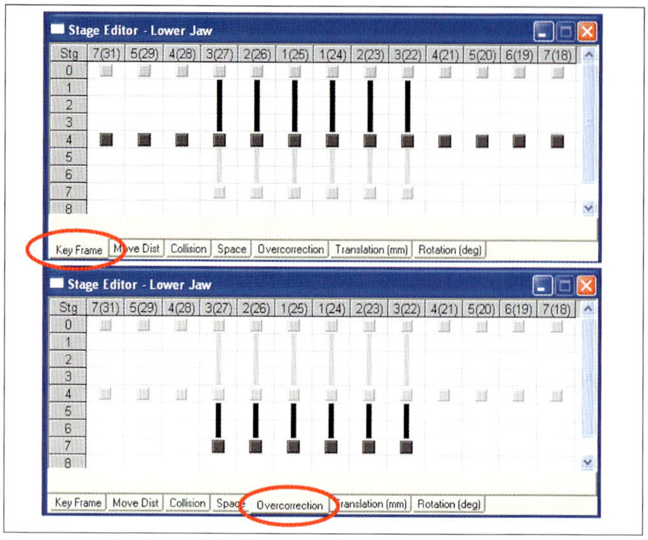

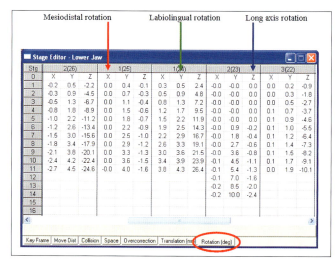

FIG 12-6 Overcorrection stages as displayed in Key Frame Editor (*top*) and the Overcorrection (*bottom*) windows.

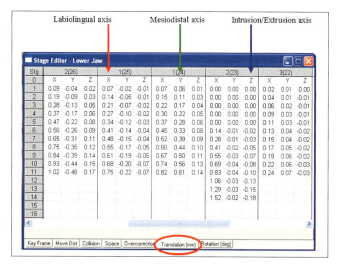

FIG 12-7 Translation window (linear movements and color correlation with widget axes).

FIG 12-8 Rotation window (angular movements and color correlation with widget axes).

Space

The Space window is similar to the Collision window, except that it measures the interproximal space between the teeth (Fig 12-5). Once the teeth overlap, the space continues to read 0.00 mm. The numbers are always displayed in blue, to differentiate them at first glance from the collision numbers, which are black. Thus, an ideal contact would read "0.00" in both the Collision and Space windows. Realistically, it is not always possible to ensure good contacts at the end of the treatment. The Space window is usually used when the technician wants to make sure that the spaces required between the teeth in certain setups are equally distributed per the clinician's request.

Overcorrection

The Overcorrection window is used to stage overcorrection movements at the end of the regular treatment sequence (Fig 12-6). Overcorrection is usually performed in three stages and is designed to compensate for aligner lag and to ensure that the teeth can be moved to their final position as depicted in the virtual setup. Overcorrection is not performed in the initial setup unless it is requested and specific instructions are given by the clinician. It is always performed during case refinements (when it is clear which movements need refinement) to ensure that these movements get expressed clinically.

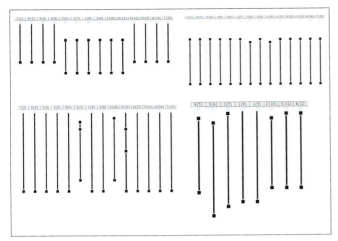

FIG 12-9a Common low-anchorage patterns.

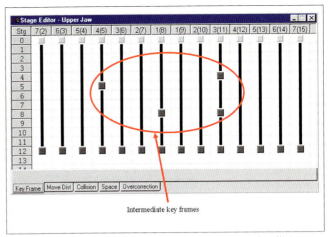

FIG 12-9b Adjusting at intermediate stages to avoid collisions.

Translation

The Translation window shows the distance that each tooth moves along the three linear axes depicted in the movement widget. These axes are the x-axis, which measures labiolingual movements along the red linear axis and is displayed under the X column; the y-axis, which measures mesiodistal movements along the green linear axis and is displayed under the Y column; and the z-axis, which measures intrusion and extrusion movements along the blue linear axis and is displayed under the Z column. The axes in the widget are shaped like arrows; if the movement is performed along the direction of the arrow's point, the number will be positive; if the movement is performed in the opposite direction, the number will be negative. A tooth can move in all three planes of space at the same time (Fig 12-7).

Rotation

The Rotation window shows the rotation that is applied to each tooth along the three rotation axes depicted in the movement widget. These rotation axes are the X rotational axis, which measures mesiodistal rotation along the red rotation axis and is displayed under the X column; the Y rotational axis, which measures labiolingual rotation along the green rotation axis and is displayed under the Y column; and the Z rotational axis, which measures rotation along the tooth's long axis along the blue rotation axis and is displayed under the Z column. If the direction of the movement is clockwise, the number will be negative; if the direction of movement is counterclockwise, the number will be positive. A tooth can rotate in all three planes of space at the same time (Fig 12-8).

Anchorage

Cases can be staged using a low-anchorage pattern or a high-anchorage pattern. This is determined based on the information contained in the doctor's prescription and diagnosis form, as well as the internal staging protocols that the technicians follow.

Low-anchorage pattern

A low-anchorage staging pattern, also known as an equal staging pattern or an "X" pattern, occurs when all the teeth move concurrently throughout the sequence (Figs 12-9a and 12-9b). The maximum velocity for tooth movement is 0.25 mm/stage, and usually all or most of the teeth are moving through all the stages at various speeds, depending on the total distance each tooth has to move. Low-anchorage patterns are usually used in Type I space closure cases, mandibular incisor extraction cases, and expansion and crowding cases where no distalization is needed. To avoid intra-arch collisions throughout the sequence of movements, intermediate key frame points can be used to manage any overlap between the teeth that may develop; these are usually added every five stages or so to ensure that the collisions remain within the protocol guidelines throughout the whole sequence. Rotations should be kept under 2 to 3 degrees per stage.

High-anchorage pattern

A high-anchorage pattern, sometimes referred to as a "V" pattern, is used when intra-arch anchorage needs to be

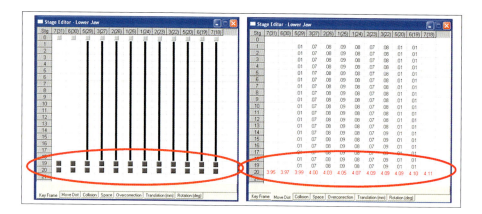

FIG 12-14 Surgical setup (mandibular repositioning). Key Frame Editor view (*left*) and Move Distance view (*right*). After stage 19, the mandible is being repositioned manually. No aligner will be made for stage 20.

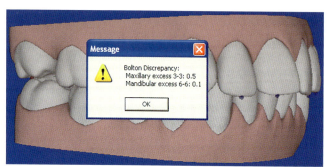

FIG 12-15 Bolton analysis in Treat software.

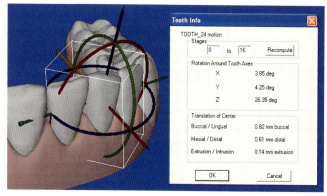

FIG 12-16 Tooth Motion Information window.

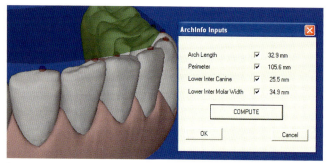

FIG 12-17 Arch Information window.

Tooth Motion Information

The Tooth Motion Information window provides a review of the clinical information on the linear movements that are being applied to the selected tooth, plus the rotation around its long axis. The measurements that are displayed include the amount of intrusion or extrusion movement, the amount of labial or lingual movement, and the amount of mesial or distal movement that are being performed, as well as the amount and direction of rotation that is being applied to the tooth around its long axis. These measurements are derived from the different axes of movement shown on the widget used to move each tooth in each particular axis (Fig 12-16).

Arch Information

When one of the arches is selected in the Treat software, the Arch Information tool allows the technician to visualize descriptive information such as arch length, perimeter, intercanine width, and intermolar width (Fig 12-17).

Attachments

Attachments are used to create a better hold for the aligner to move the teeth. They are used when the anatomy of the teeth does not provide enough undercuts for the aligner to grab the teeth solidly, to enhance the retention of the aligners to provide enough anchorage for certain movements to be expressed clinically, and to allow the aligners to apply forces in directions that they cannot otherwise achieve because of the biomechanics of the movement and the way they apply forces to the teeth. In both Treat and ClinCheck, the attachments are displayed as red

FIG 12-18 Attachment types and placement. Attachments may be requested in horizontal or vertical orientation.

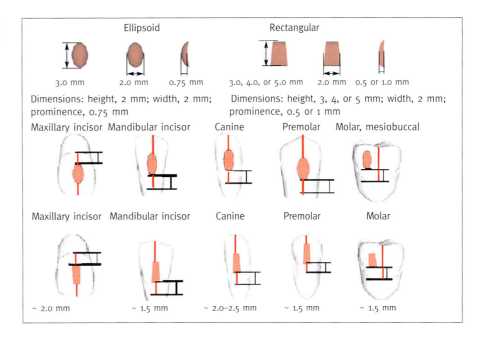

shapes. They can be placed manually or automatically, per the Invisalign attachment protocol.

Currently, ellipsoid and rectangular attachments are available (Fig 12-18). Other designs are being researched, but these are not yet available to treat regular commercial cases. Clinicians can request the type and placement of attachments and can override the aligner protocol. If no requests are made, Align will only place the attachments based on what the protocol calls for. More on attachments is covered in chapter 9.

Comments

The Notepad menu item allows the technicians to write individualized comments for the clinician to review in ClinCheck or for internal use while the case is being worked on. The Notepad window has two areas, an upper area titled Comments to Customers and a lower area called Notes. Anything typed in the Comments to Customers section will be uploaded via the ClinCheck for the clinician to review; comments typed in the Notes area do not get uploaded and are intended for internal use. These comments range from preset comments designed to alert the clinician about certain aspects of the treatment to clarifications about the treatment and explanations of the reasons certain decisions were made in the course of the setup.

113

chapter 13

OVERCORRECTION: PRINCIPLES AND CONSIDERATIONS

by
Eric Kuo, DDS

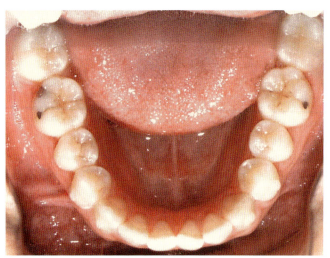

FIG 13-1a Distal-in rotation of the mandibular central incisors is needed.

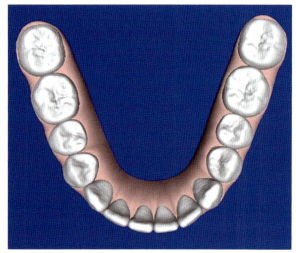

FIG 13-1b Treatment goal.

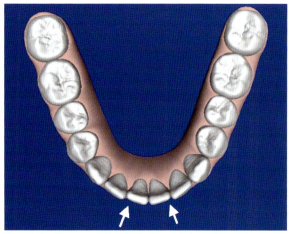

FIG 13-1c Overcorrection built in to help achieve the treatment goal.

When the final alignment of the teeth comes close to the goal but is not exactly as planned, it may be possible to program movement into additional aligners to create the extra force needed to achieve the desired outcome. Aligners built with overcorrection may be used to impart the forces needed to more effectively move the teeth to the target positions. An important point of clarification is that aligner overcorrection is not the same as "overcorrection" in fixed appliances whereby the teeth are set in an overcorrected position with the anticipation of relapse into the straight position at a later date. With aligner overcorrection, the aligner is built with tooth positions set past "ideal" so as to overcome any misalignment that would result if the teeth were to fall short of the goal.

For example, if a patient needed additional rotation of the mandibular central incisors after wearing the initial series of aligners (Fig 13-1a), additional orthodontic force on the distofacial surfaces would be needed to achieve the desired outcome (Fig 13-1b). Building overcorrection into the aligners (Fig 13-1c) may be used to improve alignment of the teeth.

Common Indications for Overcorrection

Overcorrection is most commonly used for minor incisor rotations, minor in-and-out discrepancies, minor residual spaces, and minor incisor deep bite.

The greatest challenge when planning for overcorrection is accurately predicting which teeth require overcorrection and which do not. For example, consider the mandibular incisor crowding shown in Fig 13-2a. The areas indicated by the white arrows are most likely to require additional correction to achieve the goal shown in Fig 13-2b. Consequently, adding 5 degrees of rotation beyond "ideal" may help ensure that the desired result is achieved by the last aligner. However, what if only two of the areas end up needing additional rotation, but overcorrection is built into all three areas? Building the last aligners with overcorrection in all three areas could result in making the areas with correct alignment incorrect as a result. Another possibility would be to build overcorrection into each area to account for the different combinations so that any correct areas could be omitted if the teeth are aligned correctly. Because the number of possible combinations that could result is rather large, however, this approach would not be cost-effective. In the above example, overcorrection aligners for 1 only, 2 only, 3 only,

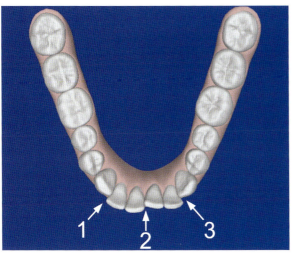

FIG 13-2a Overcorrection is likely to be needed in the three areas indicated by *arrows*.

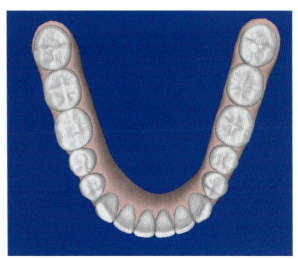

FIG 13-2b Treatment goal.

1+2, 1+3, 2+3, and 1+2+3 would have to be made in order to capture all the different possible scenarios.

Because of the current inability to determine up front which teeth may require overcorrection and which will not, overcorrection is believed to be most effective when the overcorrection stages are created not at the onset of treatment but rather when the teeth are closer to the goal, such as at the time of case refinement. Near the end of treatment, it is more obvious which areas are not correcting according to plan. These are the areas most likely to require overcorrection to achieve the desired result, and it is much easier for the clinician to pinpoint the specific teeth that require overcorrection at the time of refinement than it is to speculate at the beginning which teeth may and which may not need it.

The exception to this recommendation is perhaps in generalized space closure cases, where an additional tightening of the interproximal contacts during the last three stages (sometimes referred to as *virtual c-chain* because the movements on ClinCheck appear similar to the movements of teeth when an elastic chain is placed) can be an effective way to help avoid minor interproximal spaces at the end of the initial aligner sequence. For example, the patient in Fig 13-3a is likely to have light contacts between the teeth where spaces are initially present if the teeth are moved to the setup in Fig 13-3b, where they are positioned so that they are lightly touching interproximally. Figure 13-3c shows the overcorrected position superimposed over the tooth position in Fig 13-3b, whereby the overcorrected position is designed to tighten any light interproximal contacts that may remain. The overcor-

rection occurs in three aligners, and the clinician can stop dispensing additional aligners once the contacts are adequately tightened.

Another important consideration is to plan overcorrection movements that are within the aligner's capabilities. For example, it would not be particularly useful to build extrusion overcorrection movements if the initial extrusion movements result in aligner disengagement from the tooth that is to be extruded. Having more extrusion built into the aligner will not make the tooth extrude any further if the aligner is already disconnected from the tooth to be extruded.

Alternative to Overcorrection: Detail Pliers

An alternative to overcorrection aligners for managing alignment discrepancies at the end of treatment is the use of Invisalign detail pliers (Fig 13-4) to generate additional orthodontic forces in the aligners. The plunger and recessed stop at the tip of the detail pliers create a permanent bump in the aligner, and unlike pliers that require heat to reshape the clear aligner appliances,[1] the detail pliers can be used at room temperature. Simply squeezing the pliers in the area of the aligner where additional force is needed creates a protrusion of 0.25 to 0.75 mm that can deliver additional force to the misaligned tooth for further correction. If reinforcement of the dimple is needed to prevent the plastic from collapsing, a filler material such as ClearLoc light-cure adhesive (Align Technology)

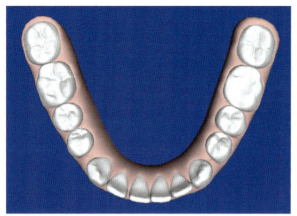

FIG 13-3a Initial position.

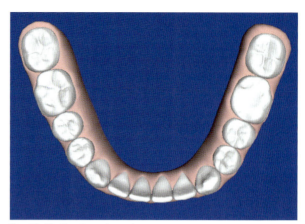

FIG 13-3b Treatment goal.

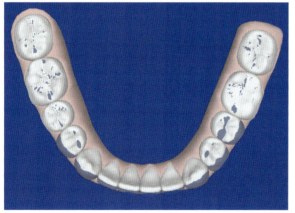

FIG 13-3c Overcorrection (*dark blue*) required to achieve goal shown in Fig 13-3b.

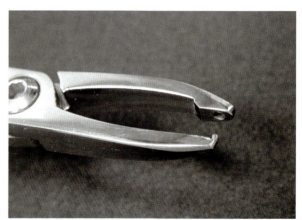

FIG 13-4 Detail pliers.

may be used for support. In the event that a dimple is positioned in the wrong location of the aligner, an "eraser" pliers can be used to flatten out the formed dimple (Fig 13-5).

Detail pliers can be used to correct minor rotations, in-and-out discrepancies, and light interproximal contacts simply by varying the position in the aligner where they are placed (Figs 13-6 to 13-8). The assumption is that the pressure point will help conform the teeth to their intended position(s) already existing in the aligner; hence, so long as the aligner shape coincides with the desired position, the aligner does not need to be cut or altered to accommodate the new tooth position. In other words, if the desired goal is not the same as that approved in ClinCheck, the dimple pliers cannot be used to move the teeth beyond the tooth positions built into the aligner without first altering the aligner.

Preventive Strategies

A well-thought-out preventive strategy for avoiding overcorrection and detail pliers can lead to a more efficient treatment outcome and a more positive treatment experience. Three important considerations to help reduce the need for overcorrection are as follows:

1. **Set proper tooth-movement expectations.** Avoid aligner-incompatible tooth movements unless these movements are to be accomplished with ancillary orthodontic treatment in conjunction with aligners. Movements such as vertical extrusion and rotation of cylindrical-shaped teeth can be more effective when aligners are used in conjunction with auxiliaries such as elastics and sectional fixed appliances, respectively.

2. **Closely monitor any needed reproximation.** Any reproximation planned as part of the treatment should be performed in a timely and accurate manner. The aligner's

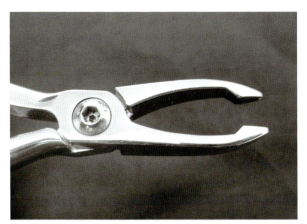

FIG 13-5 Eraser pliers.

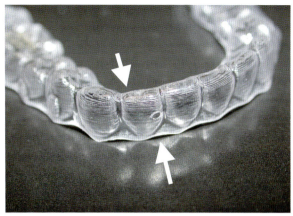

FIG 13-6 Distal-out, mesial-in forces (*arrows*) generated by the dimples for the purpose of rotating the mandibular right lateral incisor.

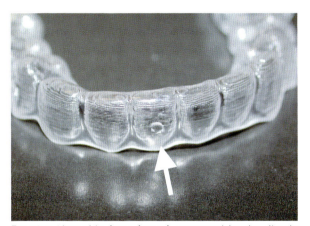

FIG 13-7 Lingual-in force (*arrow*) generated by the dimple for the purpose of moving the mandibular right central incisor lingually.

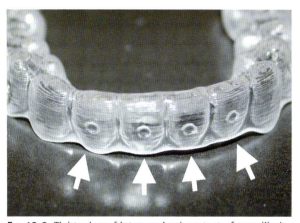

FIG 13-8 Tightening of interproximal contact of mandibular incisors through lingual-in forces (*arrows*) generated by dimples.

fit will be compromised if the teeth are not of the correct dimension, so the amounts of reproximation performed must be accurately determined. Proper timing of any needed reproximation is also important, as delaying reproximation beyond the time indicated in the patient's reproximation form (derived from the ClinCheck approved by the clinician) will prevent the teeth from moving correctly. The amount of reproximation performed can be confirmed using thickness gauges and can be documented in the patient's chart.

3. **Align first before closing spaces.** As with fixed appliances, aligners should be used first to align the teeth before retracting them to close any remaining interproximal spaces. If reproximation is needed, the teeth should also be aligned first to create more optimal access to interproximal surfaces. Unlike with fixed appliances, however, leveling should not be done initially, especially not if dental extrusion is desired, because if the aligner disengages from the tooth early on, any

additional movements "downstream," such as rotation and inclination, may be compromised.

Reference

1. Hilliard K, Sheridan J. Adjusting Essix appliances at chairside. J Clin Orthod 2000;34:236–238.

chapter 14

THREE-DIMENSIONAL SUPERIMPOSITION TOOL

by
C. Van Nguyen, DDS and Jihua Cheng, PhD

What preceded the need for a three-dimensional (3-D) measuring tool for orthodontic treatment was a quest for the ideal representation of patient occlusion as it relates to the craniofacial complex. Unfortunately, the Invisalign System currently is a tooth-borne system. Thus, dental relationships are assessed with the aid of various intraoral landmarks. Assessment of orthodontic treatment outcomes has traditionally been based on two-dimensional (2-D) tracings of before-treatment and after-treatment lateral cephalometric radiographs. The initial departure from this traditional approach was the use of 3-D physical dental casts to evaluate treatment outcome.[1,2] Such effort was carried out with the understanding that certain parts of the palatal rugae are stable and identifiable during periods of growth in humans.[3] Because Invisalign is treatment in 3-D, Align Technology found it necessary to develop appropriate tools to measure treatment outcome.

Currently, Align's 3-D measurement tool used to evaluate treatment outcome matches crown surfaces tooth by tooth and then selects intraoral registration points, namely teeth, to relate the before- and after-treatment positions of teeth. The resultant registration reflects how relative tooth movements have been achieved. With this methodology, it is also possible to assess the efficiency of tooth movement.

In this section, we review 3-D mathematical algorithms associated with surface matching (superimposition) that are used for treatment outcome measurement.

Technology of 3-D Imaging in Orthodontics

The need to digitally store dental casts has been a driving force in orthodontic 3-D imaging. The digital storage of dental casts provides such benefits as reduced storage space and more efficient record retrieval.

There are many ways to acquire 3-D orthodontic images. Stereophotography uses two pictures taken in different views at the same time to produce a 3-D image. This method utilizes a triangulation technique that is analogous to how humans see objects stereoscopically. The disadvantage of creating stereophotographic images is the inherent error involved in the registration of the 2-D photographs together.

Surface laser scanning, which is also a triangulation technique, is widely used and based on projective imaging technique.[4] Volumetric images, such as those from computed tomography (CT) scans, are 3-D images obtained from axial slices of the object.

Free-Form Object Registration

Geometric matching is performed through both high-level and low-level approaches. The high-level method requires preprocessing: features and segmentation must be extracted from the data sets before registration. Low-level geometric matching uses raw data—like points and triangles—to match the data sets.

The advantage of the low-level approach is that it is not affected by unreliable features extracted from the free-form data sets. The disadvantage is, of course, that it disregards the work of experts who can enhance the registration by distinguishing important and unimportant features in the scanned objects.

Low-level approaches may include maximizing the correlation between the two data sets or using minimization of the distances between points of data sets in tooth alignment. The minimization of distances method is also known as *geometric point matching*. Geometric point matching starts out with a rough match. The corresponding points of the two objects can then be brought closer together by data transformation. Subsequently, through an iteration process, the distance between these points gets smaller, thereby making the match better. Many mathematical algorithms were developed to optimize this iteration process.[5,6] Among the algorithms used to achieve geometric matching is the iterative closest point (ICP).

For facial superimposition applications, for example, the technique of choice is a low-level approach (like ICP) to record and register using several landmarks. Although the task of identifying and acquiring landmarks is necessary for registration, the most critical issue is timely production of the best fit.[4]

One early attempt to superimpose 3-D images as free-form shapes was done by Faugeras and Hebert.[7] Algorithms used in shape registration can be derived from any of the following geometric data: point sets, line segment sets, curves (implicit or parametric), faceted surfaces (triangle sets), and surfaces (implicit or parametric).[5] The algorithm described by Faugeras and Hebert used least-squares computation in the registration of 3-D point sets. A different version of this registration methodology was derived by Horn.[8] The drawback of Horn's method, however, was its basis in the assumption that there are large planar regions in the free-form shapes.[9] Another approach to least-squares computation was adopted to match fairly homogeneous curve data but did not perform well against shapes with highly irregular curves.[10]

Method of Registration

Geometric matching utilizes the minimization of the mean square value of the difference between the registrations of the two data sets. As a requirement, the initial registration state is determined. After the initial matching is established, a convergence theorem is then proven. The method to find this initial state is critical because it has to be within a certain range of the correct matching state such that a convergence can occur. In other words, the difference between registrations must get smaller after a single iteration. According to Besl and McKay, "The least square registration generically reduces the average distance between corresponding points during each iteration."[5]

Several steps are involved in the process of ICP. First, computation of the closest points between two geometric objects is set up. The distance to be minimized can be euclidean (point-to-point) or a reference to the closest point from one surface to another point on the other surface and its normal plane (point-to-plane).[6] The euclidian distance is defined as the square root of the sum of the square of all 3-D distances.

In the second step, a mean squared error between the two data sets is defined. This error is subsequently minimized when computing for a rigid transformation. *Rigid transformation* is defined as translation, rotation, or both.

In the third step, registration is applied using the best rigid transformation. After this, a number of iterations (or any other criteria—eg, a matching error) is carried out to achieve the desired match.

Superimposition of 3-D Images in Orthodontics

There are four main methods of superimposing before- and after-treatment images to assess discrepancy and quantify the results of orthodontic treatment.

The first method involves the matching of tooth-by-tooth geometry via best surface match. The before- and after-treatment arches are registered by a number of points; this superimposition technique involves tooth-by-tooth matching and registration via least-moving teeth. As registration markings are not stationary, superimposition allows the clinicians to see the relative positions of each tooth during treatment. This method, therefore, only shows how much movement has been achieved between two moving objects. For example, Align's superimposition tool shows how much an anterior tooth retracts relative to a posterior tooth, but does not indicate how many millimeters a tooth moves anteroposteriorly relative to the craniofacial landmark sella. For any specific movements (eg, intrusion of anterior teeth), performance trends can also be obtained using the superimposition tool. It is not surprising that, "as teeth do not have simple geometric features, the comparison of tooth positions in two different impressions is not straightforward."[11]

The second method also attempts to measure tooth movements within either the maxillary or mandibular arch using intraoral landmarks. Unlike the previous method, this method uses soft tissues for registration. The basic premise for this approach is that palatal rugae—specifically, the medial aspects—are stable during the growth period.[3] The problem that Align Technology encountered is in determining how to locate these palatal rugae and consistently register maxillae without having difficulty with the vertical dimension (ie, the arches tend to register very well anteriorly, but posteriorly they become separated because of a lack of registering ruga points). Despite repeated efforts to overcome this drawback, the problem persists unless other registration points are identified in the posterior region of the maxilla. Superimposition of before and after images depends on the availability of rugae, which are present only on the palate. For the mandibular arch, the lack of stable intraoral features presents another problem. Currently, there is no good set of registration points identified. The effort of superimposition based on intraoral soft tissues is thus assumed to be an estimation only.

The third method involves alignment of the dental arches via 2-D extraoral landmarks that are stable during growth in the craniofacial structure. The relationship of the dentition can be intra-arch or extraoral. This approach is similar to cephalometric superimposition of tooth movements. There have been many attempts to register 2-D cephalometric radiographs taken from different angles to generate a 3-D image of the craniofacial structure. The tools used in this type of registration have their limitations, and the method of registering 2-D images into 3-D has some inherent error.[12,13] Nevertheless, this approach is useful in

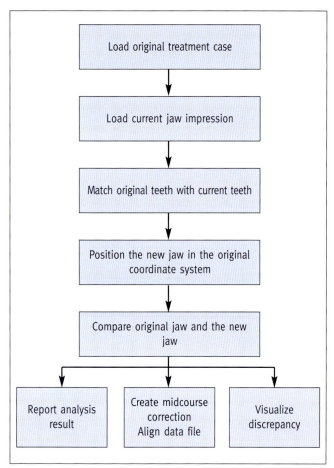

FIG 14-1 Process sequence.

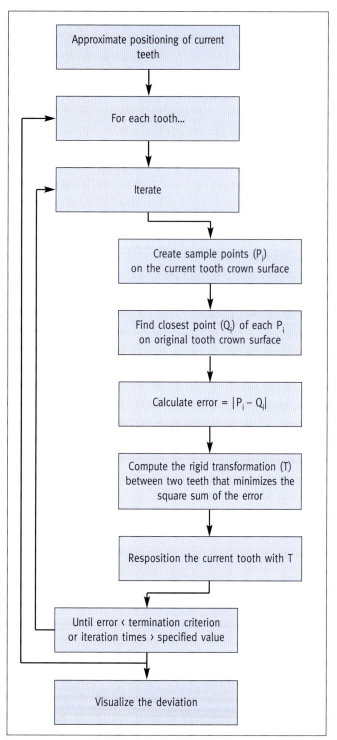

FIG 14-2 Process for matching original teeth with current teeth.

the development of a 3-D superimposition method to assess tooth movement because registration points can be selected from the cranial base, which is considered stable. Currently, researchers at the University of the Pacific (UOP) are assessing the accuracy of this methodology in treatment outcome analysis. A version of this technique that orients the 3-D dentition onto the lateral cephalometric radiograph is under development at UOP. This method was described as the manipulation of a virtual outline of the occlusal surface belonging to either the maxillary or mandibular cast so that it best fits the image of the teeth shown on the lateral cephalometric radiograph. A frame of reference was defined such that the x- and y-axes lie in the midsagittal plane of the head and the z-axis is perpendicular to both axes.[14]

The fourth method for assessing tooth movement involves volumetric 3-D images, which can be obtained by technologies developed by such companies as Hitachi, QR srl, Image Science International, and Morita. The NewTom 9000 (QR srl) scanner, for example, utilizes a cone-shaped beam approach that reduces the overall exposure dosage.[15] Limitation of the exposure dosage, however, diminishes the clarity and preci-

sion of the volumetric images.[14] The NewTom 9000 may need to be used in conjunction with panoramic or periapical radiographs, which suggests that this technology is not yet ready to replace other strategies for obtaining comprehensive 3-D images for the evaluation of tooth movement. It is safe to assume that other imaging devices (iCAT, Imaging

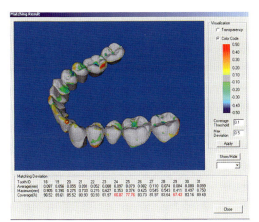

FIG 14-3 Visualization of tooth matching by color code.

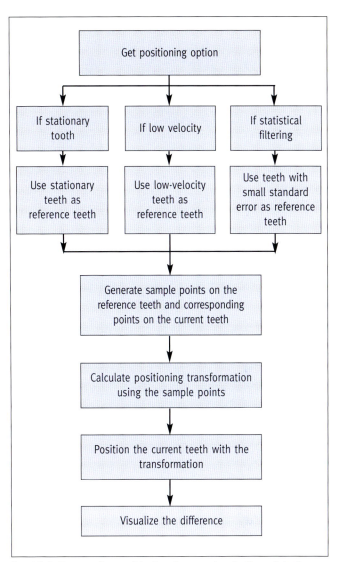

FIG 14-4 Process for positioning the new jaw in the original coordinate system.

Sciences International, or Hitachi) are plagued by a similar problem.

The volumetric technique yields far more data than does traditional 2-D cephalometric radiography. This gap in the amount of information may necessitate some conceptualization to superimpose the before- and after-treatment images in 3-D. For example, the cranial base landmark basion may need to be redefined in a 3-D image. The challenges of this are twofold: (1) the methodology of superimposition based on an abundance of 3-D features, and (2) the difficulty in recognizing these features.

Superimposition Tool

When a case deviates from the approved treatment plan, reprocessing is required (Figs 14-1 to 14-4). This involves a new impression, setup, ClinCheck approval, and new aligners. The clinician will want to determine the reasons why the teeth deviated from the expected target positions. In this process, the superimposition tool can perform several functions:

1. Allows a new scan of a midcourse correction (MCC) case that can be used in a best-fit comparison with the original approved treatment. A best-fit comparison of the overlapped models can reveal discrepancies between treatments.
2. Can be used to position the corrected teeth together with the original teeth based on the reference stage and reference teeth. The reference teeth can be specified manually or automatically.
3. Allows the discrepancies between the original and corrected tooth positions to be quantified and visualized (Figs 14-5 and 14-6).

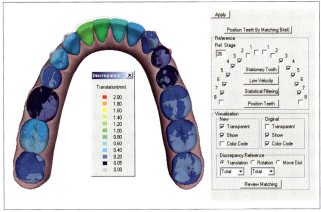

FIG 14-5 Visualization of discrepancy.

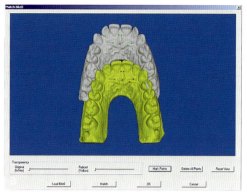 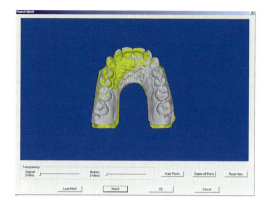

Fig 14-6 (a and b) Rugae matching.

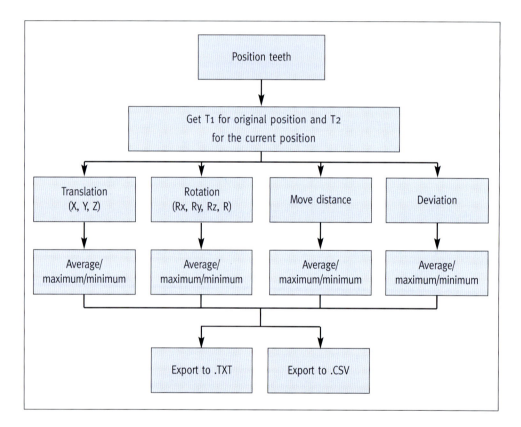

Fig 14-7 Report of analysis result. T = rigid transformation

4. Can generate a report with information focusing on the discrepancies in the location of the teeth in the original treatment and the new impression (Fig 14-7). The report is helpful in the evaluation of MCC cases.

5. Can be used to create an MCC Align data file (ADF) based on teeth matching, positioning teeth by matching original bite zero (3-D jaw model without segmentation used for initial treatment) and reboot bite zero (the same, used for MCC treatment), or by specified reference stage and teeth and target stage (Fig 14-8). Ideally, the MCC Align data file gets the treatment back on track, thus precluding the need to completely redo the case. This prevents waste of materials and allows

for the use of most of the original aligners, which are augmented by any additional aligners created to correct the deviation.

Retrospective Study of Performance Index of Aligners

Align Technology was the first company to introduce a computer-designed removable orthodontic appliance. Clearly, the effectiveness of this appliance in patient care must be established by evidence-based reports. Some of these reports are described below.

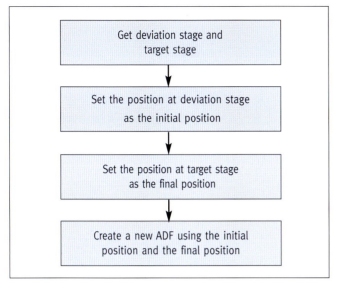

FIG 14-8 Creation of midcourse correction Align data file (ADF).

Methodology

Sixty arches (30 maxillary and 30 mandibular) were randomly selected from 38 patients. Superimposition was used to match treatment files of each arch. Treatment files contained the digital models of the patient's teeth and gingiva, which were created from an impression that had been scanned and digitized.

When matching is performed, the progress scan is superimposed over the initial scan to yield a match percentage based on tooth anatomy and position. If the initial alignment of teeth is severely irregular, the outcome of the matching is not as good and, consequently, there is a greater chance of a larger measurement error in superimposition.

After teeth in the two arches are matched, Superimposition asks for a reference to relate the maxillary and mandibular arches. When the Statistical Filtering option is selected, Superimposition measures the amount of movement for each tooth by first eliminating as reference the ones that move more than one standard deviation above or below the mean of movement of all teeth. Movement is determined by the difference in position between the cur-

This study focused on analyzing retrospective data to compare how well aligners perform relative to traditional orthodontic treatments. Concurrently, the aim was to explore the range and predictability of each possible movement. Clinicians can thus estimate which tooth movement within a certain range has a better chance of being achieved (Fig 14-9).

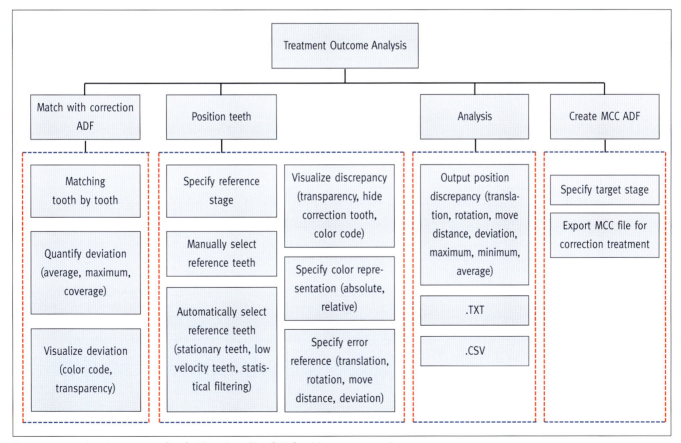

FIG 14-9 Functional summary. (ADF) Align data file; (MCC) midcourse correction.

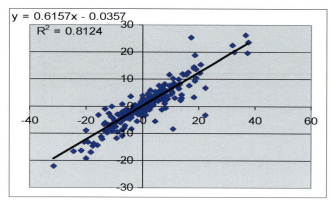

FIG 14-10 Scatter graph showing incisor rotation (degrees).

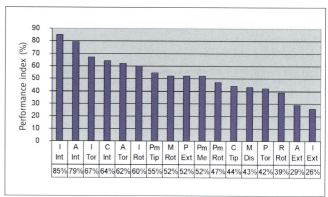

FIG 14-11 Performance index. (I) incisor; (A) anterior; (C) canine; (Pm) premolar; (M) molar; (P) posterior; (R) round teeth (canines and premolars); (Int) intrusion; (Tor) torque; (Rot) rotation; (Tip) tipping; (Ext) extrusion; (Me) mesialization; (Dis) distalization.

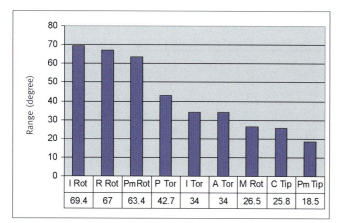

FIG 14-12 Average planned range of rotation (Rot), torque (Tor), and tipping (Tip). (I) incisor; (A) anterior; (C) canine; (Pm) premolar; (M) molar; (P) posterior; (R) round teeth (canines and premolars).

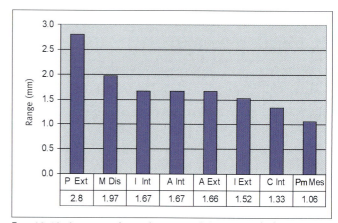

FIG 14-13 Average planned range of intrusion (Int), extrusion (Ext), distalization (Dis), and mesialization (Me). (I) incisor; (A) anterior; (C) canine; (Pm) premolar; (M) molar; (P) posterior.

rent stage and the previous one. The remaining slow or nonmoving teeth are then selected as references to measure the movement of each tooth.

A treatment stage is selected to indicate when clinical observation and simulated treatment progress deviate. The difference (of each of six movement components X, Y, Z, Rx, Ry, Rz) between the initial and progress positions is reported by Superimposition as "Achieved," whereas the "Goal" is determined by the simulation.

The amount of movement "Achieved" is plotted against that of "Goal" in scatter graphs, and trend lines are generated. Scatter graphs are then shown to demonstrate where all scattered data points are. Trend lines are generated to show the performance of the aligners. Trend lines are linear and present the best-fit straight lines for all scattered data. The performance of the aligners is represented as the slope of a trend line. The y-axis intercept signifies the amount of incidental movement that occurs when the aligners are worn. Predictability is obtained by R2, which is obtained from the regression computation of "Achieved" and "Goal" data. A scatter graph is shown in Fig 14-10.

Summary of findings and conclusion

The following groups of teeth were examined in this study: incisors, canines, premolars, molars (excluding third molars), anterior teeth, posterior teeth, and round teeth (canines and premolars). A list of tooth movements of the selected 60 arches is shown in Table 14-1. The following findings are presented in Figs 14-11 to 14-13.

1. The performance indices and coefficient of correlation of incisor intrusion and anterior intrusion show that these movements are likely to achieve the treatment goal.
2. Canine intrusion, incisor torque, incisor rotation, and anterior torque performance are average in terms of performance.

3. Premolar tipping, premolar mesial movement, molar rotation, and posterior expansion are less likely to attain the treatment goal.
4. Anterior and incisor extrusion, round teeth and premolar rotation, canine tipping, molar distalization, and posterior torque are unlikely to achieve the treatment goal.

The performance trends presented in the results do not deviate significantly from what has been common knowledge among clinicians. The exception is posterior expansion, which is thought to be a high performance movement when clinicians use aligners.

Prospective Study of Stage-by-Stage Aligner Performance

Methodology

The evaluation of progression was achieved primarily by superimposing the original treatment with the progression scan (Fig 14-14). The Superimposition tool was used to find the discrepancy between the planned movement and the actual result.

Data preparation

The following steps were used to prepare the data: the individual scans were examined, and the scans were cut. If there were attachments on the scan, the scan was detailed to remove the attachment.

Tooth matching

In the first step of the superimposition, the tooth-matching result was displayed. If any tooth showed unusually poor matching, the tooth was excluded from the reference teeth selection.

Reference teeth selection

The Superimposition tool requires the user to select the references during positioning of the jaw. Static teeth/low-velocity teeth were selected as reference teeth whenever possible. In instances of unusual discrepancy, statistical filtering was employed.

Progression of individual teeth

The same Superimposition method was applied to each stage scan: the planned movement was derived from Stage Editor. The actual outcome was derived from the analysis

TABLE 14-1 Orthdontic movements	
A Ext	Anterior extrusion
A Int	Anterior intrusion
A Tor	Anterior torque
B Mes	Premolar mesialization
B Rot	Premolar rotation
B Tip	Premolar tipping
C Int	Canine intrusion
C Tip	Canine tipping
I Int	Incisor intrusion
I Ext	Incisor extrusion
I Rot	Incisor rotation
I Tor	Incisor torque
M Dis	Molar distalization
M Rot	Molar rotation
P Exp	Posterior extrusion
P Tor	Posterior torque
R Rot	Round teeth (canines and premolars) rotation

report. If there was a big rotation, the coordinate system at the initial stage and the one after the movement were changed accordingly. The reported vectors may not be consistent; however, the observed teeth have single primary direction of motion. Thus, the coordinate system change has not affected the superimposition significantly. Because each individual stage motion is created from an individual jaw positioning, there may be fluctuation of values.

Lag

Lag represents how much the actual treatment is progressing behind the planned movement. The superimposition analysis reports the comparison of the current stage to every stage. The closest stage is selected by comparing the amount of the discrepancy. Lag is defined by the difference between the closest planned stage and the current stage. The stages that exhibit unusual lag characteristics are reported.

Movement direction

The orientation of the planned and the actual move vectors are compared. If the motion is primarily in a single direction, (eg, y direction), the y direction motion is compared. The scale perpendicular directional motions are compared to the tangential motion.

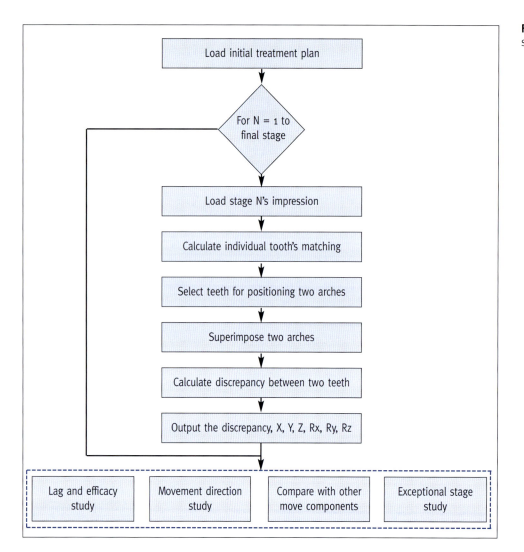

Fig 14-14 Process of progression study. (N) given stage.

TABLE 14-2 Tooth movement lag: Canine linguobuccal translation.

Stage	11	12	13	14	15	16	17	18	19	20	21	22	23	24	25	26	27	28
Closest	11	12	13	14	15	15	16	18	18	19	21	22	22	24	25	25	25	26
Lag*	0	0	0	0	0	1	1	0	1	1	0	1	1	0	0	1	2	3

*Average lag = 10/18 = 0.56 stages.

TABLE 14-3 Tooth rotation lag: Lateral incisor mesiodistal translation

Stage	16	17	18	19	20	21	22	23	24	25	26	27	28
Closest	16	16	16	17	17	17	18	18	19	20	21	21	23
Lag*	0	1	2	2	3	4	4	5	5	5	5	6	5

*Average lag = 47/13 = 3.62 stages.

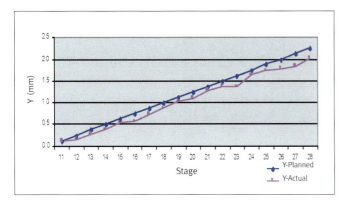

FIG 14-15 Progression study of maxillary left canine linguobuccal translation (Y).

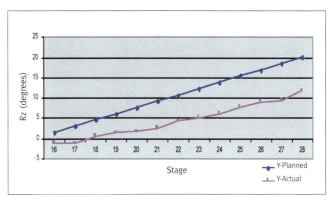

FIG 14-16 Progression study of maxillary left lateral incisor mesiodistal rotation (Rz).

Efficacy

The actual achieved motion is divided by total planned motion. The efficacy is analyzed in a single direction of motion.

Example of linguobuccal translation progression

For each stage, tooth movement has a lag. The average lag is 0.56 stages (Table 14-2). During the treatment, the maxillary left canine is moving along the y-axis as planned. The final achieved stage most closely matches planned stage 26. The achievement is 89.8% (2.02 mm/2.25 mm) (Fig 14-15). The lag at final stage is 0.23 mm.

Example of mesiodistal rotation progression

For each stage, the tooth rotation has a lag. The average lag is 3.62 stages (Table 14-3). During the treatment, the maxillary left lateral incisor is rotated around the z-axis as planned. The real final stage most closely matches planned stage 23 (Fig 14-16). The achievement is 56.2% (11.9 /20.1 degrees).

Summary

Clinically, it is safe to assume that one will get about 80% of the tooth movement seen on ClinCheck images. Thus, it is practical for the clinician to think in terms of overcorrection, and even rely on case refinement to achieve the ultimate result.

References

1. Hoggan BR, Sadowsky C. The use of palatal rugae for the assessment of anteroposterior tooth movements. Am J Orthod Dentofacial Orthop 2001;119:482–488.
2. Richmond S. Recording the dental cast in three dimensions. Am J Orthod Dentofacial Orthop 1987;92:199–206.
3. Almeida MA, Phillips C, Kula K, Tulloch C. Stability of the palatal rugae as landmarks for analysis of dental casts. Angle Orthod 1995;65:43–48.
4. Hajeer MY, Millett DT, Ayoub AF, Siebert JP. Applications of 3D imaging in orthodontics: Part I. J Orthod 2004;31:62–70.
5. Besl PJ, McKay ND. A method for registration of 3D shapes. IEEE Trans Patt Anal Machine Intelligence 1992;14:229–256.
6. Chen Y, Medioni G. Object modeling by registration of multiple range images. Int J Image Vision Comput 1992;10:145–155.
7. Faugeras OD, Hebert M. The representation, recognition, and locating of 3D objects. Int J Robotic Res 1986;5(3):27–52.
8. Horn BKP. Closed-form solution of absolute orientation using unit quaternions. J Opt Soc Amer A 1987;4:629–642.
9. Arun KS, Huang TS, Blostein SD. Least square fitting of two 3D point sets. IEEE Trans Patt Anal Machine Intelligence 1987;9:698–700.
10. Schwartz JT, Sharir M. Identification of partially obscured objects in two and three dimensions by matching noisy characteristic curves. Int J Robotic Res 1987;2(1):29–44.
11. Beers AC, Choi W, Pavlovskaia E. Computer-assisted treatment planning and analysis. Orthod Craniofac Res 2003; (suppl 1): 117–125.
12. Baumrind S. Integrated three-dimensional craniofacial mapping: Background, principles, and perspectives. Semin Orthod 2001; 7:223–232.
13. Curry S, Baumrind S, Carlson S, Beers A, Boyd RL. Integrated three-dimensional mapping at the Craniofacial Research Instrumentation Laboratory/University of the Pacific. Semin Orthod 2001;7:258–265.
14. Baumrind S, Carlson S, Beers A, Curry S, Norris K, Boyd RL. Using three-dimensional imaging to assess treatment outcomes in orthodontics: A progress report from the University of the Pacific. Orthod Craniofac Res 2003;6(suppl 1):132–142.
15. Hatcher DC, Aboudara CL. Diagnosis goes digital. Am J Orthod Dentofacial Orthop 2004;125:512–515.

chapter 15

VIRTUAL INVISALIGN PRACTICE

by
David Chenin, DDS

Virtual Invisalign Practice (VIP) is a robust portion of the Invisalign website (invisalign.com). It is customized with all of the patient information from the treating clinician's practice and requires a secure log-in. VIP contains features that allow the treating clinician to quickly and easily access complete patient and order information on his or her own Invisalign cases. Thus, VIP is the means by which a treating clinician accesses his or her three-dimensional (3-D) virtual treatment setups and the method by which Align and the treating clinician can communicate with one another about specific cases. Additionally, VIP allows access to the latest clinical information and practice development material regarding Invisalign.

To access VIP, certified clinicians must first connect to www.invisalign.com. Once connected, they access VIP by going to the "Doctor" page and entering their assigned username and password. The username and password are only available to certified clinicians and provide security to the clinician's patient information in accordance with the guidelines outlined by the Health Insurance Portability and Accountability Act (HIPAA). Once the username and password have been entered, the clinician is connected directly to the VIP home page, where all of his or her patient information can be accessed. For additional privacy, clinicians can also log in directly to a patient file to provide maximum confidentiality during a consultation. This is achieved by providing the patient's first and last name (ie, John Smith) or by entering the patient case number along with the username and password.

Once a clinician gains access to VIP, he or she is directed to a personal VIP home page, which provides a quick overview of issues that require attention (Fig 15-1). Displayed here is a link to the clinician's list of patients; patients that require an action to be taken are highlighted. The Patient List page provides the clinician with a sortable listing of patients that can be organized according to parameters of the clinician's choice (Fig 15-2). The default is a list of patients with "action required," but the clinician can sort the patient list in other ways such as "currently in treatment," "by name," "with patient number," etc. Also displayed at the bottom of the home page are important notices from Align regarding the clinician's practice.

By clicking on a specific patient, the clinician is directed to the Patient File page, which provides all patient-specific information (Fig 15-3). It includes multiple orders (past and present ClinCheck modifications) for a given patient. The status of the current order is shown in blue, and an abbreviated order history section is shown in gray. From this page, the clinician may view the All History page, which details all current and past orders. Patient icons (for Patient Files, ClinCheck, Images, and Treatment Forms) allow the clinician to navigate and access all patient information (eg, radiographs or prescription and diagnosis forms) that has been uploaded online.

In the left navigation box titled "Tools and Forms," clinicians may click on Case Forms to access a new treatment form for a patient. This area allows clinicians to fill out an online prescription form and upload photographs and radiographs to Align's secure database (Fig 15-4).

Another feature, called Doctor Profile, can also be modified online. Doctor Profile permits clinicians to change their password or security question/answer, review the existing billing and shipping addresses on file, and make updates and additions quickly and easily. In addition, clinicians can indicate how they would like to manage communication with Align for matters such as billing.

Finally, clinicians can establish or edit their treatment preferences, which are used by Align to set up cases. Treatment preferences, along with the information supplied in the prescription and diagnosis form, are used by Align technicians to provide a ClinCheck that more closely meets the clinician's expectations.

In the left navigation box titled "Clinical Information," clinicians can access a wide range of clinical information to help achieve excellent clinical results. Ancillary products (eg, buttons, elastics, interproximal reduction kits, etc) can also be ordered from this location (Fig 15-5). For reference, clinicians can read the Invisalign glossary. This glossary is not designed to be all-inclusive, but is intended for use as a tool for dental professionals as they learn about the Invisalign treatment modality. Case studies are also available (Fig 15-6). In the Case Studies section, representative cases of patients treated with Invisalign are shown in detail. From diagnosis to final results, each case provides comprehensive information on treatment planning, ClinCheck, and finishing—three integral elements for getting consistent, quality treatment outcomes with Invisalign. Each case includes extensive clinical commentary, interactive ClinChecks, and full records and forms. Another feature of the Clinical Information area is the community forum, which is designed to encourage discussion and the sharing of knowledge within the Invisalign community. A valuable part of the Clinical Information area is that it provides an opportunity for clinicians and staff to earn continuing education credits online at no cost by reading case studies or helpful clinical techniques.

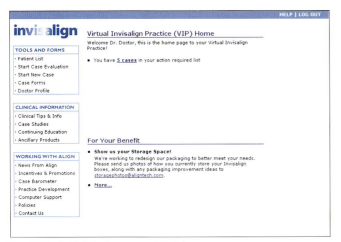

FIG 15-1 A clinician's personal VIP home page.

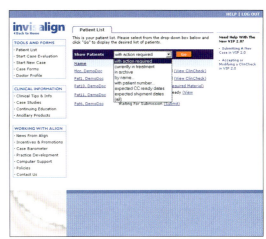

FIG 15-2 Patient List page.

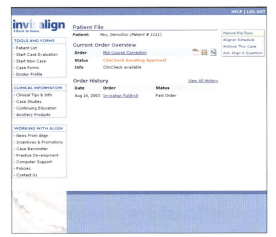

FIG 15-3 Patient File page.

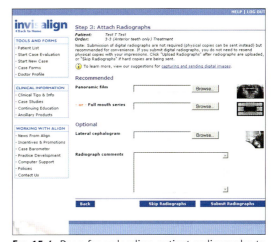

FIG 15-4 Page for uploading patient radiographs to Align.

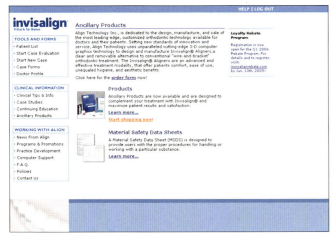

FIG 15-5 Ancillary products can be viewed and ordered.

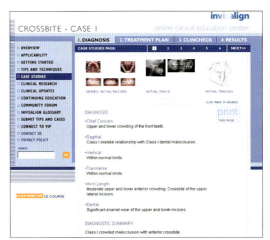

FIG 15-6 Case Studies page, used to view records of other Invisalign cases.

In the left navigation box entitled "Working with Align," clinicians can click on Incentives & Promotions to access a new informational area dedicated to practice development (see Fig 15-5). Additionally, clinicians can find computer-related information to help their practices stay current with the latest technologies that Align uses to communicate with clinicians. For example, recommended computer specifications are published to help clinicians make decisions about the purchase of new computer equipment.

Features valuable to Align, the clinician, and the clinician's staff or patients are added or improved every week. As a result, many other features found in VIP that have not been discussed here may be valuable to the clinician's practice. In many ways, the VIP site functions as part of the patient's chart.

Computer-Oriented Dental Measurements

by
Vadim Matov, PhD

This chapter introduces a novel measurement system implemented in the Align Technology software that is based on computer-oriented dental irregularity metrics (CODIM). Unlike the traditional measurements performed on plaster casts, measurements from CODIM are performed on three-dimensional (3-D) computer dental models produced by scanning impressions or casts or intraorally. Such models allow the introduction of a much wider variety of measurements than does the traditional manual approach.

The goal of CODIM is to provide a complete, objective, and consistent characterization of the dental irregularities captured by 3-D computer modeling. While CODIM comprises all traditional orthodontic measurement, it has the following distinctions:

- Measurements are much more accurate and detailed.
- Metrics incorporate measurements that can only be obtained through 3-D computer modeling (ie, they cannot be obtained using traditional instruments and protocols).
- Most of the measurements from CODIM are performed automatically, which makes them independent of the clinician's preferences or the skills of the technicians performing them.

Measurements from CODIM are implemented as a plug-in to two proprietary software programs integral to the Invisalign System: Treat and ToothMeasure. The measurement software, most notably ToothMeasure, provides the functionality to support the following:

- Automatic diagnosis of malocclusion with complete analysis of dental irregularities
- Evaluation of treatment plans with detection of difficult movements
- Automatic selection of arch forms for final position setup
- Validation of staging
- Collection of dental statistics for data mining

In this chapter, a new algorithmic approach to dental measurement that constitutes the basis of CODIM is introduced. The main component of this algorithmic approach is the rigorous "form measurement" definition, which is translated into software error-free.

In addition to incorporating measurements of the teeth and gingiva from 3-D dental models, CODIM utilizes several other measurements. These may be split into three groups: (1) shape of individual teeth, (2) alignment of the teeth of the same arch (intra-arch measurements), and

(3) bite characteristics (interarch measurements). We will focus our discussion primarily on intra-arch and interarch measurements, as these are most relevant to the alignment process. The images in this chapter were created using ToothMeasure 1.0.

Dental References

In addition to the scanned geometry of the teeth and gingiva, the following set of objects is essential for the evaluation of irregularity of tooth positions. These objects are derived from the geometry and location of the teeth and serve as references for the measurements. For example, the tip of the incisor (incisor angulation) is measured (according to Andrews[1]) as the angle between the facial axis of the clinical crown (FACC) and a line below it perpendicular to the occlusal plane (called a *normal*), as seen from a facial view of the tooth. Both the FACC and the occlusal plane are references.

The main references used in CODIM are occlusal plane, FACC curve, facial plane of the clinical crown, facial axis point, middle plane of clinical crown, facial axis line, facial normal line, wire curve, arch form curve, and arch form template.

Occlusal plane

The occlusal plane is constructed for the mandibular arch. For well-aligned teeth, this is the plane that passes through the tips of the central incisors and the cusps of the first molars. For average position of the mandibular teeth, the occlusal plane sits on top of all mandibular teeth (except the canines) and passes through at least three points, two of which are the tips of the incisors (Fig 16-1).

Facial axis of the clinical crown

The facial axis of the clinical crown is the curve on the facial part of a tooth's clinical crown between the occlusal and gingival extremities. For incisors, canines, and premolars, the FACC curve is the midline of the facial part of the clinical crown. For molars, the FACC curve goes along the buccal groove. Endpoints of the FACC curve are called the occlusal and gingival points, correspondingly (see Figs 16-1 and 16-2).

Facial axis point

The facial axis point (FA point) is the midpoint of the FACC curve. For anterior teeth, the FA point is the center of the facial part of the clinical crown of the tooth (see Fig 16-2).

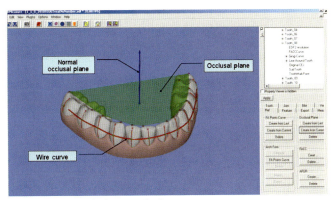

FIG 16-1 Occlusal plane and wire curve.

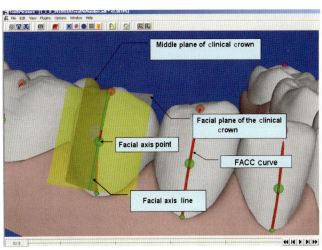

FIG 16-2 Tooth references.

Middle plane of the clinical crown

It is important to remember that the FACC curve is not a linear segment between its endpoints but rather a curve on the facial surface of the tooth. This curve is close to a middle plane of the clinical crown (MPCC) of the tooth (in nonpathologic cases), which is transversal to the facial surface of clinical crown. (see Fig 16-2).

Facial axis line

The facial axis line (FA line) is tangent to the FACC curve at the FA point. For regularly shaped anterior teeth, the FA line passes through the FA point in the direction of the FACC curve, but otherwise has no other common points with the tooth (see Fig 16-2).

Facial plane of the clinical crown

The facial plane of the clinical crown (FPCC) is tangent to the facial surface of a clinical crown at the FA point. As with the FA line, the facial plane passes through the FA point but otherwise has no common points with the tooth (see Fig 16-2).

Facial normal line

The facial normal line (FN line) is perpendicular to the FA line on the facial plane at the FA point.

Wire curve

The wire curve is a smooth curve passing through the FA points of all teeth of the same arch (see Fig 16-1).

Arch form curve

The arch form curve is a particularly important reference. It provides a measurement of how well the teeth are aligned within the same arch with respect to rotations along the vertical axis and prominence. The arch form curve in 3-D can be constructed in several different ways. In early versions of the ToothMeasure software, the arch form curve was constructed in one of two ways:

- The wire curve was made symmetric and convex from the occlusal view.
- One of the arch form templates (see below) was scaled to fit the case under consideration.

Arch form curve template

The arch form curve template is one of several typical arch form curves collected from the Align Technology database of treated and approved cases. Although the arch form curves differ from patient to patient, they can be grouped into clusters of arch forms of similar shape. One arch form curve that is representative of each cluster becomes an arch form template. Arch form templates are used as arch form curves for new patients after they are appropriately scaled to the patient's arches.

Intra-arch Measurements

Intra-arch measurements are measurements applied to the teeth of the same arch. These measurements provide numeric values that characterize the alignment of teeth within the arch, as well as individual characteristics of the teeth. Intra-arch measurements can be divided into several groups: tooth shape characteristics, tooth angular position with respect to the references (tip, torque, rotation), tooth linear position with respect to the references (prominence, level), crowding and spacing, degree of anterior teeth alignment, and degree of posterior teeth alignment.

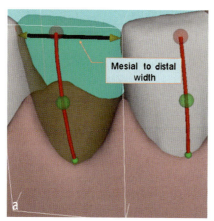 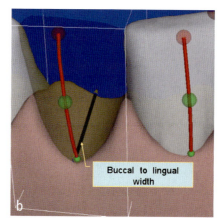

FIG 16-3 Mesial-to-distal (*a*) and buccal-to-lingual (*b*) widths.

All intra-arch measurements are described below except for the last two groups, which will be described after relevant tooth anatomic features are introduced.

Tooth shape characteristics

The measurements for individual teeth capture the basic features of crown shapes. There are common characteristics for different types of teeth. Tooth shape characteristics are important since the efficacy of the aligners depends on the aligner's grip, which in turn depends on the shape of the crown (as well as on the level of crowding).

The following common tooth characteristics are measured by ToothMeasure and other Align Technology software applications: mesial-to-distal width, buccal-to-lingual width, and crown height.

The *mesial-to-distal width* of a tooth is the distance between the horizontal points of the tooth projected onto the FPCC. This distance is measured in the direction of the normal middle plane. In other words, the mesial-to-distal width is the width of a tooth as it seen from the facial direction (Fig 16-3a).

The *buccal-to-lingual width* value is the distance between the innermost and outermost points of the tooth projected onto the MPCC. This distance is measured in the direction of the normal facial plane. In other words, the buccal-to-lingual width is the width of a tooth's profile (Fig 16-3b).

Crown height is the length of the crown measured in the direction of the FACC line; it is the height of a tooth's clinical crown.

Tooth angular position

The following measurements reflect the angular position of each tooth relative to the references: crown angulation (tip), crown inclination (torque), and crown rotation (around the

tooth axis). Note that tooth angular characteristics make sense only with respect to the references. They are meaningless for a tooth taken in isolation.

Crown angulation (tip) is the angle between the FA line and the upward normal to the occlusal plane. The angle is measured as projected onto the FPCC. See Fig 16-4, where the normal to the occlusal plane has been translated to FA point.

Crown inclination (torque) is the angle between the FA line and the upward normal to the occlusal plane. The angle is measured in projection onto the MPCC. See Fig 16-5, where the normal to the occlusal plane has been translated to FA point.

Crown rotation is the angle between the FN line and the arch form curve. The angle is measured in projection onto the occlusal plane. See Fig 16-6, in which the tangent line to the arch curve is represented by a red arrow.

Tooth linear position

The following measurements reflect the linear position of each tooth relative to the references: crown level, crown prominence, and curve of Spee. As with tooth angular position, tooth linear position measurements make sense only with respect to references and are meaningless for a tooth taken in isolation.

The *crown level* is the distance from the occlusal endpoint of the FACC curve to the occlusal plane. The distance is measured along the normal to the occlusal plane in the direction from the dental arch. Crown level is associated with the curve of Spee, which reflects how far from planar position the tips of the teeth are.

Crown prominence is the distance from a tooth's FA point to its arch form curve. The distance is measured after both FA point and arch form curve are projected onto the occlusal plane. This measurement can have a positive

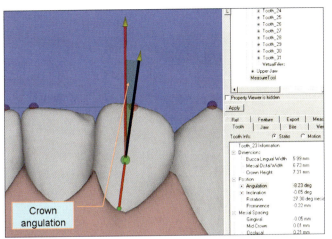

FIG 16-4 Crown angulation.

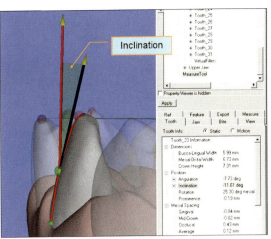

FIG 16-5 Crown inclination.

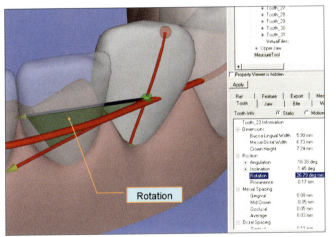

FIG 16-6 Crown rotation.

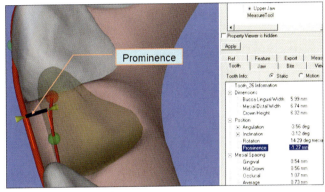

FIG 16-7 Crown prominence.

or negative value. A positive crown prominence value corresponds to FA points located outside the arch form curve, whereas a negative value corresponds to points inside the curve (Fig 16-7).

The *curve of Spee* is a smooth curve that connects the tips of the teeth of the same arch, where the tip is a point closest to the occlusal plane.

Crowding and spacing

Crowding is a measure of tooth overlap as viewed from the buccal direction. Elimination of crowding is one of the primary goals of orthodontics—a goal that requires precise and comprehensive measurements. Spacing is a measure of the distance between adjacent teeth. Note that crowding and spacing are not opposite notions: teeth can be crowded and spaced at the same time. For example, two teeth can overlap when viewed from the buccal direction and yet also be far apart when viewed from the occlusal direction (Fig 16-8). Crowding values can be neg-

ative. Negative crowding corresponds to a gap between the teeth. Crowding and spacing are measured for all pairs of adjacent teeth.

The measurement of crowding and spacing for a pair of adjacent teeth is illustrated below. These measurements are called *local crowding* and *local spacing* to distinguish them from *global crowding*, which is the sum of all values of local crowding of the teeth of the same arch.

Local crowding is measured as follows: the mesial and distal extreme points of each tooth are projected onto the arch form curve. After projection, the mesial and distal extreme points of a tooth are considered as the endpoints of the interval along the arch form curve. These intervals for two adjacent teeth can overlap or be spaced apart. In the case of overlap, the length of the overlap between the intervals is a measure of local positive crowding (Fig 16-9).

If the two intervals are apart (which corresponds to a gap between the teeth), then the length of the interval between them is a measure of local negative crowding (Fig 16-10).

141

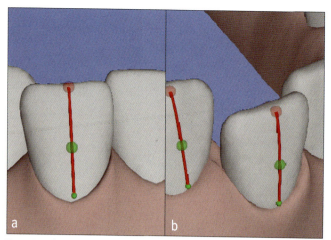

FIG 16-8 (a and b) Crowding and spacing as viewed from buccal and occlusal directions.

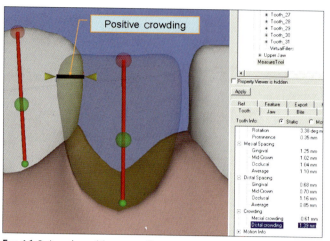

FIG 16-9 Local positive crowding.

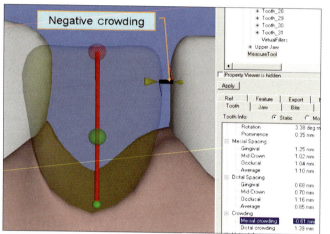

FIG 16-10 Local negative crowding.

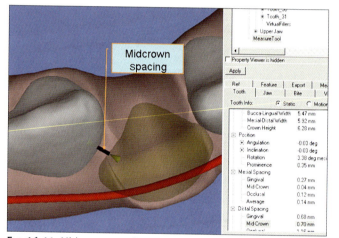

FIG 16-11 Midcrown spacing.

Local spacing is computed as follows: each tooth is split into several slices along its long axis. Each value in the set is the shortest distance between the corresponding slices of the adjacent teeth. In ToothMeasure 1.0, the number of slices is preset to three and the spacing values are called gingival spacing, midcrown spacing, and occlusal spacing (Fig 16-11).

Anatomic Dental Features

Dental features allow computing of the characteristics of alignment of teeth within one arch (intra-arch alignment), as well as characteristics of bite or the degree of malocclusion between the arches (interarch alignment).

For measurement purposes, two types of features are considered: pointed features and elongated features. Pointed features are described by the center point of a tooth and the region around this point. Cusps are an example of a point-ed feature. Elongated features are described by a tooth's center curve and the region around it. Grooves and ridges are examples of elongated features. Dental anatomy and morphology have classified several hundred different dental features. Not all of these features are required for measurements. The following pointed features are used for measurement of malocclusion and misalignment: canine cusps, buccal/lingual premolar cusps, mesiobuccal/lingual molar cusps, and distobuccal/lingual molar cusps. Elongated features used for these measurements include incisor and canine ridges, central premolar grooves, and central and buccal molar grooves. Figure 16-12 illustrates the mandibular arch with all relevant features marked.

In addition to pointed and elongated features, a third type of anatomically distinctive feature plays an important role in the measurement of malocclusion. This feature represents different regions of a tooth. For orthodontic measurements, we use only occlusal and interproximal regions. Figure 16-13 illustrates occlusal regions of the maxillary arch.

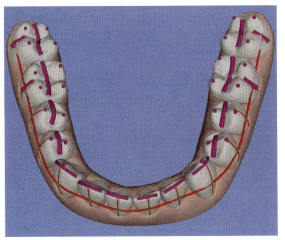

FIG 16-12 Mandibular arch features.

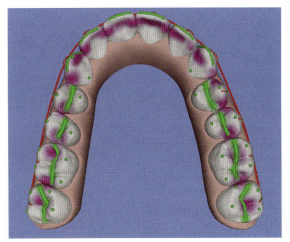

FIG 16-13 Occlusal regions of the maxillary arch.

Intra-arch Alignment Characteristics

The measurements used in ToothMeasure to characterize the alignment of teeth within one arch are described below. These measurements differ from the ones described above in two important aspects: direct utilization of anatomic features and global (versus local) alignment characteristics.

The quality of global intra-arch alignment is measured by anterior alignment characteristics, posterior alignment characteristics, and interproximal contacts.

Anterior alignment characteristics are defined by incisor ridge angles, which are the angles between the ridge and the tangent to the arch form curve. The angle is measured after both the incisor ridge and the arch form curve are projected onto the occlusal plane. The tangent to the arch form curve is computed at the closest point to the midpoint of the ridge (Fig 16-14).

Mandibular posterior alignment characteristics are expressed in terms of left and right perimeter curves. The perimeter curves are smooth curves that connect the left or right mesiobuccal and distobuccal cusps of the molars and the corresponding (ie, left or right) buccal cusps of the premolars. Perimeter curves constitute the outer boundary of the arch in the posterior region. Mandibular posterior alignment characteristics measure the alignment of the perimeter curves relative to the arch form curve. Mathematically, the value of the mandibular posterior alignment characteristics is (Dl – Ds)/Dl, where Dl and Ds are the longest and shortest distance between the corresponding perimeter curve and the arch form curve.

Maxillary posterior alignment characteristics are expressed in terms of left and right core curves. The core curves are smooth curves connecting the left or right cen-

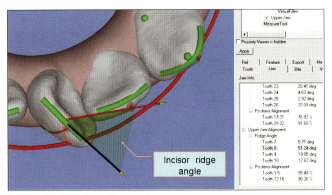

FIG 16-14 Anterior alignment.

tral grooves of molars and premolars. Perimeter curves constitute the "middle curve" of the arch in the posterior region. Maxillary posterior alignment characteristics measure the alignment of the core curves relative to the arch form curve. The value of each of two maxillary posterior alignment characteristics is (Dl – Ds)/Dl, where Dl and Ds are the longest and shortest distance between the corresponding core curve and the arch form curve.

Interproximal contacts are a measure of the spacing between adjacent teeth (see the description above).

Interarch Measurements (Bite Characteristics)

Interarch measurements describe the relative position of the maxillary and mandibular dental arches. Their values reflect different aspects of the quality of the bite. Interarch measurements implemented in ToothMeasure fall into the following groups: occlusal contacts, occlusal relationship, anterior relative position, and relative discrepancy.

143

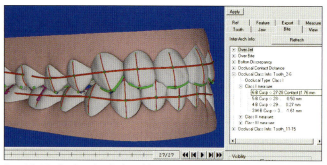

FIG 16-15 Occlusal relationship.

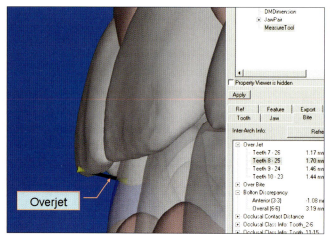

FIG 16-16 Overjet.

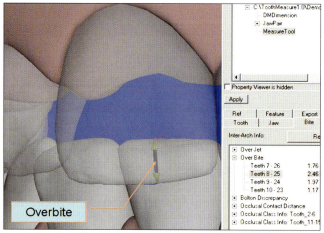

FIG 16-17 Overbite.

Measurements in these groups capture all commonly used bite characteristics and augment them with computational algorithms, providing a level of accuracy and detail that is impossible with traditional manual measurements.

Occlusal contacts

Occlusal contact of the mandibular premolars or molars is the set of distances of the buccal cusps to the central groove of the opposing tooth. Similarly, occlusal contact of the maxillary premolars or molars is the set of distances of the lingual cusps to the central groove of the opposing tooth. Occlusal contact of the mandibular anterior teeth (incisors and canines) is the set of distances from the ridges to the occlusal surfaces of the maxillary anterior teeth.

Occlusal relationship

Occlusal relationship measurements evaluate the magnitude of deviation from Class I, Class II, or Class III relationships. The measurements for a particular class of malocclusion compare a patient's relative interarch relationships to an ideal position for this class. After all the measurements are performed, the class of the bite is determined by proximity of the measured values to the ideal values for this class. Note that bite can be of a different class on the left and on the right.

Class I occlusal relationships comprise the following measurements, all of which are measured along the arch curve:

- Distance from the maxillary canine cusp tip to the embrasure contact between a mandibular canine and the adjacent premolar
- Distance from the buccal cusp of the maxillary first premolar to the interproximal contact between the mandibular premolars
- Distance from the buccal cusp of the maxillary second premolar to the interproximal contact between the mandibular premolar and first molar
- Distance from the mesiobuccal cusp of the maxillary first molar to the buccal groove of the mandibular first molar
- Distance from the mesiobuccal cusp of the maxillary second molar to the buccal groove of the mandibular second molar.

Class II occlusal relationships comprise the following measurements, all measured along the arch curve:

- Distance from the mesiobuccal cusp of the maxillary first molar to the embrasure or interproximal contact between the mandibular second premolar and the first molar
- Distance from the mesiobuccal cusp of the maxillary second molar to the embrasure or interproximal contact between the mandibular first molar and the second molar.

Class III occlusal relationships comprise the following characteristics and measurements:

- Mandibular premolars are extracted
- Distance from the buccal cusp of the maxillary second premolar to the buccal groove of the mandibular first molar (measured along the arch curve)

It is important to understand the distinction between occlusal contact and occlusal relationship. Occlusal contacts measure how close the occlusal regions come together in a vertical direction, whereas occlusal relationship measures the distance between the intended occlusal contacts along the arch curve (Fig 16-15).

Anterior relative position

The group of anterior relative position measurements comprises overjet and overbite. Different sources provide different definitions for overbite and overjet. Below are the definitions used within ToothMeasure.

Overjet is defined for each of the mandibular incisors as well as for the mandibular anterior region as a whole. For an incisor, overjet is the distance from the midpoint of the incisor's ridge to the surfaces of the maxillary incisors. The distance is measured perpendicular to the mandibular arch form curve and parallel to the occlusal plane (Fig 16-16). The overall overjet is the average of the overjets of the two central incisors.

Overbite is defined for each of the mandibular incisors and for the mandibular anterior region as a whole. For an incisor, overbite is the proportion of vertical overlap with the maxillary anterior region to the height of the incisor's crown. This proportion is computed as the ratio of the distance between the midpoint of the incisor's ridge and the closest point on the ridges of the maxillary incisors to the incisor's crown height. The distance is measured in a vertical direction that is perpendicular to the occlusal plane (Fig 16-17). The overall overbite is the average of the overbites of the two central incisors.

Relative discrepancy

Relative discrepancy comprises midline discrepancy and Bolton discrepancy. Discrepancies express the misfit of maxillary and mandibular arches with respect to their sizes.

Midline discrepancy is the distance between the midlines of the mandibular and maxillary arches as measured along the arch. This measure shows how far the teeth have to be moved laterally to establish a common midline.

Bolton discrepancy measures the mismatch of the perimeter of the arches. Bolton discrepancy has two values: 3-to-3 and 6-to-6. A 3-to-3 Bolton discrepancy is defined as follows: Let R be the ratio of the mandibular 3-to-3 perimeter to the maxillary 3-to-3 perimeter. If $| R - 0.772 | < 0.001$, then 3-to-3 Bolton discrepancy is considered to be zero; otherwise 3-to-3 Bolton discrepancy is equal to the product of the maxillary 3-to-3 perimeter and $(1.0 - R/0.772)$. If Bolton discrepancy is greater than zero, then its value shows 3-to-3 maxillary excess; otherwise it shows 3-to-3 mandibular excess.

The formula for 6-to-6 Bolton discrepancy is similar to the one for 3-to-3, except for the constants. A 6-to-6 Bolton discrepancy is defined as follows: Let R be the ratio of the mandibular 6-to-6 perimeter to the maxillary 6-to-6 perimeter. If $| R - 0.913 | < 0.001$, then 6-to-6 Bolton discrepancy is considered to be zero; otherwise 6-to-6 Bolton discrepancy is equal to the product of the maxillary 6-to-6 perimeter and $(1.0 - R/0.913)$. If Bolton discrepancy is greater than zero, then its value shows 6-to-6 maxillary excess; otherwise it shows 6-to-6 mandibular excess.

Conclusion

Besides its value in software implementation, computer-oriented dental irregularity metrics (CODIM) has much broader applications as one of the possible standards of exchange for dental data. Standard dental indices like Peer Assessment Rating (PAR) and the Objective Grading System for Dental Casts and Panoramic Radiographs can be computed from the measurement provided by CODIM. Moreover, since these computations are human independent, calibration of the person collecting the measurements is not required.

Reference

1. Andrew LF. Straight Wire: The Concept and Appliance. San Diego: L. A. Wells, 1989:14.

PERFORMANCE CHARACTERISTICS OF THE INVISALIGN SYSTEM

chapter 17

Mechanics of Tooth Movement with Invisalign

by
Andrew Beers, PhD and Trang Duong, DDS

Biomechanics in orthodontics is the study of the response of periodontal apparatus to forces applied to it. The direction, degree, distribution, and duration of mechanical forces affect the periodontal response. Orthodontic tooth movement is the net result of the reaction of supporting periodontal apparatus. It is understood, however, that forces acting upon the periodontal tissues are complex and vary by the minute.[1,2] It is indeed very difficult to visualize, let alone to define, the total force system generated by the orthodontic appliances, as multiple teeth are interconnected by the orthodontic appliance in a dynamic environment.

Control of Tooth Movement

Fundamentally, tooth movement is controlled by a selective combination of forces. Any orthodontic appliance will produce an assortment of effects. Some effects are advantageous and produce the desired end result, whereas many others are undesirable, can lead to uncontrolled tooth movement, and add problems during treatment.[1,2] An understanding of such interactions allows the clinician to properly place forces and use auxiliaries that can minimize or eliminate the unwanted reactive forces.[3]

Every orthodontic appliance generates loads through different means. The Invisalign aligner is no different in this respect. This chapter and those that follow examine the mechanics of the Invisalign System and discuss it based on what is known about the mechanics of traditional fixed orthodontic appliances.

Tooth Movement with Fixed Appliances

Any type of orthodontic tooth movement requires force application. Much can be found in the literature describing the initial forces generated by fixed appliances upon their insertion. Yet, there is no consensus on the optimal force magnitude for orthodontic tooth movement; forces ranging from 2 to 30 kPa, however, have been reported. In general, translation, root torque, rotation, and extrusion require heavy forces of 50 to 150 g; tipping requires medium forces of 50 to 75 g; and intrusion requires light forces of 10 to 25 g.

Ideal force levels for orthodontic tooth movement should be high enough to stimulate cellular activity without occluding blood vessels in the periodontal ligament. The simplest form of orthodontic tooth movement is tipping upon application of a single force. Subsequently, the tooth rotates around its center of resistance. Translation, on the other hand, requires application of two or more force systems. These two systems work to balance the ratio between the moment produced by the force applied to move the crown and the counterbalancing moment produced by the couple used to control root position. The simplest way to determine how a tooth will move with fixed appliances is to determine the ratio between the moment created when a force is applied to the crown of a tooth and the counterbalancing moment generated by a couple within the bracket. In the orthodontic literature, the relationship between the force and the counterbalancing couple is termed the *moment-to-force ratio* (M/F). Moment-to-force ratios of 1 to 7 produce controlled tipping, whereas ratios of 8 to 10 result in bodily movement, and ratios greater than 10 affect the root torque.

In addition to the forces created by the archwire configuration, frictional resistance between the archwire and the bracket slot should be considered. To generate moments of a couple in orthodontics so as to control root position, rectangular wires are used; the wires need to be twisted (placed in torsion) in the bracket slot. Almost every force applied in the oral environment is complex because it is under the influence of biologic variation and the effects in three planes of space.[4] Because of these numerous and unknown contributing factors, exact force systems in fixed appliances have never been reported.

With Invisalign, the system is even more complicated because there is no exact point of force application. The aligner covers the entire surface of the crown: the point of force application depends on the anatomy of the tooth, the properties of the material, the fit or adaptation of the aligner over the tooth, and the amount of activation programmed into the aligner. Much is still to be understood. Chapter 18 discusses such forces generated in vitro.

Challenges of Studying Biomechanics with the Invisalign Appliance

The design of the Invisalign aligner makes studying its mechanics a formidable challenge. At first approximation, it appears straightforward because the position and orientation of each tooth are specified over the course of the treatment. The forces associated with a planned treatment can be either measured or simulated by a computer system without the need to further involve the patient. Furthermore, these planned forces can be compared to the results of the actual treatment because the set of Invisalign appliances fully specifies where the teeth should be at each stage of the treatment. But there are several challenges in understanding the mechanics of the aligners. The most obvious challenge is that, like many removable appliances, it is not rigidly affixed to the teeth on which it operates. This could lead to more complex interactions between the aligner and the teeth, such as slipping motions where the contact points between the aligner and the teeth change dynamically. This can also make the exertion of what we conceptually think of as "pulling" forces more difficult.

Another challenge arises from the complex shape of the appliance itself. It fits snugly over the teeth and derives its ability to apply forces almost anywhere on a tooth from this snug fit. But it is difficult to conceptualize where exactly the appliance contacts the teeth, and from there what net forces and moments result from all of those contacts. This situation is further complicated by the wide variety of actual tooth shapes, which makes the understanding of the interaction between the aligner and the teeth a patient-specific task. Also, each successive appliance is a different shape, and understanding the interaction between tooth and appliance in one stage does not necessarily provide insight into the next.

A further complication results from how the appliance is made and used. ClinCheck images prescribe the resultant individual tooth positions with each aligner wear. The plastic appliances are then manufactured accordingly. While the computer-modeled tooth positions could provide an understanding of the force interactions, it must also be considered that any deviations the teeth make from the ClinCheck-predicted locations may change the force systems between the aligner and the tooth. For example, if the tracking is lost, then the ill-fitting aligner will apply intrusive forces. As seen above, intrusion requires very light forces. Unfortunately, once intruded, the tooth cannot be recaptured in the aligner without the use of auxiliary force modules, such as vertical elastics and the like.

It is clear that such questions as "What is the optimal force level per aligner?" and "How can the complex surface-and-force interactions be studied?" need to be answered to enhance aligner performance and reduce reliance on the clinician for a successful treatment outcome.

References

1. Proffit W, Fields H. Contemporary Orthodontics, ed 3. St Louis: Mosby, 2000:295–325.
2. Burstone C. Orthodontics as a science: The role of biomechanics. Am J Orthod Dentofacial Orthop 2000;117:598–600.
3. Kusy RP. The future of orthodontic materials: The long-term view. Am J Orthod Dentofacial Orthop 1998;113:91–95.
4. Demange C. Equilibrium situations in bend force systems. Am J Orthod Dentofacial Orthop 1990;98:333–339.

chapter 18

APPLICATIONS OF MECHANICS WITH INVISALIGN

by
Heng Cao, PhD and Trang Duong, DDS

Conceptual Models

Unlike with fixed appliances, the forces that move teeth with aligners are generated by the aligner material. Moreover, these forces are highly controlled for the distance teeth are to be moved. It is generally accepted that the aligner tray generates roughly 50 g of force upon initial placement. In time, this force level decreases, but teeth still move into the positions shown by the Treat software.

Actual tooth position is defined as the position of the tooth in the mouth, whereas the beginning position captured in the polyvinyl siloxane (PVS) impression is called the *initial position*. In contrast, the planned position of the teeth is defined as the *virtual position*, which is determined using Treat. Naturally, these virtual positions are determined by the clinician with the consent of the patient within the framework of what is biologically possible.

The final position of the teeth can be achieved in individual small movements called *stages*. After each stage, the teeth are at a position closer to the final position. For reasons of the flexibility of the aligner material and the variation in the response of supporting periodontal apparatus, tooth movement lag (ie, the actual position of teeth being behind the planned position) has been shown to occur. Since the planned position is always ahead of the actual position, there would be a displacement between the two in a reference Cartesian coordinate system. This discrepancy exerts a certain amount of force along some direction on certain teeth. The interaction between the force the aligner exerts on the teeth and the resultant reaction of the teeth is shown in Fig 18-1.

Because of the variability of wear time and the material properties of the aligner, the force exerted by the aligner is not constant. It actually decreases significantly during the 2-week wear time. The instantaneous response to the force is seen mainly in the periodontal ligament (PDL) and gingiva. The viscoelastic properties of the PDL (see chapter 19) dampen and alleviate the force. The rapid decline in the aligner force shown is due to this dampening effect (Fig 18-2).

The relationship between the shock-absorbing capacity of the PDL and the physical properties of bone explains the nature of tooth movement. When the PDL is compressed to its minimal volume, the reaction then comes from bone tissue. The remodeling of bone is relatively slower than the deformation of soft tissue because bone tissue is more rigid. The reaction from bone, therefore, is continuous for hours and even days. Simultaneously, the stress relaxation that occurs in the aligner material also reduces the force magnitude. After an aligner is worn for one stage (normally 2 weeks), the teeth move to a new position. Because of the variability in the response of the teeth and the changes in the stress relaxation of the aligner material, the forces placed on the teeth will change over the course of the 2 weeks.

Tooth Movement Model

To understand how aligners work to move teeth and how to improve the efficiency and efficacy of the appliance, it is necessary to understand how teeth move spatially and temporally with aligners. A model was developed to evaluate how tooth movement occurs with aligners. The model assumes that forces and torque applied on the teeth by the aligner can be determined by experimental and finite element analysis (FEA) and was designed to understand the characteristics of the Invisalign appliance and improve its performance. The primary goal of the model was to evaluate the deviation of the actual tooth position from the prescribed treatment goal. The model was not designed to answer questions on a biologic level (such as what happens within the PDL or to the bone remodeling or gingival remodeling processes), but rather to enable researchers to learn from existing data and current tech-

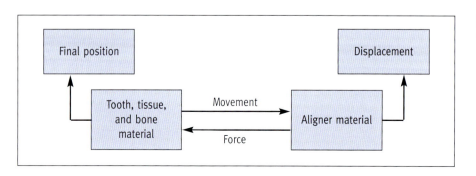

FIG 18-1 Conceptual model of the aligner-dental system.

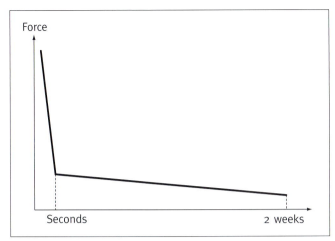

FIG 18-2 The force from the aligner changes with time.

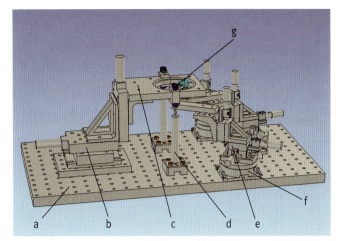

FIG 18-3 Force measurement device. (a) Board in which all components are attached; (b) translation table that holds the platform; (c) platform where the tooth models are fixed; (d) support structures that add rigidity to the platform; (e) translation table connected to the force gauge (sensor), which moves the sensor in x, y, and z directions; (f) rotation table fixed on the board and connected to the translation table (rotates along an upright axis); (g) force gauge (sensor).

nology. A secondary goal was to validate the methodology of the tooth movement model as a basis for future force studies. This model is based on previously established models of force measurements for tooth movement.

Finite Element Analysis Model

Developed in the late 1940s, finite element analysis is a technique created to help aerospace engineers design aircraft structures. Through the application of computer technology, FEA became useful as a tool for a variety of other engineering tasks. This technique is based on the premise that an approximate solution to any complex engineering problem can be reached by dividing the problem into smaller and more manageable (finite) elements. Using finite elements, complex partial differential equations that describe the behavior of certain structures can be reduced to a set of linear equations that can be easily solved using standard matrix algebra. FEA is used in a variety of engineering disciplines and also in dental and medical research.

With fast-advancing computer technology, FEA is now extensively applied in biomechanics to study the effects of forces on biologic systems. This method was used to simulate the force-displacement interaction between the dentition and the aligner. With this model, researchers can collect data on force distribution on the teeth and aligner surface consequent to a given displacement. The variability and complexity of tooth geometry and surrounding biologic tissue material, however, make simulation of the dental-aligner interaction extremely difficult. Additionally, tooth geometry and tissue properties vary

from individual to individual and also from tooth to tooth within the same person.

Stresses That Develop in the Aligner During Thermoforming

FEA was used to predict the stress and strain on aligners and to estimate the final result of orthodontic movement using the tooth-movement model. Aligners are made from a 0.030-mil polyurethane material called Ex30. The blank material is made from a 5 × 5–inch sheet that is thermopressed over a stereolithographic (SLA) model of the teeth. Following thermal heating, the aligners are peeled off the model, trimmed, polished, and disinfected. In the thermoforming process, residual stress can be introduced into the material. The residual stress can change the mechanical behavior of the aligners and affect the force response under displacement, fatigue, and stress relaxation.

Although experimental data are available for the stress-strain relationship of Ex30 samples, no data are available on the stress-strain relationship of Ex30 once the aligners are formed over the tooth models. The complexity of the aligner geometry makes testing more difficult than for a flat single piece of material; however, using FEA it is possible to simulate how the material will react in the shape of an aligner.

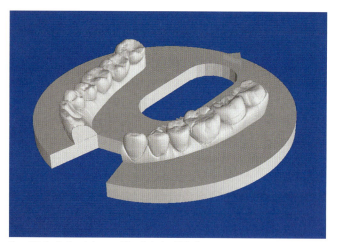

Fig 18-4 Cutout jaw with disk in STL format.

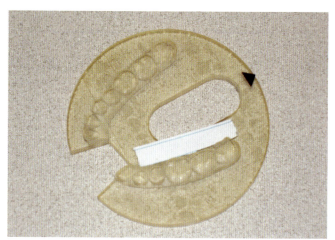

Fig 18-5 SLA model built from the STL model in Fig 18-4.

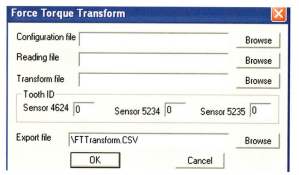

Fig 18-6 Interface of force transformation plug-in in Treat.

Forces Generated by the Aligner

The force response of an aligner under displacement depends on both the material properties and the geometry of the aligner. Material properties can be obtained by running material characterization tests such as tensile, compressive, and indentation tests. When the material properties are kept constant, the variation of geometry of the aligner affects the response to displacement. For example, changes in the thickness of the aligners produce different force responses to the same displacement.

It is difficult to measure the force response of an aligner directly on each tooth of a jaw. For one, the force gauges currently available are too big for this purpose. Second, the aligner contacts the tooth with the inner surface area and not the outer surface area, which creates further difficulty. Currently, there are no sensors that can monitor the pressure field in real time and fit between the aligner and the teeth. Third, because of the variability of the geometry of the teeth and the various malocclusions, the measurement device has to have various degrees of freedom to fit into

the different geometries. Once the aligners are placed on the models, the problem of rigidly fixing the system arises. The difficulties with this, and how it affects the measurements, are discussed later in this chapter.

Force Measurement Device

To measure the force response of an aligner with a certain displacement, a special force measurement device was developed (Fig 18-3). Treatment is arranged into a series of stages. At each stage, only a small movement is designed and achieved. The force measurement device can be used to measure force vectors and torque vectors in the x, y, and z directions on three adjacent target teeth at each stage.

The fundamental design first requires creation of stereolithography (STL) files for the models on which measurements will be made; Fig 18-4 shows the STL file in Treat software. Subsequently, an SLA model is built based on the computer file. Figure 18-5 shows the SLA model built from the STL file shown in Fig 18-4. The aligners are then made from those SLA models using the thermoforming machine (see chapter 3).

The next steps in the process are to set up the force measurement device, which includes bonding target teeth, setting up data acquisition software, and initializing target teeth to their original position with respect to the reference jaw model at stage n. After this, measurements at stage n + 1 are made. Finally, vectors from the sensor coordinate are transformed to tooth coordinate systems. Figure 18-6 shows the interface of the Treat plug-in that performs the transformation.

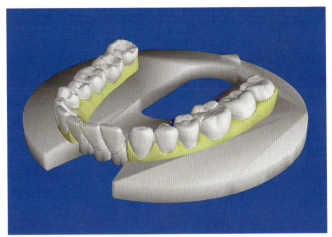

FIG 18-7 Model of measurement jaw and target teeth.

	Translation (K)	
Tooth[†]	Kx (N/mm, 100 g/mm)	Kz (N/mm, 100 g/mm)
Central incisor	19.78	51.06
Lateral incisor	30.38	52.28
Canine	25.64	85.5
First premolar	16.02	28.38
Second premolar	15.82	43.42
First molar	16.95	33.9

TABLE 18-1 Stiffness of aligner on teeth at room temperature and humidity*

*The values listed are much higher than what is normally expected in treatment protocols.
[†]All teeth tested were in the maxillary left quadrant.

To measure the force, a stage 0 model—which shows the initial position of the teeth—is used. The target tooth is then moved along the translation table along a certain direction. The tooth movement is recorded by the micrometer on the translation table (Fig 18-7).

From the experimental data it was found that when a single tooth is moved, a simple single force on the target tooth is not generated. Instead, forces on the adjacent teeth are also generated. In physics, this opposite and reactive force is known as *Newton's third law of motion.* Indeed, programmed movements on one tooth produce a force on other teeth as well. This principle also holds for fixed appliances and is well-known. When more than one tooth is moved, all these forces are simultaneously active. Some of the forces are additive, whereas others counteract each other. Because of this principle, it is extremely difficult to get a clear idea of the total force and direction. If the problem is examined through FEA, however, it is possible to develop a clear picture of what happened on the continuum of the aligner.

Stiffness of the Aligner

Aligner stiffness is the ratio of force to displacement along a certain direction on the aligner. The force measurement on initial tooth movement was performed using the device described above.

A central target tooth, which can be any tooth in the arch, is moved through adjustments made to the translation table connected to it. The total translation for each central target tooth is 1.25 mm, which is divided into 10 steps when turning the micrometer on the translation table. Only the translations along the x (buccolingual) and z (occlusal) directions were done because the flexibility of the measurement device in the y (mesiodistal) direction was too high to sustain loading. Table 18-1 presents stiffness data for several teeth. Further study is needed to determine the coefficient to convert the stiffness to those under body temperature and humidity.

Variation in Thickness of Gingiva

It is easy to understand that changing the aligner thickness changes the stiffness and therefore transmits different amounts of force. One of the factors that affects the thickness of the aligner is the height of the virtual gingiva, which is defined as the vertical distance between the lowest point on the frontal gingival line and the bottom of the gingiva in the Treat software. To test this postulate, an experiment was designed in which two groups of 10 aligners were made based on two SLA models. Aligners from both SLA models were identical except for the height of the virtual gingiva—which was twice as high in the second group (Fig 18-8). Once made from the SLA models, the aligners were weighed on a precision scale. Because the aligners were trimmed along the gingival line, which was the same for both SLA models, the surfaces of the aligners from both groups were considered the same. Therefore, the ratio between different weights of aligners is equivalent to the ratio of thickness. The study found that increasing the gingival height of the SLA model causes a reduction in aligner thickness. The mean weight of aligners with a 4-mm gingival height was 1.630 g (±0.036), and those with an 8-mm gingival height weighed 1.531 g

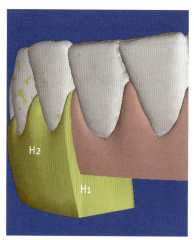

FIG 18-8 Height (H) of gingiva used in two experimental groups.

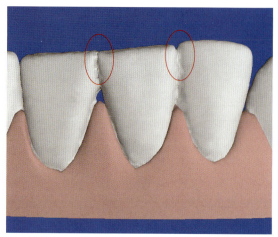

FIG 18-9 Interproximal contact.

(±0.055). In addition, the two groups of aligners were used to measure the force response to the same displacement. One measurement was taken for each aligner in each group. The mean force is summarized in Table 18-2. As Table 18-2 shows, aligners formed on SLA models with higher gingiva generated less force, given the same displacement on the target teeth. Therefore, aligners built on higher gingival models have lower stiffness values.

Variation of Force Measurement

A study was designed to assess whether the variation in force measurement on different cases and setups could be estimated. If there is an error in estimation, what is it? The force measurement was grouped into different setups, which focused on various factors that might affect the variation of measurement. These factors are interproximal con-

tact, complexity of tooth geometry, attachment, movement, and aligner thickness.

Where does the variation in force measurement results come from? First, variation exists in the aligners. No two aligners are identical, even if they were made for the same dental arch. Second, when an aligner is placed on the arch, its engagement is important. One aligner can be engaged on teeth slightly differently every time; that difference causes different force readings each time. Third, the target teeth do not occupy the same position in every trial—in other words, the device does not fit the target teeth position perfectly. The frictional contact between two adjacent target teeth can prevent them from returning to their original position after the position is disturbed by removing the aligner from the arch. Additionally, creep in the aligner contributes to measurement variations. After the aligner has been in place on an arch for some time, the aligner material loses its original strength, which results in the application of less force on the teeth. After the aligner is removed, the aligner material recovers its strength partially, depending on how long it was worn and how long it rests.

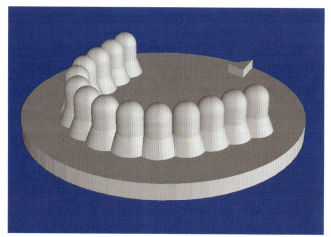

FIG 18-10 Bullet teeth on arch form with disk.

TABLE 18-2 Force (N) from aligners formed on SLA models with different gingival heights

	Sensors		
Gingival height	No. 4624	No. 5234	No. 5235
8 mm	1.68	2.22	1.25
4 mm	2.20	3.35	2.58

TABLE 18-3 Force reading (F) on three target teeth* with interproximal contact

	Fx (N)	Fy (N)	Fz (N)
Sensor no. 4624			
SD	0.22	0.16	0.17
Mean	1.08	0.29	0.22
Sensor no. 5234			
SD	0.46	0.26	0.36
Mean	1.78	−0.30	0.28
Sensor no. 5235			
SD	0.26	0.27	0.17
Mean	0.60	−0.88	−0.35

*Sensor nos. 4624, 5234, and 5235 refer to the sensor series numbers connected to the target teeth.

TABLE 18-4 Force reading (F) on three target teeth* without interproximal contact

	Fx (N)	Fy (N)	Fz (N)
Sensor no. 4624			
SD	0.34	0.26	0.10
Mean	1.04	0.10	0.28
Sensor no. 5234			
SD	0.57	0.14	0.20
Mean	1.87	−0.33	0.40
Sensor no. 5235			
SD	0.30	0.31	0.32
Mean	0.51	−0.76	−0.10

*Sensor nos. 4624, 5234, and 5235 refer to the sensor series numbers connected to the target teeth.

In the following experiment, 10 aligners were made on one model for each testing purpose to alleviate the creeping effect. In every trial, a different aligner was used. If the measurement involved 20 trials, different aligners were used for the first 10 trials and then recycled from the first aligner for the next 10 trials. These data are presented in Tables 18-3 to 18-10.

Interproximal contacts

One SLA model was built with an interproximal contact (Fig 18-9). Ten aligners were formed on this SLA model. With the interproximal contact, force measurements were taken 10 times, each time using different aligners. The interproximal contacts between the target teeth were then removed mechanically using a diamond strip. The same 10 aligners were used to take measurements without the interproximal contact. Test of equivalent variance and Wilcoxon signed rank test were made between these

groups to determine if they had equivalent variance. As presented in Tables 18-3 and 18-4, the data showed that the variance of the two groups was equivalent, which indicates that the interproximal contact does not contribute to the variation of measurement results.

Complexity of tooth geometry

Tooth geometry refers to the surface and curvature of the tooth. The variability in the geometry of a tooth is infinitely more complex than the geometry of any man-made mechanical part. Thus, if a tooth is thought of as a bullet that is aligned along the arch form, the tooth and arch geometry are substantially simplified (Fig 18-10). When an attachment is added, however, tooth geometry becomes more complex.

An experiment was conducted to examine the difference between a tooth in a bullet arch and a tooth in a typodont. In each testing arch, only the center target tooth

TABLE 18-5 Force measurement (F) on bullet tooth arch

	Fx (N)	Fy (N)	Fz (N)
Mean	4.03	0.42	1.03
SD	0.72	0.38	0.38
S/M*	0.18	0.90	0.37

(S/M) Ratio of standard deviation to mean force.

TABLE 18-6 Force measurement (F) on the typodont arch

	Fx (N)	Fy (N)	Fz (N)
Mean	4.25	0.24	0.53
SD	0.94	0.47	2.51
S/M*	0.22	1.96	4.75

(S/M) Ratio of standard deviation to mean force.

TABLE 18-7 Force measurement (F) on the typodont arch with attachment on the target tooth

	Fx (N)	Fy (N)	Fz (N)
Mean	1.99	0.15	1.59
SD	0.39	0.25	1.28
S/M*	0.20	1.67	0.81

(S/M) Ratio of standard deviation to mean force.

TABLE 18-8 Force measurement (F) on target tooth with rotation along z-axis

	Fx (N)	Fy (N)	Fz (N)
Mean	−1.32	−0.53	−2.04
SD	0.42	0.56	2.50
S/M*	−0.31	−1.07	−1.22

(S/M) Ratio of standard deviation to mean force.

TABLE 18-9 Force measurement (F) on target tooth with rotation along y-axis

	Fx (N)	Fy (N)	Fz (N)
Mean	−1.69	−0.30	1.83
SD	0.44	0.48	0.86
S/M*	−0.26	−1.57	0.47

(S/M) Ratio of standard deviation to mean force.

TABLE 18-9 Force measurement (F) on target tooth with translation along x-axis

	Fx (N)	Fy (N)	Fz (N)
Mean	−4.25	0.24	−0.53
SD	0.94	0.47	2.51
S/M*	−0.22	1.96	−4.75

(S/M) Ratio of standard deviation to mean force.

had the same amount of movement, along the buccal and lingual directions. Measurements from 20 consecutive trials were made. The mean and standard deviations of forces were then calculated on the center target tooth (Tables 18-5 to 18-7).

Standard deviation to mean (S/M) is the ratio of standard deviation to mean force reading, which indicates how consistent the data are within each category. The smaller the ratio, the more consistent the data. For example, the comparison of S/M of Fx in Tables 18-5 and 18-6 indicates that the force measurement on the bullet arch is more consistent than that on the typodont arch. In the Force Measurement Device section, we mentioned the force transformation plug-in that can transform the force measurement from the force gauge coordinate system to the tooth coordinate system. The force gauge coordinate system is fixed on the force gauge itself, and the force gauge

coordinate system consists of x-, y-, and z-axes, a typical coordinate triad. The tooth coordinate system is also composed of x-, y-, and z-axes. The x direction is the buccolingual direction; the y direction is the mesiodistal direction; and the z direction is the extrusion-intrusion direction. Therefore, each tooth has its own coordinate system. The data are presented to show how the repeatability of the data and variance compare between the data groups.

Theoretically, the addition of an attachment and consequent increase in the geometry of the tooth would produce an increase in the variation of the measurements. Interestingly, however, a comparison of Tables 18-6 and 18-7 shows that the addition of an attachment did not increase the variability of the results. Although the addition of an attachment increased the complexity of the geometry, it also introduced a good grip on the aligner, which helped to snap the aligner in a repeatable way. This might explain why the measurement results were contradictory to expectations.

Movement

When the movement on a target tooth is rotation or translation, the rotation is carried by the aligner shape. Each time an aligner is placed on the jaw manually, the aligner position on the jaw slightly changes. This contributes to the variation in the force reading. Because rotation requires engagement of the tooth and the aligner, measurements for rotation showed higher variation compared to translation (Tables 18-8 to 18-10).

Summary and Future Studies

This chapter introduced the initial steps of studying the mechanics of tooth movement with the Invisalign appliance. The core of tooth mechanics research is the tooth movement model and the aligner FEA model. Generally, many techniques and methods in mechanical engineering have been and will continue to be applied to dental systems. The force measurement device serves as a workbench to validate the aligner FEA model. Once the aligner FEA model is developed, more tests can be performed to develop a better understanding of how the aligner moves the tooth and to optimize the aligner design.

Future studies are focused on the development and perfection of devices to measure the movement and forces generated with aligners. The first step is to improve the force measurement device to make the readings more consistent and accurate. The second is the development of FEA modeling of the aligner to better understand the forces generated with aligners. Last, our vision is to develop tooth movement models using the aligner to understand the effects of periodontal response under these forces.

chapter 19

BIOLOGIC ELEMENTS OF TOOTH MOVEMENT

by
Orhan C. Tuncay, DMD

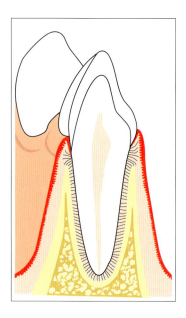

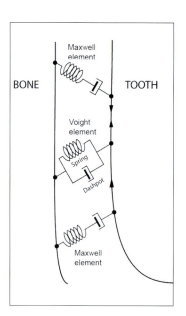

Fig 19-1 (*left*) Anatomy of periodontal support. (Modified from Lindhe et al[3] with permission.)

Fig 19-2 (*right*) Maxwell and Voight elements alternate between live and dead forms upon force application and its removal. These spring and dashpot parallel and serial configurations explain the viscoelastic properties of periodontal ligament upon loading.

Tooth movement is a product of periodontal remodeling that occurs as a result of an applied mechanical force. The origin of the mechanical force is irrelevant. When the mechanical force is exerted by a stomatognathic system applied to move teeth into a desired alignment, it is termed *orthodontic tooth movement*. In the absence of an orthodontic goal, however, such factors as occlusal force, habits, and posture can all move teeth, sometimes into a state of pathology.

It has long been suggested that orthodontic forces might damage the periodontium. It was first demonstrated in 1979 that extrinsic forces applied to move teeth elicit an inflammatory response from the periodontal tissues.[1] Typically, orthodontic forces create a wound deep in the periodontal tissues. The nature of this wound is hypoxia.[2] Recovery from this hypoxic condition in certain regions of the periodontal ligament (PDL) requires removal of bone. The inflammatory response is essential to bone remodeling. It can be argued that it is not the mechanical forces themselves that move teeth, but rather the remodeling of the periodontal tissue that creates the spaces into which teeth can be pushed by orthodontic appliances.

Understanding the clinical behavior of periodontal tissues is a prerequisite to the successful application of mechanical forces to move teeth efficiently and without undesirable sequelae. Our current knowledge of periodontal remodeling comes from experiments conducted to simulate fixed appliance effects: heavy forces, necrosis, a switch from normoxia to hypoxia or hyperoxia. These are the events that take place to heal the wounds created by the experimental orthodontic forces. In contrast, the bio-

logic responses to Invisalign mechanics are different, as there is no periodontal wound to be healed.

Anatomy of Periodontal Structures Affected by Tooth Movement

The periodontal tissues have been defined as the "attachment apparatus," but they do more than hold the teeth in place. They are instrumental in determining tooth motility. The dentoalveolar structures, composed of teeth and the periodontium, are intrinsically dynamic structures. More important, however, the development of periodontal tissues is synchronous with the development of teeth. They are interdependent; one cannot exist without the other.

Gingiva

The masticatory mucosa includes the gingiva and the hard palate. The gingiva surrounds the teeth. Its final shape is determined by the position of the teeth during the growth and development of the oral structures. A fully developed gingiva can be categorized into three different sections (Fig 19-1). The region where the gingiva meets the tooth is known as the *free gingival margin*. Further apically, the tissue is called the *alveolar mucosa*. It is separated from the lining of adjacent oral structures by a demarcation zone called the *mucogingival junction*. Healthy gingiva is tightly attached to both the underlying bone and the tooth surface.

The gingival surface exposed to the oral cavity is keratinized. The keratin-producing cells are often devoid of nuclei. Additionally, the cells of this keratinized layer are tightly bound by a series of cytoplasmic processes called *desmosomes*. For purposes of orthodontic treatment, this tight bonding of gingival tissues is particularly significant in that it affects both the rate of tooth movement and the intra-arch stability of corrected tooth positions. Gingival remodeling is a significant factor in tooth movement.

Periodontal ligament

The PDL cuddles the tooth. It is composed of thick connective tissue and is highly vascularized. Its dependence on a constant blood supply is comparable to that of highly vascularized organs such as the heart and brain.[2] In addition to vascular cells, the PDL contains fibroblasts, osteoblasts, cementoblasts, osteoclasts, and epithelial cells. Nerve fibers are also present. Loose connective tissue fibroblasts present during development form the collagen fibers that attach to the cementum surface and the lamina dura of the alveolar bone. These fibers are classified according to their directional and positional arrangement: apical, oblique, horizontal, and alveolar crest fibers that go toward the crown.

The PDL space has an hourglass shape. It is narrowest at the midroot areas. The PDL width is approximately 0.25 mm (0.2 to 0.4 mm). Although narrow, it cushions the tooth when it is subjected to masticatory action or orthodontically generated mechanical forces. The viscoelastic properties of the PDL can be described by serial- or parallel-connected spring and dashpot elements[4] (Fig 19-2). Mechanical forces are selectively transmitted to the adjacent bone according to the duration and intensity of their initial application.

During periods of tooth movement, collagen fibers of the PDL are also affected. Normally, the collagen adjacent to the bone is less mature than the collagen next to the cementum. Thus, the collagen in the alveolar bone might remodel rapidly and the cemental surface fibers might not be affected at all. This arrangement may be responsible for the integrity of the PDL during orthodontic tooth movement.

Forces are transmitted to the tooth via the cementum layer. Cementum is a mineralized tissue that covers the root surface. It contains no blood or lymph vessels and is devoid of innervation. It serves to connect the tooth surface to the PDL; fibers attach to the cemental surface. Because the PDL does not have blood vessels, interruptions of the blood supply within the PDL are likely to affect cemental viability. This may be particularly true if the interruptions are sustained for a lengthy period.[5]

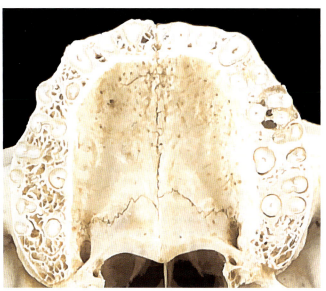

FIG 19-3 Basal bone is considerably wider in the posterior segments. Yet, the wider bone remodels more readily. (Reprinted from Lindhe et al[3] with permission.)

Alveolar bone

This special bone forms in response to the presence of the tooth. It is contiguous with the corpus maxilla and the mandible. The alveolar process develops in response to the formation and eruption of the teeth. Like all other bones in the body, alveolar bone has an outer layer of cortical bone and an inner trabecular structure. It is a thin band in the incisor region but thickens considerably around the molars (Fig 19-3). This design might relate to the forces these teeth will be subjected to throughout an individual's life. Oddly, alveolar bone is more readily remodeled around the posterior teeth than the anterior teeth.

The behavior of trabeculae has been studied extensively in orthopedics. Depictions of the load-bearing capacity and characteristic of the femoral head, for example, have been highly publicized (Figs 19-4a and 19-4b). In the alveolar bone, the response of trabecular structures (Fig 19-5) to orthodontic forces has not been investigated. It has been determined, however, that the alveolar trabeculae do not remodel—as had been theorized (Fig 19-6a and 19-6b).

Haversian canals form around the blood vessels. This structural characteristic might be linked to the calcification process.[6]

Osteoblasts are responsible for new bone modeling. These bone-forming cells densely populate the outer and inner lining membranes, the endosteum and periosteum, respectively. The alveolar bone is constantly remodeled as dictated by the functional demands placed on it (ie, the

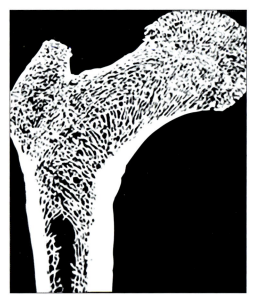

FIG 19-4a The femoral head section depicts the typical trabecular arrangement.

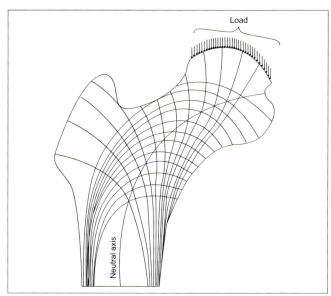

FIG 19-4b Diagram of force systems within the femoral head.

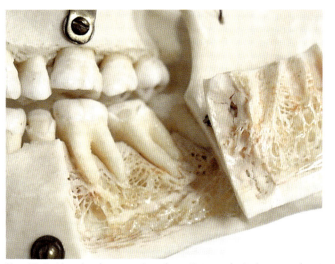

FIG 19-5 Alveolar bone trabeculae. Not much is known about their behavior during orthodontic tooth movement.

Blood supply

Gingival tissues receive their blood supply from various sources. This ensures uninterrupted nutrient supply despite the numerous insults intraoral tissues normally receive. It is interesting to note that the main vascular supply of the free gingiva from the supraperiosteal blood vessels anastomose with those from the alveolar bone and the PDL. Blood supply to the periodontal tissues is crucial: 50% of the PDL space, for example, is blood vessels by volume (Fig 19-7). Periodontal tissues receive their nutrient supply not only through the hydraulic force of arterial pressure but also through osmotic pressure. The difference between the two results in the transportation of substances from the blood vessels to and from the extravascular space.[3]

Periodontal Structures Subjected to Mechanical Forces

Perhaps alongside dental health, dental cosmetics has been in the minds of human beings since they first formed civilized societies. It was Aurelius Cornelius Celsus (25 BC to AD 50) of the Augustan age who wrote that finger pressure can move teeth into alignment.[8] Ever since, dental professionals have endeavored to find methods and implements for moving teeth into alignment that involve minimal effort, maximal comfort for the patient, and maximal efficiency.

The history of orthodontics is replete with the invention of novel appliances. It started with Edward H. Angle,

eruption or movement of teeth). The resorptive process is always associated with osteoclasts. During orthodontic tooth movement, the relationship between the lining membranes and the outer-layer tissues of the alveolar bone might be important. The tight connection of the gingiva to the periosteum could dictate the amount and rate of new bone deposition. Gingival tissue remodeling has been reported to be significant in tooth movement.[7] One could posit that the two determinants of alveolar bone remodeling during tooth movement are (1) gingival resistance to remodeling and (2) interruption of the vascular supply as a result of the squeezed PDL.

FIG 19-6a Schematic arrangement of alveolar bone trabeculae at rest.

FIG 19-6b Theoretical rearrangement of alveolar trabeculae upon application of orthodontic forces (*large and small arrows*). Unfortunately, fractal analyses of radiographic images do not support the notion that these trabeculae rearrange to withstand the external forces maximally. *Circular arrows* represent the tipping direction of the tooth.

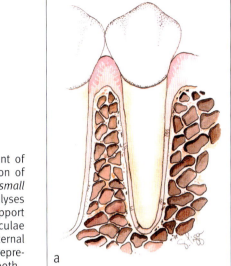
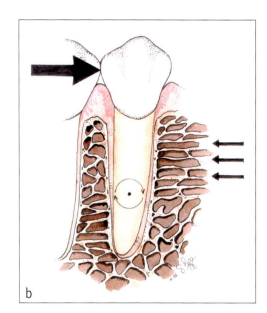

who was under contract with the SS White Company in Philadelphia to invent new appliances. Like today's novelists and musicians, who are under contract to regularly produce hit songs and best-selling novels, Angle was expected to deliver a regular stream of innovative orthodontic devices. Orthodontics, being the tradition-laden specialty that it is, has seen a multitude of appliances.

But it is clear that teeth are dumb.[9] They cannot distinguish the source of mechanical force. They move whenever and by whatever appliance applies pressure to them. This reaction is a complex process governed by the frequency, intensity, and duration of the applied force.

In earlier days, tooth movement in its most primitive form was explained as a pressure-tension hypothesis. That is, pressure causes resorption and tension deposition. Histologically, on one side of the root the PDL was compressed, and on the other side the fibers appeared to be stretched. Hence, the pressure-tension hypothesis was born. But evidence that compression causes resorption and that tension causes deposition does not exist. In the long bones, the opposite is true: pressure elicits deposition and tension elicits resorption. Even more fundamental than this debate, however, is the lack of evidence that mechanical forces applied to the teeth affect the bone at all. If this were the case, no implant would ever be successful. Indeed, one could apply significant force onto an implant, in various directions, and bone around the implant would not allow it to move. Ankylosed tooth is another example: it too will not move no matter how great a force is applied. Then what are the conditions that would cause the bone to remodel? Arguably, it has to be the soft tissues.[10]

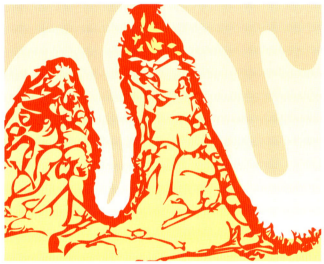

FIG 19-7 India ink perfusions have demonstrated that periodontal ligament is 50% blood vessels by volume.

Application of orthodontic forces results in subtle changes in the morphology and organization of periodontal tissues. It is known that in the initial stages of tooth movement, periodontal cells are compressed. It has been speculated that blood and extracellular fluid are forced from the periodontium into marrow spaces.[2,4,11] Escape of tissue fluids may lead to the creation of hypoxic regions or changes in tissue pH. Selective localized changes in the supply of blood to complex tissues such as alveolar bone and PDL cells are likely to produce profound changes in cellular metabolism. It has been suggested for 20 years that, in highly vascularized tissues, this type of change can result in increased dependence on glycolysis or inhi-

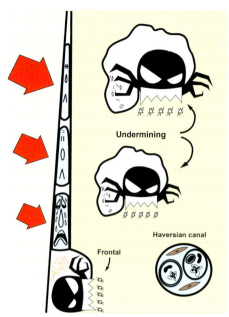

Fig 19-8 Squeezed periodontal ligament triggers undermining resorption in marrow spaces and frontal bone resorptive activities in socket walls.

TABLE 19-1 Tooth movement achieved in felines with and without administration of inflammatory mediators	
Treatment protocol	**Tooth movement (mm)**
NSAID	1.12
No medication	2.34

bition of both glycolytic and respiratory activity.[12] In the dentoalveolar complex, these effects may vary according to the cells' need for oxygen and their ability to adapt to an environment of low oxygen tension.

Periodontal Ligament and Alveolar Bone Under Stress

The PDL forms a cushion around the root of the tooth. It is, therefore, the initial site affected by any mechanical force applied to the tooth. If the magnitude of the applied force exceeds the dampening capacity of the PDL, which is approximately similar to the arterial blood pressure, then the ligament is squeezed. The dampening capacity is determined not only by the cells, vascular elements, or collagen fibers that populate the ligament space, but also by the glycosaminoglycans that hold the interstitial water. Accordingly, both the magnitude and the duration of the applied force are important. High magnitude–low duration perturbations force the PDL to behave like a solid material. Sustained high-magnitude forces, on the other hand, elicit significant injury within the PDL in the form of necrosis. The necrotic tissue forms in response to the occluded blood vessels and the hypoxic condition that result. This necrotic tissue is eventually removed as newly formed blood vessels grow into the area. When teeth are moved

with fixed appliances, formation of a necrotic zone within the PDL is inevitable. In contrast, animal studies have shown that it is possible to apply sustained or intermittent forces of very low magnitude to elicit a remodeling response without inflicting injury. Tiny beads bonded onto premolar teeth have been shown to effect tooth movement simply through the pressures exerted on them from the cheek or the tongue.[13]

The injured PDL takes time to heal. Indeed, until the necrotic tissue is removed, the tooth does not move. While the healing takes place, alveolar bone reacts to the presence of the necrotic tissue with resorption in the marrow spaces. In time, as vascular activity removes the necrotic region, walls of the socket next to the compressed PDL are also resorbed. The first resorptive process is commonly known as *undermining resorption*, and the latter as *frontal resorption* (Fig 19-8). Eventually, these two resorptive regions connect to form the large space into which the tooth can move. Clearly, remodeling of the PDL under forces generated by fixed appliances is nothing more than a wound-healing process. Accordingly, conditions present in any kind of wound healing anywhere in the body are likely to occur in the periodontal tissues as well. In its simplest form, wound healing is an inflammatory response. Thus, mediators of inflammation need to be examined as they may affect the remodeling process. These mediators are also involved in the pain associated with tooth movement.

Most of our knowledge of periodontal remodeling comes from animal studies. Many of the published animal studies are done over a 14-day period. Unfortunately, the periodontal tissue complex is such that within the 14-day period just about anything could be "proven." Once the investigation is extended to 21 or 28 days, the differences in cellular activity or the rate of tooth movement seen earlier tend to disappear. Experimental designs that span over 3 to 4 weeks are technically difficult because of high attrition rates. Animals are hard on delicate orthodontic appliances. Long-duration experiments better differentiate the artifactual and real effects of the experimental variable.

It was first shown in 1980 that the rate of tooth movement is regulated by inflammatory mediators.[1] Administration of the aspirinlike drug indomethacin to laboratory

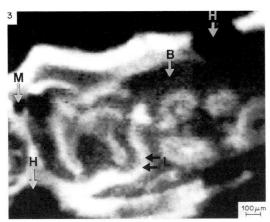

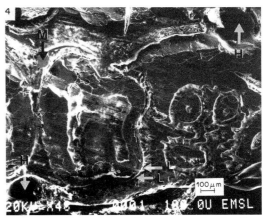

FIG 19-9a NAD/NADH distribution in the transversely sectioned rat maxillary dentoalveolar complex. (M) metallic marker; (B) bone; (H) hole; (L) periodontal ligament.

FIG 19-9b The corresponding anatomy for the fluorescence images above. (M) metallic marker; (H) hole; (L) periodontal ligament.

animals slowed the rate of tooth movement by 50%. Pooled measurements for tooth movements were 1.12 mm for felines that received indomethacin and 2.34 mm for those that received no medication (Table 19-1).

Indomethacin inhibits the synthesis of prostaglandins (PGs). This finding corroborated the suggestions pertinent to bone loss in inflammatory periodontal disease. Interestingly, patients with chronic arthritis who take aspirin daily exhibit less periodontal bone loss than age-matched controls, even if they are unable to maintain a regimen of good oral hygiene.[14] Direct injections of PGs into the dental papilla increase the rate of tooth movement, but because PGs are also pain mediators, patients experience significant pain. If teeth are not moving predictably, the experienced clinician will know to ask if the patient is on a daily aspirin regimen. All nonsteroidal anti-inflammatory drugs (NSAIDs) work the same way. In addition to these problems with NSAIDs, inhibitors of bone resorption such as biphosphonates (Fosamax) also slow the movement of teeth. Although these medications are known to inhibit tooth movement by affecting the remodeling process, they have not been explored for their potential to prevent relapse.

The orthodontist's inability to precisely control the force magnitude with fixed appliances necessitates a discussion of the metabolism of tissues subjected to extreme changes in blood supply. The energy status of the cells that make up a tissue or organ governs a wide range of metabolic, biosynthetic, and secretory functions. In a mixed structure, such as the dentoalveolar complex, measurement of energy metabolism by biochemical methods is a formidable challenge, as it is impossible to dissect and collect individual tissues without disturbing their metabolic status. It has

been possible, however, to measure the metabolic state of the dentoalveolar structures using a technique called *microfluorimetry*.[6] The basis of this technique is that the mitochondrial oxidative activity is reflected in the redox status of the respiratory chain: areas of high oxidative activity within a given tissue contain low levels of nicotinamide adenine dinucleotide (NADH), whereas the tissues that are glycolytic have high NADH levels. Scanning microfluorimetry records the fluorescence of this reduced pyridine nucleotide. The data gathered with this technique reveal that the vascular structures such as the alveolar bone, the pulp, and the PDL exhibit a high oxidative state and the gingival tissues a low oxidative state (Figs 19-9a and 19-9b).

These findings do not differ in a scan from the apical to the coronal. But it was clearly shown that the PDL is hypoxia-sensitive, similar to the heart, kidney, and brain. Alveolar bone, on the other hand, appears to be more resistant to a reduction in oxygen supply. Thus, it can be suggested that during the course of orthodontic tooth movement (and possibly periodontal disease), changes in oxygen supply to discrete regions of the periodontium may trigger alterations in cellular energy metabolism and consequent remodeling. This point was further strengthened by the studies of nitric oxide (NO) synthesis in the PDL during tooth movement.[15]

Up until a decade ago, NO was considered merely an environmental pollutant. It was not until NO was recognized as an endothelial relaxing factor that its importance in biologic systems began to emerge.[16] Since then, evidence has revealed an involvement of NO in a wide array of key physiologic processes, including regulation of vascular tone, platelet aggregation, host defense, inflammation, neurotransmission, learning and memory, penile erec-

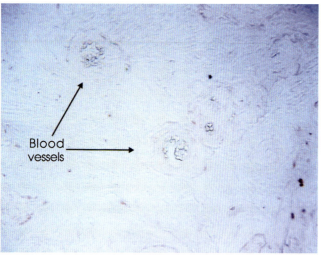

FIG 19-10a Immunochemically stained periodontal ligament blood vessels at rest (original magnification x100; immunohistochemical staining for anti-NOS). (Reprinted from Borgan et al[15] with permission.) .

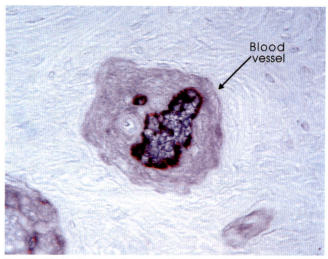

FIG 19-10b Periodontal ligament blood vessels under strain. Note the intense NOS staining (original magnification x100; immunohistochemical staining for anti-NOS). (Reprinted from Borgan et al[15] with permission.)

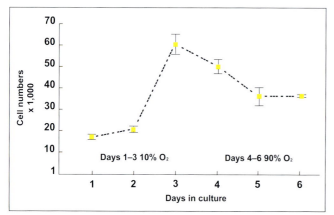

FIG 19-11a Osteoblast proliferative activity in crossover low and high O$_2$ saturations in culture media.

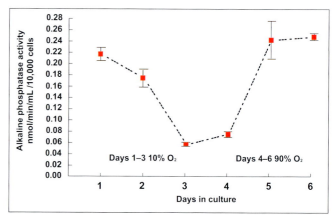

FIG 19-11b Alkaline phosphatase activity in the osteoblasts in low and high oxygen availability.

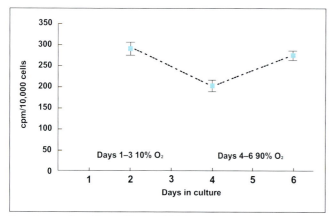

FIG 19-11c The effect of low and high oxygen in the culture medium on total collagen synthesis. (cpm) counts per minute.

tion, gastric emptying, hormone release, cell differentiation, cell migration, and apoptosis. Some of these processes have similarities to those that take place during tooth movement. The half-life of NO in a physiologic milieu is 1 to 10 seconds. It is difficult, therefore, to study NO production directly in an in vivo setting. An alternative is to study the localization of nitric oxide synthase (NOS) enzymes, which endogenously produce NO.

Studies to identify the sites of NOS activity in the periodontal tissues of stationary and orthodontically moved teeth have revealed significant differences. The periodontal tissues of stationary teeth exhibited hardly any immunohistochemical staining for NOS (Fig 19-10a). In contrast, NOS activity in the PDL blood vessel walls was strikingly increased in teeth that had undergone orthodontic tooth movement (Fig 19-10b). Even after the orthodon-

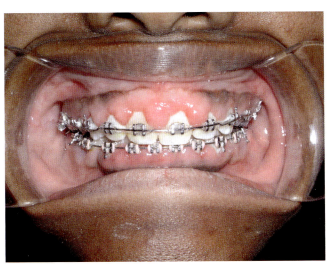

FIG 19-12 Overgrown gingival tissues inhibit tooth movement.

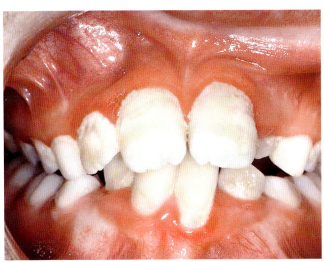

FIG 19-13 Inflamed and fragile gingival tissues will offer very little resistance to tooth movement and will remodel readily.

tic appliance activity had decayed (in 28 days), NOS activity could still be detected in the connective tissues surrounding the roots. The NOS-stained tissues included the interradicular bone. These data strongly support the argument for the importance of vascular activity within the periodontal complex during orthodontic tooth movement.

Alveolar bone may not be as sensitive to oxygen availability as the brain, kidney, heart, or the PDL, but can it still be affected to some extent? There is significant evidence that bone growth and repair exhibit such dependence. The presence of an oxygen gradient in epiphyseal growth cartilages[6,17–19] or in fracture hematoma[20] has been shown to play a role in bone growth and repair. These observations have been supported by the report that chondrocytes of distinct maturational level (proliferating and calcifying) exhibit differences in oxygen consumption and in energy-charge ratio.[2] Furthermore, the initial foci of calcification are in intimate contact with blood vessels,[20] and the calcifying cells exhibit higher NADH/NAD ratios than do their counterparts that are more distant to the vascular canal.[21] In tooth movement, the compressed PDL blood is squeezed out, causing the vessels to collapse. On the tension side, however, they dilate. Eventually, collapsed vasculature is reestablished and the bone resorbed. The dilation of blood vessels on the tension side appears to be conducive to new bone deposition.[22,23] These reports indicate that the functional state of calcified tissue cells is intimately associated with vascular canals, and form the rationale for the hypothesis that during tooth movement alveolar bone remodeling is triggered by changes in oxygen availability.

The regulation of osteoblast function by oxygen tension has been studied in vitro.[24] In low ambient oxygen tension, cellular proliferation increases, whereas alkaline phosphate (AP) activity, collagen synthesis, and media partial pressures for oxygen and carbon dioxide (pO_2 and pCO_2, respectively) decrease. In contrast, hyperoxic conditions suppress cellular proliferation and produce concomitant increases in AP activity, collagen synthesis, and pO_2 and pCO_2. When the conditions are reversed—that is, when hypoxic cells were put in a hyperoxic environment—their metabolic activities were abruptly reversed. It was shown, therefore, that in the absence of humoral, intercellular, or tissue architectural considerations, oxygen availability can serve as a trigger for bone remodeling (Figs 19-11a to 19-11c).

Gingival Response to Tooth Movement

To the clinician, alveolar bone appears to be subject to the dictates of PDL vascular activity. But if bone is not critical, why do teeth move very slowly? The potential resistance of gingival tissues was explored.[7] When the gingiva was eliminated, teeth moved faster. If bone limited the rate of tooth movement, elimination of gingival tissue would not slow tooth movement. This finding does not come as a surprise to the expert clinician. It is nearly impossible to close an extraction site into which a gingival invagination has developed. The expert orthodontist always asks the oral surgeon to preserve the buccal cortical plate by not squeezing it as conventionally taught in dental schools. The positionally intact cortical plate prevents invagination.[25] The clinician cannot move the teeth to close residual spaces if gingival tissue is present. As with an invagi-

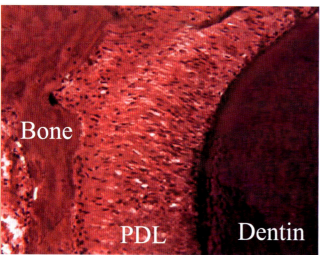

FIG 19-14a Normal periodontal ligament (PDL) architecture. (Reprinted from Nicozisis et al[29] with permission.)

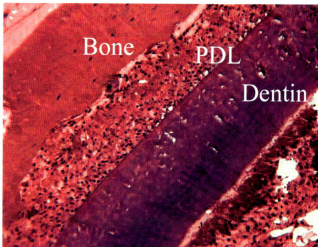

FIG 19-14b Relaxin-treated specimen. Note the loss of organization of periodontal ligament (PDL) fibers. (Reprinted from Nicozisis et al[29] with permission.)

nation, a true frenum diastema is nearly impossible to close unless it is eliminated by surgical dissection. Also known are the inhibitory effects of overgrown gingival tissues in patients taking medications such as Dilantin (phenytoin) or cyclosporine. Gingival overgrowth can also occur idiopathically; some patients react to the presence of fixed appliances with overgrowth (Fig 19-12). Both types of overgrown gingival tissues share one common characteristic: resistance to remodeling.

Resistance to remodeling may only be an issue with fixed appliance treatment. That is, matters such as diastema closure and gingival invagination do not generally occur when the teeth are moved with aligners. Aligners permit precise, controlled movement of teeth; the gingival tissue conforms to the gentle forces generated by the Invisalign System. The tissue contour looks excellent, exhibiting no signs of inflammation at the gingival margins. Since the gingival tissue does not contain any elastin (except in conjunction with the blood vessels), its remodeling rate appears to correlate well with the rate of tooth movement with an aligner.

In stark contrast, inflamed gingival tissue is fragile and loose, offering little resistance to tooth movement (Fig 19-13). In such cases, the orthodontist knows the teeth can be moved quickly and the treatment brought to an end. Of course, the combined effect of inflamed gingiva and mechanical force could cause a reduction in crestal bone height. Nonetheless, in this scenario the only determinant of tooth movement is the degree and depth of injury inflicted by the fixed orthodontic appliance. In practical terms, tooth movement rate in such conditions is deter-

mined by the rate of alveolar bone remodeling. Theoretically, the alveolar bone remodels more efficiently if the PDL is not injured and the formation of necrotic areas is avoided.

To summarize, efficient tooth movement can be achieved if the following conditions are met: (1) the periodontal ligament is not necrosed, (2) the gingival tissues offer no resistance, and (3) the vascular activity is abundant.

The first condition can be met if orthodontic force does not squeeze the PDL more than its thickness. Teeth move with the slightest of sustained forces; the Invisalign System is designed to apply such a force. With the Invisalign System, tooth movements are highly controlled and incremented as in the ClinCheck. In an effort to increase vascular activity noninvasively, ultrasound is applied to the gingival tissues of the orthodontically moving teeth. Ultrasound has been shown in rabbit models to accelerate the healing of fractured bones by increasing vascular activity. Mechanical forces (specifically, tooth brushing and orthodontic tooth movement) have been shown to affect gingival blood flow.[26,27] Unfortunately, clinically applied ultrasound has not been shown to yield faster tooth movement.[28] Although mechanical perturbation did not influence the rate of tooth movement, hope for a physiologic adjunct persists. Indeed, how the hormone relaxin might modulate the remodeling of the periodontal connective tissue has been investigated in an exploratory study.[29]

Relaxin is produced by pregnant females. It relaxes the pubic symphysis to widen the birth canal for parturition.

Clinically, relaxin has been tested as a possible treatment for scleroderma, but it also exerts effects on other parts of the body—especially the joints, ligaments, and regions containing collagen and fibroblastic activity. For example, temporomandibular joint (TMJ) problems disproportionately afflict female patients. A role of the female reproductive hormones has been proposed in the onset and progression of these diseases, but no direct evidence links female reproductive hormones to TMJ disorders. Relaxin alone, or in combination with beta-estradiol, has been implicated in the degradative remodeling of the fibrocartilaginous disc.[30]

It was shown in organ culture that the suturelike structures (cranial sutures or the PDL) possess receptors to relaxin. Interestingly, these receptors are also present in males. Addition of relaxin to the culture medium resulted in explicit changes in the collagen fibril arrangement of the PDL: from being dense and highly organized with a perpendicular direction between tooth and bone to randomly organized, loose, and devoid of any directionality between the tooth and bone (Figs 19-14a and 19-14b). Additionally, protease activity was increased in the relaxin-treated cultures.[29] In recent years, several studies have provided increasing evidence that relaxin can also act on several of its targets by increasing the expression and activity of NOS isoenzymes, thereby promoting the generation of NO.[31]

The future is exciting, as a switch from Platonic thought to Hippocratic is within our grasp.[32] If tissue behavior could be modulated (as opposed to building different and smaller brackets), orthodontics will truly become a biology-based field of study and practice. Invisalign provides the element of controlled force application, but it is the hope that the gingival tissue compliance will be enhanced by a routine topical application of relaxin.

Cementum

Cementum is a mostly acellular layer that covers the root. Only around the apex can a cellular cementum be seen. The PDL connects to the tooth via the cemental layer. Cementum is not directly involved in determining the rate of tooth movement; nevertheless, cementum is a source of concern to the clinician because it often resorbs during tooth movement, taking the dentinal portion of the root with it. Indeed, orthodontic treatment is known to be the most common cause of apical root resorption. Factors

responsible for external apical root resorption (EARR) are not well understood. Clearly, these factors can be patient- or treatment-related. It was recently reported that variations in the interleukin (IL)-1β allele 1 cytokine is strongly associated with an increased risk of EARR.[33] Patients homozygous for IL-1β allele 1 have a 95% chance of developing root resorption greater than 2 mm. Clearly, individual susceptibility cannot be predicted by the methods commonly available to the practitioner today.

Treatment-related mechanics, however, can be controlled. It is essential to understand these mechanic-related factors. Unfortunately, the published literature is not uniform and well controlled. Most of our knowledge of the mechanisms of root resorption comes from animal studies, which are of limited clinical utility because of limitations related to their design. Usually, animal studies examine short-term experimental conditions with the significant magnification of scanning electron microscopy and report seemingly significant conclusions. Undoubtedly, such conclusions are scientifically accurate, but actual clinical shortening of the root is rarely the experimental condition. Thus, we are perplexed to explain the treatment-related elements of EARR. These can be the frequency and magnitude of force application, duration of each force or overall treatment, or the direction in which these forces are applied. Whether orthodontically induced root resorption is a factor or not, the maxillary central incisor resorbs more than any other tooth during the course of orthodontic treatment.[33–35] The characteristics of the supporting bone may also be a factor. It has been postulated that tooth movement in dense bone requires greater or longer force application and consequently results in more root resorption.[27] In a rodent model, teeth were shown to move faster and develop EARR in animals that had a calcium-deficiency–induced decrease in bone density.[36] Similar experiments in dogs also showed slower tooth movement in denser dentoalveolar complexes.[37] Proximity of the root to the cortical bone has been suggested as a potential factor, but this could never be proven. A recent study could not demonstrate that the density and morphology of the dentoalveolar complex were significant factors in the etiology of EARR.[38]

A meta-analysis of treatment-related factors considered the distance the apex of the maxillary central had moved.[5] Total apical displacement might represent a better marker for overall treatment duration. Also, there is no way to move a maxillary apex any considerable distance using fixed appliances without forming extensive necrotic regions within the PDL. Perhaps this is why the maxillary centrals resorb the most. The meta-analysis revealed that root resorption was strongly correlated with total apical displacement and the time it took for the apex to traverse the distance. Thus, it can be concluded that in predisposed individuals distance is critical. Greater distances take longer and create extended regions of hypoxia within the PDL, which could ultimately affect the cemental layer.

But how important is root resorption for the health of the tooth? Severe root resorption is distressing to the orthodontist. When confronted with root resorption, at what point should the treatment be terminated? The perceived significance of root resorption may, in fact, be overstated. Only minor inconveniences have been suggested even in the most severe cases of resorption. There have never been any reports of iatrogenic tooth loss as a result of severe orthodontic root resorption. The worst outcome has been hypermobility.[39]

The amount of periodontal attachment loss following root resorption has been computed in a theoretical model.[40] Results indicated that 4 mm of root resorption translates to 20% total attachment loss and that 3 mm of apical root loss equals only 1 mm of crestal bone loss. After the initial 2-mm apical root loss, calculations revealed that every additional 2-mm root loss equaled only 1 mm of crestal bone loss.

The seriousness of dentists' perception was reported[41]; the reaction of general practitioners (GPs) and different specialty groups to morphed images of 10% to 50% root resorption was widely varied. GPs were the most concerned about root resorption. Although most practitioners believe that 50% root resorption is significant and detrimental to the longevity of the tooth, extraction followed by prosthetic replacement was never viewed as a viable option. There was no agreement among practitioners as to when orthodontic treatment should be terminated. Overall, GPs were the most conservative, suggesting termination after 35% root loss. History of trauma, genetic disposition, and root morphology are the most cited predisposing factors. Lengthy treatment times were of greater concern to GPs than to orthodontists. With the exception of orthodontists, dentists believe excessive force is detrimental to the root, but no one is able to define what excessive force is. Overall, dental school curricula overstate the causes of root resorption. This study suggested that many dental professionals base their opinions on myths and are largely inconsistent in their assessments.

Summary

Our current understanding of mechanical force effects on the periodontal tissues comes from experiments that simulate fixed appliance therapies. Thus, for more than a century, we have had studies of the effects of rather heavy forces. From the discussions in this chapter, it can be concluded that fixed appliances inflict serious injury to the supporting periodontal tissues. An increased blood supply—but not as a result of wound healing—is important for the maintenance of tissue integrity and the promotion of accelerated tooth movement. Activations of the orthodontic appliance in increments of the width of the PDL are best.

References

1. Chumbley AB, Tuncay OC. The effect of indomethacin (an aspirin-like drug) on the rate of orthodontic tooth movement. J Dent Res 1986;89:312–314.
2. Tuncay OC, Shapiro IM. A possible role for hypoxia in cellular energy metabolism of calcified tissues. In: Norton LBC (ed). Biology of Tooth Movement. Boca Raton: CRC Press, 1988:249–261.
3. Lindhe J, Karring T, Araújo M. Anatomy of the Periodontium. In: Lindhe J, Karing T, Lang NP (eds). Clinical Periodontology and Implant Dentistry. Oxford: Blackwell Munksgaard, 2003:3–49.
4. Bien S, Ayers H. Responses of rat maxillary incisors to loads. J Dent Res 1965;44:517–520.
5. Segal GR, Schiffman PH, Tuncay OC. Meta analysis of the treatment-related factors of external apical root resorption. Orthod Craniofac Res 2004;7:71–78.
6. Tuncay OC, Haselgrove JC, Frasca P, Piddington C, Shapiro IM. Scanning microfluorimetric measurements of redox status in the rat dento-alveolar tissues. Arch Oral Biol 1990;35:113–118.
7. Tuncay OC, Killiany DM. The effect of gingival fiberotomy on the rate of tooth movement. J Dent Res 1986;89:212–215.
8. Weinberger BW. Orthodontics: An historical review of its origin and evolution. St Louis: Mosby, 1926.
9. Tuncay OC. Teeth are dumb [editorial]. Cases Commentaries Orthod Technol [annual newsletter] 2003.
10. Tuncay OC, Villa G. Why not try to move on ankylosed tooth orthodontically?[in Italian]. Mondo Ortod 1990;15:475–480.
11. Sah R, Grodzinsky A. Biosynthetic response to mechanical and electrical forces. In: Norton LBC (ed). Biology of Tooth Movement. Boca Raton: CRC Press, 1988:335–347.
12. Hochachka P. Defense strategies against hypoxia and hypothermia. Science 1986;231(4735):234–241.
13. Weinstein S. Minimal forces in tooth movement. J Dent Res 1967;53:881–903.
14. Feldman R, House J, Chauncey H, Goldhaber P. Inhibition of alveolar bone loss in humans by aspirin. J Dent Res 1980;29(special issue A).
15. Brogan J, Kang K, Koyama E, Tuncay O. Localization of nitric oxide synthase in the periodontal tissues of orthodontically moved and stationary teeth. Prog Orthod 2002;3:12–16.
16. Moncada S, Palmer RM, Higgs EA. The discovery of nitric oxide as the endogenous nitrovasodilator. Hypertension 1988;12:365–372.

17. Kakuta S, Golub E, Haselgrove J, Chance B, Frasca P, Shapiro I. Redox studies of the epiphyseal growth cartilage: Pyridine nucleotide metabolism and the development of mineralizatlon. J Bone Miner Res 1986;1:433–440.

18. Brighton C, Heppenstall R. Oxygen tension in zones of the epiphyseal plate, the metaphysis and diaphysis. An in vitro and in vivo study in rats and rabbits. J Bone Joint Surg Am 1971;53:719–728.

19. Shapiro IM, Boyde A. Microdissection—Elemental analysis of the mineralizing growth cartilage of the normal and rachitic chick. Metab Bone Dis Relat Res 1984;5:317–326.

20. Brighton C. Principles of fracture healing. In: Murray JA (ed). Instructional Course Lectures. St Louis: Mosby, 1984:60–62.

21. Shapiro IM, Golub EE, Chance B, et al. Linkage between energy status of perivascular cells and mineralization of the chick growth cartilage. Dev Biol 1988;129:372–379.

22. Khouw F, Goldhaber P. Changes in vasculature of the periodontium associated with tooth movement in the rhesus monkey and dog. Arch Oral Biol 1970;15:1125–1132.

23. Rygh P, Bowling K, Hovlandsdal L, Williams S. Activation of the vascular system. Am J Orthod Dentofacial Orthop 1986;89:456–468.

24. Tuncay OC, Ho D, Barker MK. Oxygen tension regulates osteoblast function. Am J Orthod Dentofacial Orthop 1994;105:457–463.

25. Rivera Circuns AL, Tulloch JF. Gingival invagination in extraction sites of orthodontic patients: Their incidence, effects on periodontal health, and orthodontic treatment. J Dent Res 1983;83: 469–476.

26. Atkins S, Tuncay O. Gingival blood flow. Miss Dent Assoc J 1993;49(2):27–29.

27. Rygh P, Reitan K. Ultrastructural changes in the periodontal ligament incident to orthodontic tooth movement. Trans Eur Orthod Soc 1972;393–405.

28. Guajardo G. A clinical study of the effect of ultrasound application on the rate of tooth movement [thesis]. Philadelphia: Temple University, 1995.

29. Nicozisis JL, Nah-Cederquist HD, Tuncay OC. Relaxin affects the dentofacial sutural tissues. Clin Orthod Res 2000;3:192–201.

30. Kapıla S, Xie Y. Targeted induction of collagenase and stromelysin by relaxin in unprimed and beta-estradiol-primed diarthrodial joint fibrocartilaginous cells but not in synoviocytes. Lab Invest 1998; 78:925–938.

31. Nistri S, Bani D. Relaxin receptors and nitric oxide synthases: Search for the missing link. Reprod Biol Endocrinol 2003;1(1):5.

32. Tuncay OC. Taking stock: Hippocratic and Platonic thoughts on orthodontic tooth movement. Orthod Craniofac Res 2004;7:162–164.

33. Newman WG. Possible etiologic factors in external root resorption. J Dent Res 1975;67:522–539.

34. Kaley J, Phillips C. Factors related to root resorption in edgewise practice. Angle Orthod 1991;61:125–132.

35. Sameshima GT, Sinclair PM. Predicting and preventing root resorption: Part II. Treatment factors. Am J Orthod Dentofacial Orthop 2001;119:511–515.

36. Goldie RS, King GJ. Root resorption and tooth movement in orthodontically treated, calcium-deficient, and lactating rats. Am J Orthod 1984;85:424–430.

37. Midgett RJ, Shaye R, Fruge JF Jr. The effect of altered bone metabolism on orthodontic tooth movement. J Dent Res 1981;80:256–262.

38. Otis LL, Hong JS, Tuncay OC. Bone structure effect on root resorption. Orthod Craniofac Res 2004;7:165–177.

39. Killiany D. Root resorption caused by orthodontic treatment: An evidence-based review of literature. Semin Orthod 1999;5:128–133.

40. Kalkwarf KL, Krejci RF, Pao YC. Effect of apical root resorption on periodontal support. J Prosthet Dent 1986;56:317–319.

41. Lee KS, Straja SR, Tuncay OC. Perceived long-term prognosis of teeth with orthodontically resorbed roots. Orthod Craniofac Res 2003;6:177–191.

chapter 20

PROPERTIES OF ALIGNER MATERIAL EX30

by
Robert Tricca, PhD and Chunha Li, PhD

A survey of the literature indicates that a multitude of materials has been used throughout the history of dentistry. The role of biomaterials in orthodontics was reviewed comprehensively by Kusy.[1] Indeed, the use of biomaterials in dentistry dates back to the Etruscans (100 to 400 bc), who fashioned dental space retainers from gold bands and calves' teeth. Pierre Fauchard (1678–1761), a French surgeon considered by many to be the "Father of Orthodontics," worked with gold and silver while developing orthodontic appliances such as the bandolet, an appliance designed to expand the dental arch. In the late 1800s and early 1900s, a plethora of materials became available for the fabrication of orthodontic appliances (ie, loops, ligatures, spurs—including platinum, stainless steel, gum rubber, vulcanite, and various metal alloys such as brass). Occasionally, wood, ivory, zinc, and copper were also used.

While the introduction of novel orthodontic materials slowed dramatically from the early 1930s through 1960, it was during this period that stainless steel gained in popularity as the wire material of choice, ultimately leading to the abandonment of the noble metal alloys by the 1960s. Stainless steel exhibited superior mechanical properties and outstanding corrosion resistance and was available at reasonable cost. More advanced materials emerged in the 1960s and 1970s. Cobalt-chromium alloys were introduced in the 1960s. Research efforts at the Naval Ordnance Laboratory led to the discovery of nitinol, an alloy of nickel and titanium, in 1962. Later generations of nickel-titanium (NiTi) alloys would feature superelasticity and shape-memory effects. Toward the end of the 1970s, meta-stable titanium alloys based on beta-stabilized titanium were introduced. The 1980s saw further diversification in orthodontic materials with the development of ceramic appliances.

More recently, a novel computer-aided design/computer-assisted manufacture (CAD/CAM) approach has been developed that utilizes a clear thermoplastic to accomplish orthodontic tooth movement. For the Invisalign System, a series of clear, plastic tooth-positioning devices, or aligners, are fabricated with programmed movements. The use of thermoplastic materials to facilitate tooth movement represents a significant departure from the past (except as noted in chapters 1 and 3) and present for the practicing orthodontist. While thermoplastics have the potential to offer distinct advantages (eg, clarity, removability, ease of use, etc), their chemistry presents challenges when used in the oral cavity. The aim of this chapter is to investigate the properties of thermoplastics, as well as the experimental techniques used for determining their applicability for use in the oral cavity.

An Overview of Thermoplastic Polymers

Thermoplastics are based on linear or slightly branched polymers, which have strong intramolecular covalent bonds and weak intermolecular van der Waals bonds. At elevated temperature, it is easy to "melt" these bonds and cause the molecular chains to flow over each other. During this process, the thermoplastic material does not undergo any chemical changes. When cooled, however, the molecular chains solidify into new shapes. The process of softening with heating and hardening may be repeated. One example of this is the recycling and reprocessing of thermoplastic scrap.

In their solid form, thermoplastic materials fall within two classes of molecular arrangement: amorphous or semicrystalline. At a microscopic level, the long polymer chains of amorphous thermoplastics are randomly ordered in space. Amorphous thermoplastics do not exhibit exact melting points (T_m). Yet, when heated to a characteristic temperature called the *glass transition temperature* (T_g), they become less brittle and more flexible. In contrast, the long polymer chains of crystalline thermoplastics tend to be packed together in an orderly way, similar to the way atoms are arranged in a metallic crystal. Crystalline thermoplastics exhibit well-defined melting points and glass transition temperatures. Some thermoplastic materials may contain crystalline and amorphous regions. An example of this is high-density polyethylene (HDPE), a hydrocarbon thermoplastic polymer that exhibits a well-defined melting point as well as a glass transition temperature.

Polymer crystallinity is a factor that has a significant influence over polymer properties. For instance, the degree of crystallinity determines if a polymer is opaque or transparent. Similarly, the presence of a well-defined glass transition temperature affects the ease with which a polymer may be thermoformed. Both of these material properties should be considered when evaluating thermoplastics for the Invisalign System.

Properties of Aligner Materials

Mechanical properties

As an aligner is fitted on a patient's dentition, a force develops in areas with programmed tooth movement. The force results from the displacement of the aligner material; it is this force that causes tooth movement. Programmed tooth movements may vary from relatively simple movements (such as tipping of a tooth in one dimension) to more complex movements that involve bending motions coupled with rotational movements. The extent of aligner displacement and the resultant forces and moments produced on the teeth depend upon the movement programmed into the aligner, the material thickness, and the intrinsic material stiffness.

Aligners are subjected to both short-term and long-term loading forces. For example, an aligner is subjected to a short-term load when a patient fits an aligner on his or her teeth. Once fitted to teeth, aligners are subjected to intermittent long-term loads while being worn between meals and overnight. These longer-term loads are caused by programmed tooth movements and the biomechanical forces generated from the musculoskeletal system in the oral cavity.

A thermoplastic polymer is the structural material used in the fabrication of aligners. Understanding the mechanical properties of polymers is therefore critical if we are to assess the performance of a particular thermoplastic material as a means for accomplishing tooth movement. Mechanical properties may be investigated by studying how a material deforms when subjected to an applied force. By varying the nature of the deformation and the duration of the applied force, we can learn much about the mechanical properties of a thermoplastic.

Forces applied over a short duration

The generation of stress-strain curves is a useful approach in the evaluation of a material's mechanical properties. Numerically, stress in any direction at a given point in a material is simply the force or load that happens to act in that direction at that point divided by the area on which the force or load acts. If stress at a certain point is s, then

$$\text{Stress} = s = \text{load/area} = P/A$$

Similarly, strain is a measure of how far apart the atoms at any point in a solid are being pulled apart (ie, by what proportion the bonds between the atoms are stretched).

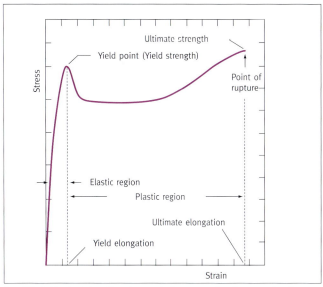

FIG 20-1 Typical tensile stress-strain curve for thermoplastic.

When generating a stress-strain curve, it is important to keep in mind the nature of the deformation. Three important modes of deformation for aligners are tension, bending, and torsion, and therefore these deformations should be evaluated when testing aligner materials. American Society for Testing Materials (ASTM) test D638-96, Standard Test Method for Tensile Properties of Plastics, is one of the most widely used and fundamental of all material tests and describes methodology for determining material properties while the material is subjected to tensile forces. A typical tensile stress-strain curve for a thermoplastic material under tension is shown in Fig 20-1. Data were generated using an Instron testing machine in which one end of the test specimen is clamped in a loading frame and the other subjected to a controlled load or force. From this simple curve we can learn much about the mechanical properties of this material.

Material modulus

The most important and fundamental characteristics of any material are the moduli. The modulus is defined as the ratio between the applied stress and the corresponding material deformation. For materials evaluated under tension, the constant of proportionality is the modulus of elasticity or Young's modulus, denoted E:

$$\sigma = E\pi$$

where σ is stress and π is strain. Young's modulus is a unique characteristic for a given material and is considered by scientists and engineers as a measure of material "stiffness." For aligners, a material should possess sufficient stiffness to generate forces and moments on teeth; however, if the material modulus is too high (very high stiffness), then the patient will experience difficulty with the insertion and removal of the aligners. Similarly, a material with a very low modulus may not provide sufficient force to move teeth.

Elastic region
In the low strain portion of the curve (small deformations), many materials obey Hooke's law to a reasonable approximation, so that stress is proportional to strain. In this region, the curve exhibits linear elastic behavior. If stress is removed, the material returns to its original shape and length.

Yield point
The yield point is the first point at which an increase in strain occurs without an increase in stress. In general, thermoplastics with high yield points are desirable for fabricating aligners.

Plastic region
The area between points 5 and 6 is known as the *plastic region* because the material will not return to its original shape and length after the stress is removed.

Ultimate tensile strength
Ultimate tensile strength is the maximum stress a material can withstand before rupturing.

Material toughness
Toughness is a measure of the energy a sample can absorb before it ruptures. It is found by calculating the total area under the stress-strain curve.

Elongation
Elongation is the strain that the material undergoes while being stressed. Elongation is typically measured at the material yield point or at the material break point.

Data generated from stress-strain curves on standardized samples are valuable for understanding the mechanical properties by which alternative aligner materials may be evaluated. These curves may also aid in the prediction of aligner performance for short-term loads. As an example, consider the short-term forces applied to aligners as they are removed from a patient's dentition. The duration

of these forces is short, often on the order of seconds. During this period, however, the aligner may undergo severe deformations. For short-term loads, it is critical that an aligner respond in an elastic manner if it is to return to its original shape. An understanding of elastic properties may be derived from a stress-strain curve for a particular material. In the above situation, we seek a thermoplastic material that exhibits substantial linear elastic behavior along with a high yield point.

Forces applied over a long duration
As mentioned above, for small strains or deformations, thermoplastics follow Hooke's law for elastic materials; $\sigma = E\pi$; stress σ is proportional to strain π. In reality, it is well-known that thermoplastic materials deviate from Hooke's law in various ways because they exhibit viscous (liquidlike), as well as elastic (solidlike), characteristics. Because of this behavior, scientists and engineers refer to thermoplastics as viscoelastic materials. Importantly, for these materials the relationship between stress and strain depends on time. Therefore, thermoplastic materials used in aligner fabrication exhibit viscoelastic behavior that can have a profound influence on the performance of aligners in vivo.

A fundamental time-dependent material property of thermoplastics is stress relaxation, which is defined as the gradual decrease in stress when a material is held at constant strain. Strain develops in aligners in regions with programmed tooth movement. The aligner's elastic nature allows it to deform and stretch to accommodate the programmed movement. Because of the viscoelastic nature of the aligner thermoplastic, the force generated by the programmed movement decreases as a function of time.

Stress relaxation processes are usually accelerated by the presence of moisture. The severity of this effect depends on the nature of the plastic, the amount of water absorbed, the temperature, and the severity of the loading to which the part is subjected.

Nonmechanical properties
While it is clear that material mechanical properties affect aligner performance, there are also many material nonmechanical properties that are of critical importance.

Thermal properties
Align Technology uses a thermoforming process that draws an extruded thermoplastic sheet over a stereolithographic mold to form an aligner. Since each aligner is unique, the thermoforming process is more suitable than

an injection molding process where the same part is made in a large quantity. The thermoforming process, however, is highly dependent on processing temperatures, and consequently it is critical to understand the material's thermal properties. The most obvious thermal properties of a thermoplastic are its melting or softening temperatures, and temperature variations with regard to mechanical properties, such as tensile modulus, yield strength, and hardness. The glass transition temperature may be defined as the temperature below which the polymer is "glassy" and above which it is "rubbery." "Glassy" implies brittleness, and "rubbery" suggests flexibility. It was previously mentioned that semicrystalline polymers do exhibit a melt point, whereas amorphous polymers do not. Glass transition and melt temperatures may be determined using a differential scanning calorimeter (DSC). These tests indicate when softening occurs and whether it occurs gradually or suddenly. Understanding these two material properties allows for a better understanding of the thermoforming process with respect to the uniformity of heating, the effect of temperature on a material's drawing properties and thickness profile, and the window of temperature variability that can be tolerated.

Chemical resistance

When fitted on the dentition, aligners are constantly bathed in dental fluids such as saliva and crevicular fluid at a constant body temperature (37°C). Besides water, there are many constituents of saliva. Common inorganic constituents include bicarbonate, calcium, phosphorous, fluoride, magnesium, and trace metal ions. The major organic salivary components are proteins and small peptides. The presence of moisture, salivary components, increased temperature, and the constant mechanical stresses that are simultaneously acting on an aligner can adversely affect its performance. Water is especially notorious, as it may react chemically with the polymer backbone chain through a process termed *hydrolysis* and irreversibly degrade many polymers. Polymers particularly susceptible to water degradation are polyesters, polyamides, and polycarbonates.

Optical properties

One of the features that distinguishes aligners from traditional orthodontic appliances is that they are invisible when worn. This requires that aligner thermoplastic materials have suitable optical properties. The morphology of a thermoplastic polymer has a major effect on such optical properties as refraction, absorption, reflection, and scattering of light. Highly crystalline polymers are typically opaque because they tend to scatter visible light and decrease transmission. In general, amorphous polymers exhibit good light transmittance and are either transparent or translucent. Materials evaluated for use as aligners should transmit at least 80% visible light. Examples of amorphous polymers with good optical properties are polyurethane, polycarbonate, polysulfone, and polyester.

Biocompatibility

Aligners are medical devices and consequently require biocompatibility assessment to assure safety of the device. Safety data can be obtained by testing according to certain prescribed or recommended guidelines, including guidance documents developed by the International Organization for Standardization (ISO) and the US Food and Drug Administration (FDA). These guidelines include ISO 10993, "Biological Evaluation of Medical Devices," and the guidance document released by the FDA in 1995, "Use of International Standard ISO 109333, Biological Evaluation of Medical Devices." These guidelines provide a framework to aid manufacturers in the assessment of device biocompatibility. The number and type of specific safety tests required to assess product safety and compliance are dependent on the individual characteristics of the device, its component materials, and its intended clinical use. Ultimately, it is the responsibility of the manufacturer to select and justify the specific tests most appropriate for the establishment of product safety and compliance with regulatory requirements.

It may not be necessary to conduct biocompatibility tests on a device if it is made of materials that have been well characterized chemically and physically in the published literature and that have a long history of safe use. Typically, for new devices, biocompatibility testing and evaluation are performed to determine the potential toxicity from contact of the device with the body. The device materials should not, either directly or through the release of their material constituents, produce adverse local or systemic effects, be carcinogenic, or produce adverse reproductive and developmental effects.

Experimental Methods for Evaluating Aligner Materials

There are many possible approaches for systematically screening aligner materials. One approach is shown in Fig

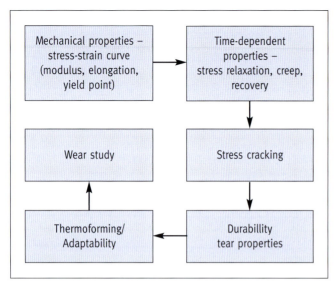

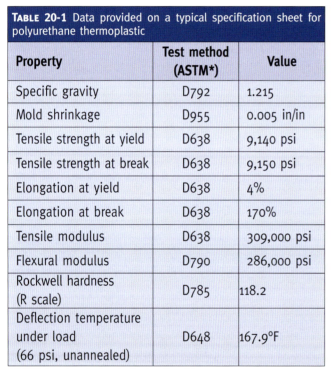

FIG 20-2 Material screening method.

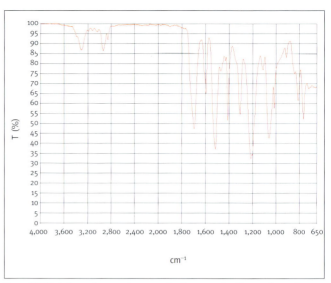

FIG 20-3 Infrared spectrum of thermoplastic polyurethane. T = Transform.

TABLE 20-1 Data provided on a typical specification sheet for polyurethane thermoplastic

Property	Test method (ASTM*)	Value
Specific gravity	D792	1.215
Mold shrinkage	D955	0.005 in/in
Tensile strength at yield	D638	9,140 psi
Tensile strength at break	D638	9,150 psi
Elongation at yield	D638	4%
Elongation at break	D638	170%
Tensile modulus	D638	309,000 psi
Flexural modulus	D790	286,000 psi
Rockwell hardness (R scale)	D785	118.2
Deflection temperature under load (66 psi, unannealed)	D648	167.9°F

*(ASTM) American Society for Testing Materials

TABLE 20-2 Typical mechanical properties of amorphous polyamide and polyester

Property	Amorphous polyamide	Polyester
Stress at yield (psi)	9,400	7,800
Strain at yield (%)	5.5	4.6
Tensile strength (psi)	21,000	8,500
Elongation at break (%)	55	85
Tensile modulus (psi)	435,000	260,000

20-2. Whenever possible, efforts are undertaken to evaluate samples under conditions encountered in vivo. This is accomplished by making modifications to laboratory equipment that allow for the use of artificial saliva and temperature conditions approximating 37°C.

If one is to seek information on a particular material, a good place to start is with the supplier data sheet. These data sheets usually contain a wealth of technical informa-tion that has been generated using test procedures developed by reputable organizations such as the American Society for Testing and Materials (ASTM). An example of the information provided on a typical supplier data sheet for a thermoplastic polyurethane is shown in Table 20-1.

Polymer chemical structure

Polymer molecular structure may be investigated using spectroscopic techniques. Probably the most important spectroscopic technique used is infrared (IR) spectroscopy, which itself includes Fourier transform infrared (FTIR) detection. The principles behind IR spectroscopy are straightforward: IR radiation is used to excite the polymer molecules, typically between 600 and 4,000 cm. The amount of IR energy absorbed depends on the type of functional groups present as well as the quantity. Absorbed energy is reflected on an IR scan as a characteristic IR band. An infrared spectrum for a thermoplastic polyurethane is shown in Fig 20-3.

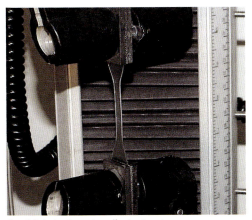

FIG 20-4 Instron tensile test setup.

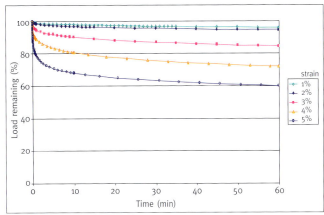

FIG 20-5 Stress relaxation properties of thermoplastic polyurethane (Ex30) at different strains (in ambient temperature and humidity).

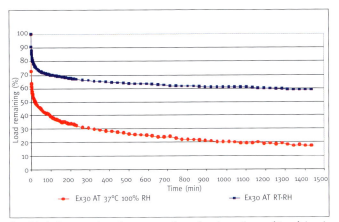

FIG 20-6 Stress relaxation properties of polyurethane (Ex30) in air and in 100% relative humidity (RH) following 5% strain. (RT) Relative temperature.

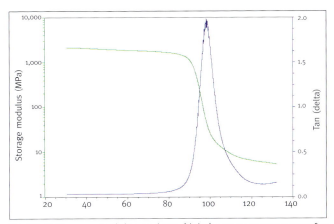

FIG 20-7 Storage modulus and tan (delta) versus temperature for thermoplastic polyurethane (Ex30).

Material mechanical properties

As discussed earlier, material short-term mechanical properties may be evaluated through the generation of stress-strain curves, which has been done for two thermoplastic materials: a polyamide and a polyester. Data were generated using an Instron testing machine in which one end of the test specimen is clamped in a loading frame and the other subjected to a controlled load or force (Fig 20-4). From this test, the various mechanical characteristics can be determined (Table 20-2).

Longer-term time-dependent material properties may be evaluated by stress relaxation and creep recovery. The stress relaxation properties for a polyurethane material are shown in Fig 20-5. The data in Fig 20-6 compare the stress relaxation properties for polyurethane in air and in 100% relative humidity. This example illustrates the adverse effect moisture can have on long-term thermoplastic properties.

Material thermal properties

Thermal analysis involves measuring a mechanical or physical property as a function of temperature or time. Common methods used in thermal analysis are differential scanning calorimetry (DSC), thermogravimetric analysis (TGA), and dynamic mechanical analysis (DMA).

DMA allows an investigator to measure both the elastic (G') and viscous (G") components of a viscoelastic polymer while it is being subjected to a sinusoidal stress. It is a standard thermal analysis tool. The example below shows a DMA evaluation undertaken to characterize material morphology and thermal properties of a polyurethane. Figure 20-7 shows the storage modulus and tan (delta) at different temperatures for a polyurethane material. The storage modulus decreases slightly with increasing temperature from 30°C to 80°C and dramatically decreases from 80°C to 105°C. The temperature at the midpoint of the curve corresponds to the glass transition temperature.

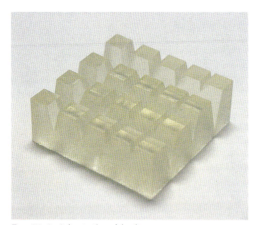

FIG 20-8 Adaptation block.

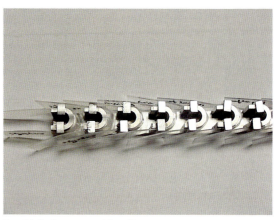

FIG 20-9 Stress cracking fixture.

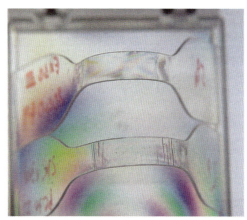

FIG 20-10 Results of stress cracking test on Ex30.

Material adaptation

A thermoforming process is used for aligner fabrication. A thermoplastic sheet is first heated and then a vacuum/pressure thermoforming process is used to form the aligner. The hot sheet is drawn down over a stereolithographic (SLA) model of the patient's dental anatomy. Pressure and vacuum forces cause the material to adapt or conform to the SLA model. A special SLA was designed to evaluate how a material conforms to a particular geometry during the manufacturing thermoforming process. In this situation, heated sheets of material are drawn over SLA molds formed with V-grooves of varying depth (ie, 4 to 16 mm) (Fig 20-8). The depth to which the material penetrates is an indication of its ability to adapt during the thermoforming process. At a defined temperature, the level of adaptation for polyurethane is known to be superior to that of polycarbonate material.

Material stress cracking

Aligner surfaces are subjected to varying deformations (ie, strains) while worn in the oral cavity. Additionally, saliva and salivary components can affect aligner material performance. The ability of an aligner material to resist stress cracking while under strain is of paramount importance. In the environmental stress cracking test, material samples are subjected to strains (2%, 5%) on a metal fixture (Fig 20-9) immersed in artificial saliva at 37°C for up to 48 hours. At the end of this time, samples are removed and dried for visual inspection (Fig 20-10). The tensile properties for each sample are evaluated using an Instron machine. Results show that neither polycarbonate nor polyurethane exhibits stress cracking after immersion for 48 hours in artificial saliva. Although tensile properties (eg, yield at strain, tensile strength, modulus, etc) for these materials decreased, both materials exhibited similar changes after immersion in artificial saliva for 48 hours.

Aligner durability

This test was designed to simulate aligner wear in vivo. In this test, aligners are subjected to cycling (ie, repeated insertion and removal steps) on a typodont attached to a fatigue tester. Two types of typodonts are utilized for this study: a lower-stage typodont based on a moderate occlusion with few attachments and an upper-stage typodont based on severe occlusion and a significant number of attachments. Typodonts with aligners are soaked in artificial saliva at 37°C for up to 2 weeks. Aligners are removed on a daily basis and subjected to 12 cycles on the fatigue tester. Aligners are checked for defects (eg, cracks, tears) at the end of each cycle. Aligners fabricated from three lots of each material performed in a similar manner over a 2-week test period.

In vivo aligner wear study

A clinical evaluation was conducted to evaluate and compare the materials while being worn in vivo. For this study, tooth movements were not programmed into aligners. A total of 14 volunteers were recruited from the company. Study participants received an oral examination and were asked to complete an informed consent form before being admitted into the study. Each participant was randomly assigned one Ex30 aligner and one Ex30-X4995 aligner (split-mouth design). They were also requested to maintain a daily diary form to keep track of the number of their aligner wear schedule. At the end of the 3-week study, participants were asked to turn in their aligners and to complete a material evaluation form covering the following categories: mouth dryness, aligner fit, aligner color, ease of aligner removal, and feeling in the mouth.

Results from this study showed no significant differences in material behavior for the following categories: mouth dryness, aligner fit, ease of aligner removal, and

feeling in the mouth. For aligner color, however, maxillary aligners based on Ex30-X4995 exhibited less discoloration (yellowing) compared to aligners made from Ex30.

Conclusion

Data presented in this chapter should help the clinician to understand the performance range and characteristics of aligners. Moreover, it should lead the operator to be more conservative while working with the ClinCheck images. But most significantly, it should make clear that longer wear times might be necessary for certain types of tooth movements.

References

1. Kusy RP. Orthodontic biomaterials: From the past to the present. Angle Orthod 2002;12:501–512.

chapter 21

Ex40 Material and Aligner Thickness

by
Trang Duong, DDS; Eric Kuo, DDS; and Mitra Derakhshan, DDS

Finishing in orthodontics requires precisely controlled force application to achieve the final alignment. With conventional fixed appliances, stiff rectangular stainless steel or titanium molybdenum alloy (TMA) wires are used to achieve these precise movements. Detailing bends are placed in the wires to achieve the final movements required for finishing. The Invisalign System shares this goal of precise control of tooth movements with fixed appliance techniques. Theoretically, the use of a thicker material increases the control of tooth movement because of the increased stiffness. Based on data from a University of Washington study on material stiffness and the case refinement, the idea of using a thicker polyurethane material (Ex40) during Invisalign treatment to reduce the case-refinement rate was explored.

Currently, Invisalign appliances are fabricated from a polyurethane material of 0.030-mil thickness (Ex30). Although generally effective through early stages of tooth movement, Ex30 appliances have led to some difficulties in achieving the desired final detailing at the end of treatment. Currently, additional case-refinement aligners—or other auxiliaries such as detail pliers, buttons/elastics, or even sectional wires—are used to finish cases. Align Technology's retention material is the same polyurethane material used to fabricate the aligners; the difference is that it has a thickness of 0.040 mil (Ex40). This chapter explores the idea of using a thicker polyurethane material (Ex40) during Invisalign treatment to reduce the case-refinement rate.

Effects of Thickness on the Elastic Properties of Polyurethane Materials

Reports on the material properties of various archwires used in orthodontics are copiously available in the literature. Regardless of the material, the elastic properties—strength, stiffness, and range—are greatly affected by changes in the geometry of the wire. Both the cross section (whether the wire is round, rectangular, or square) and length of the wire determine its properties. Studies on the material properties of archwires are conventionally done using beams. The method of support for the beam determines how the elastic properties will change. For example, in a cantilever beam supported by one end, doubling the diameter of the wire increases its strength eight

times. Regardless of how the beam is supported, however, changes in the diameter of a beam greatly affect its properties. Changes in the length of an archwire also affect its properties. For example, if the length of a cantilever beam is doubled, its strength is halved but its springiness increases eight times and its range four times. These properties usually cannot be changed with aligners because the shape and length of tooth-cupping polyurethane material are determined by arch and tooth anatomy. The thickness or diameter, however, can be changed with aligners. For example, increasing the thickness of aligners from 0.030 to 0.040 mil increases the stiffness by approximately one third.

A study was undertaken to determine if using a thicker polyurethane material (Ex40) at the end of Invisalign treatment reduced the need for additional case-refinement aligners. It was found that thicker materials worn at the end of treatment slightly improved the alignment but did not eliminate the need for additional aligners. Another study was launched to further evaluate the effectiveness of Ex40 in Invisalign treatment.

The primary objectives of this latter, randomized trial were to explore (1) the effectiveness of Ex40 aligners in the Invisalign treatment process and (2) the effect of Ex40 on the prevalence of case refinement/midcourse correction. A secondary goal of the study was to obtain descriptive data related to potential risk factors associated with wearing an Ex40 aligner. The parameters evaluated included amount of root resorption, oral hygiene, plaque, tooth sensitivity, and temporomandibular joint changes.

The patients were recruited from the Ferrara, Italy, area. There were no exclusions based on gender or race. All patients were in the adult dentition with growth completed. Any malocclusion was accepted in the study except cases requiring premolar extractions, major extrusions, rotations of round teeth, and molar uprighting. In addition, patients with periodontal disease or active caries who did not have a dentist or periodontist of record were excluded and referred for treatment. Patients with preexisting and active symptoms of temporomandibular disorders were also excluded from the study. The patients had to be willing to undergo at least one midcourse correction (but no more than two) throughout the treatment process.

Patients were randomly assigned to one of two groups on an alternating basis (ie, the first person enrolled was assigned to group 1, the second person enrolled was assigned to group 2, etc.) until 15 patients were in each group. Patients assigned to group 1 were treated with the following aligners: every fifth aligner was made out of Ex40, and the patient wore this aligner for 2 weeks and then progressed to the next aligner. The last aligner was made from Ex40. Patients assigned to group 2 were treated with the following aligners: the entire group used aligners made from Ex30 with the last five aligners in Ex40. The speed of tooth movement was the same for both groups with a maximum ranging from 0.15 to 0.20 mm of tooth movement per stage (current manufacturing guidelines). The ClinChecks for both groups were set to ideal alignment at the end of treatment with no programmed over-correction.

For group 1, one patient dropped out, two finished treatment and did not have refinement, eight went into refinement, one is under review for refinement, and three are still in the initial treatment series of aligners. For group 2, one patient dropped out, one finished treatment and did not have refinement, six went into refinement, one patient had a midcourse correction, and six are still in the initial treatment series of aligners.

Preliminary conclusions of the study indicate that there is no difference in the case-refinement rate of the two groups. Neither the use of a thicker material (Ex40) for every fifth aligner nor for the last five aligners seems to reduce the case-refinement rate. Clearly, more data are needed if the use of a thicker material might reduce the case-refinement rate.

Finishing with Invisalign

When Andrews introduced the straight-wire appliance in the 1970s, he changed the way orthodontics was practiced. His ideas greatly increased the efficiency and efficacy of fixed appliances.[1] Instead of adding first-, second-, and third-order bends for each tooth, this information was programmed into the bracket. Interestingly, when the appliance was introduced, there was a misconception that wire bending would become obsolete because the bracket would do all the work. Although the prescription bracket greatly reduced the amount of archwire bending required to treat a case, it did not eliminate the need. The clinician still placed subtle bends along the archwire or used additional finishing techniques (eg, rubber bands and positioners). Finishing still required bracket repositioning and detailing bends to achieve the desired results. Factors responsible for this included inaccurate bracket placement, variations in tooth anatomy, tissue rebound,

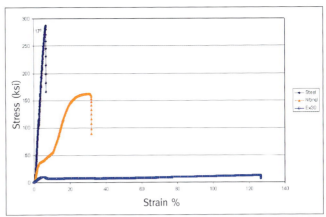

FIG 21-1 Stress-strain curve for 0.017 × 0.017–inch stainless steel and nitinol, and Ex30. Ex30 is more ductile than the metals.

and play between the bracket slot and archwire.[2,3] Rarely are cases finished with only brackets and a straight archwire.

As with fixed appliances, several factors play an important role in finishing with Invisalign and can affect the anticipated results. Because of the overlay design of the appliance, the anatomy of the tooth plays an important role and can cause minor alignment discrepancies. Variations in tooth shape (eg, irregular facial surfaces, unusual crown shapes, and unfavorable crown shapes) require additional aligners to achieve the desired alignment. Tooth movement is dependent on the response of the periodontal tissues to an applied force. Variation in the biologic response to tooth movement and the viscoelastic properties of the periodontal tissues affect the treatment outcome. This tissue behavior is similar to "slot play" in fixed appliances, in that there exists a lag period. Additionally, a secondary lag is introduced based on the material properties of the aligners.

In an effort to improve the finishing regimen and also increase the predictability of achieving the desired treatment result, a study was conducted to determine if using a thicker polyurethane material at the end of treatment reduced the need for additional case-refinement aligners. Figure 21-1 shows the stress-strain graph comparing 0.017 × 0.017–inch stainless steel versus 0.017 × 0.017–inch nitinol and 0.030-mil polyurethane material (Ex30). The graph illustrates the difference in stress-strain characteristics of orthodontic wires compared to aligners. It also indicates that aligners produce a lower level of stress for a specified strain compared to wires, and that the amount of stress delivered is fairly consistent relative to the strain in contrast to wires.

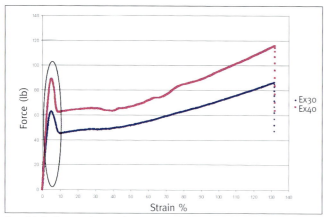

FIG 21-2 Comparison of stress-strain curves for Ex30 and Ex40 (maximum 5% yield strain). Area of stress-strain curve that pertains to aligners is circled.

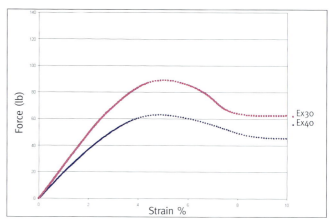

FIG 21-3 Magnification of area on the stress-strain curve that is used with aligners (circled in Fig 21-2). Increasing the thickness of the polyurethane material from 0.030 to 0.040 mil increases the stiffness by one third, which translates to a force increase of one third.

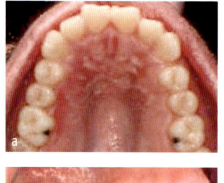

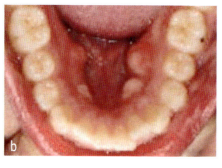

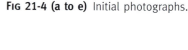

FIG 21-4 (a to e) Initial photographs.

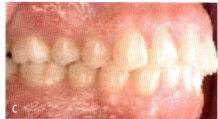

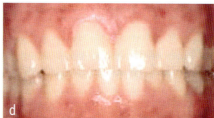

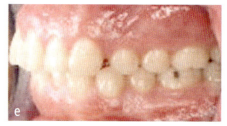

In the study, patients wore their initial series of aligners and progressed to the next set every 2 weeks. After the initial set, the patients wore a duplicate last aligner in a thicker material (Ex40) for 2 weeks. Figures 21-2 and 21-3 show the stress-strain graphs comparing 0.030 mil (Ex30) and 0.040 mil (Ex40). By increasing the thickness from 0.030 mil to 0.040 mil, the stiffness increased by approximately one third. Following this aligner, the clinician evaluated the results and determined whether additional finishing aligners were required.

Alignate impressions were made at the end of the initial set of aligners (pre-Ex40) and then after the patient wore aligners made from the thicker polyurethane material (post-Ex40). If additional case-refinement aligners were required, alginate impressions were also made at this time (case-

refinement aligners). The impressions were then poured and the models scanned. The individual time points were superimposed over the projected ClinCheck goal to determine the correlation between the goal and the actual achieved movements. Superimpositions were done using a best-fit algorithm. The maxillary and mandibular canines and incisors were evaluated via measurements of the in-and-out (labiolingual) and rotational movements.

The following case from this study did not require additional case-refinement aligners. The initial photos of this case show Class I maxillary spacing and mandibular crowding (Figs 21-4a to 21-4e). Figures 21-5a and 21-5b show the ClinCheck final position goal for the case. The treatment involved closing the maxillary spaces and alleviating the mandibular crowding through anterior interproximal reduc-

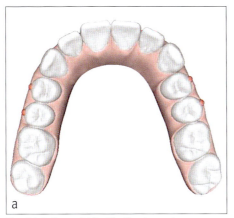

FIG 21-5 (a and b) ClinCheck goal.

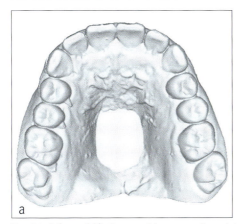
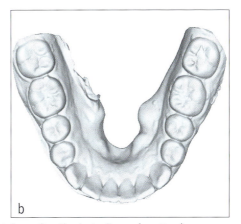

FIG 21-6 (a and b) Scanned images of models taken after the last aligner (pre-Ex40) was worn.

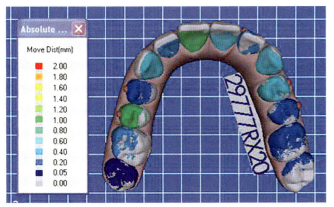
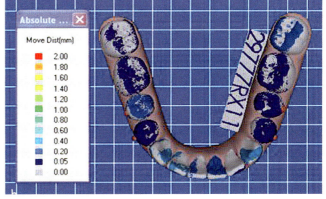

FIG 21-7 (a and b) Superimposition of pre-Ex40 models and ClinCheck goals. The legend on the left represents a color schematic of the difference (in millimeters) of the position of the teeth.

tion during treatment. The total number of aligners was 20 for the maxillary arch and 11 for the mandibular arch. After the last set of aligners (pre-Ex40) were used, alginate impressions were made and poured, then scanned into the computer (Figs 21-6a and 21-6b). The pre-Ex40 models were superimposed over the projected ClinCheck goal (Figs 21-7a and 21-7b), These figures show that, compared to the projected goal, a patient who wears only the initial series of aligners achieves a fairly good match with the actual treat-

ment result. However, some teeth were slightly short of the projected goal. Specifically, the position of the maxillary incisors was short approximately 1 mm with the projected goal. Comparison of the pre-Ex40 and the projected ClinCheck goal superimposition of the combined maxillary and mandibular anterior teeth reveals that the in-and-out movements showed a strong correlation of .94 (Fig 21-8a), while the rotation movements showed a fairly good correlation of .85 (Fig 21-8b).

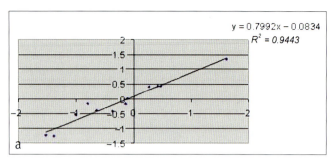

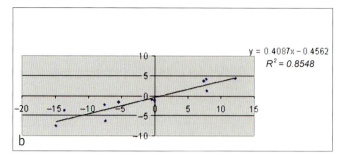

FIG 21-8 (a and b) Pre-Ex40 versus ClinCheck goal superimposition of anterior teeth for in-and-out movements (*a*) and rotation (*b*) (n = 1).

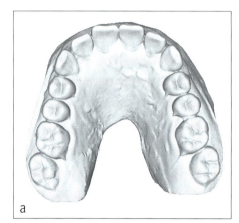

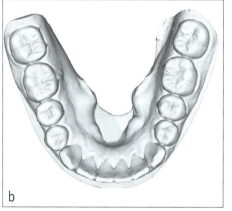

FIG 21-9 (a and b) Scanned images of models taken after aligner (post-Ex40) was worn for 2 weeks.

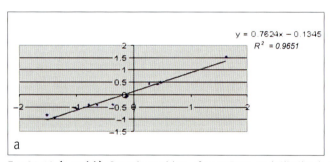

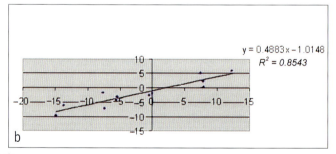

FIG 21-10 (a and b) Superimposition of post-Ex40 and ClinCheck goals.

Figures 21-9a and 21-9b show the scanned models after the patient wore Ex40 aligners for 2 weeks. When these models were superimposed over the ClinCheck goal, improved alignment compared to the pre-Ex40 models was evident (Figs 21-10a and 21-10b). The plot graph shows that the correlation improved slightly from .94 to .97 for the in-and-out movements and did not change in the rotational movements (Fig 21-11). This case shows that wearing Ex40 aligners at the end of treatment slightly improves the anterior alignment. This particular case did not require additional case-refinement aligners after wearing the Ex40 aligners, but some cases did.

Data for a pool of 14 patients were combined, and the resulting plot graphs showed a similar trend of improvement in alignment for in-and-out movements and rotation after wearing Ex40 aligners (Figs 21-12 to 21-14). However, even after wearing the Ex40 aligners, 5 of the 14 patients required additional case-refinement aligners. This data suggest that wearing Ex40 aligners at the end of treatment can slightly improve the anterior alignment. This also suggests that patients who use Ex40 aligners as retainers at the end of treatment can expect to achieve slight improvement in their alignment during the retention phase. Overall, the study showed that using a thicker aligner material at the end of treatment slightly improved alignment but did not completely eliminate the need for additional aligners.

The results from this study showed that, similar to fixed appliances, finishing with Invisalign sometimes requires

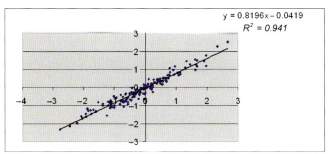

$y = 0.8196x - 0.0419$
$R^2 = 0.941$

FIG 21-11 Post-Ex40 versus ClinCheck goal superimposition of anterior teeth for in-and-out movements (n = 1).

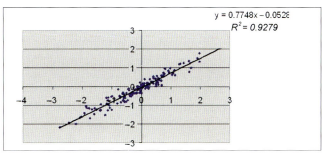

$y = 0.7748x - 0.0528$
$R^2 = 0.9279$

FIG 21-12 Pre-Ex40 versus ClinCheck goal superimposition of anterior teeth for in-and-out movements of patients (n = 14).

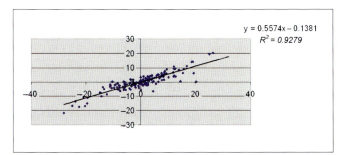

$y = 0.5574x - 0.1381$
$R^2 = 0.9279$

FIG 21-13 Pre-Ex40 versus ClinCheck goal superimposition of anterior teeth for rotational movements of patients (n = 14).

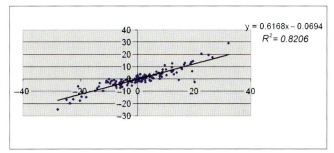

$y = 0.6168x - 0.0694$
$R^2 = 0.8206$

FIG 21-14 Post-Ex40 versus ClinCheck goal superimposition of anterior teeth for rotational movements of patients (n = 14).

additional aligners and use of auxiliaries, such as detailing pliers, to achieve the desired treatment results. The best way to determine the need for additional movements is to wait until the last aligner is delivered and then clinically examine the teeth. This is the time when the precise amount and direction of additional movement can be requested on the specified teeth. This process is more effective and efficient than trying to guess at the beginning which tooth will require additional movement—and how much—to achieve full alignment. If the last aligner fits well and the movements do not exceed three aligners, additional aligners can be ordered to achieve the last additional movements. However, if the last aligner does not fit well and the case requires movements with more than three aligners, a new impression should be made.

Detailing pliers have proved successful at achieving movements at the end of treatments that require in-and-out movements and minor incisor rotations. There is a misconception with Invisalign treatment that the appliance performs all of the work and therefore that treatment

requires simply dispensing the appliances. As with the prescription bracket, there is also a misconception that successful outcomes are based on a proper diagnosis and treatment plan and careful monitoring during treatment. Finishing a case with Invisalign may require additional aligners and other armamentaria to produce the desired treatment goals. Invisalign as a treatment modality can provide the clinician with the tools to offer patients an excellent esthetic treatment option. However, good clinical results are based on good case selection and careful monitoring during treatment.

References

1. Andrews LF. Straight Wire: The Concept and Appliance. San Diego: L.A. Wells, 1989.
2. Reitan K. Principles of retention and avoidance of posttreatment relapse. Am J Orthod 1969;55:776–790.
3. Creekmore TD, Kunik RL. Straight wire: The next generation. Am J Orthod Dentofacial Orthop 1993;104:8–20.

chapter 22

EXTRACTION TREATMENT WITH INVISALIGN

by
David E. Paquette, DDS

TABLE 22-1 Optimal forces for orthodontic movement*	
Type of movement	**Force (g)**
Tipping	50–75
Bodily movement (translation)	100–150
Root uprighting	75–125
Rotation	50–100
Extrusion	50–100
Intrusion	15–25

*Data from Proffit and Fields.[1]

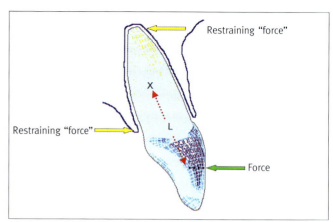

FIG 22-1 Tipping tooth movement is created by rotation of the tooth around the center of resistance. (X) Center of resistance; (L) moment arm.

Whether one is an advocate of extractions to facilitate orthodontic correction of a malocclusion or not, the fact is that even the most adamant extraction-averse orthodontist faces the occasion where extraction of one or more teeth is the only option. That said, proper control of root position and anchorage during closure of extraction spaces is the greatest challenge faced by any orthodontist. The question then becomes: Is extraction treatment with Invisalign a practical alternative to fixed appliances?

In 2000, Sims predicted that the future of orthodontics would include the abolition of bracket systems.[2] In his textbook *Contemporary Orthodontics*, Proffit stated that adult patients are often opposed to wearing conspicuous fixed appliances and would rather use a removable appliance.[1] He also described the characteristics required of an orthodontic appliance system:

"No matter what the type of orthodontic appliance, it must meet certain basic design criteria: it (1) should not interfere with function; (2) should cause no harm to the oral tissues or interfere with the maintenance of good oral hygiene; (3) should be as light and inconspicuous as possible, yet sufficiently strong to withstand masticatory forces and a reasonable amount of abuse; (4) must be firmly retained in position; (5) must be capable of exerting an appropriately controlled force in the correct direction and delivering this force for as long as possible between adjustment visits; and (6) should allow control of anchorage, so that tooth movements other than those intended are minimized.[1 p475]"

On the surface it would appear that Invisalign satisfies all these criteria.

According to Proffit,[1] removable appliances are only capable of simple tipping movements and are easily displaced by the forces required to produce controlled root movement. He concluded that the usual solution to this problem was to use fixed appliances.

When the orthodontic department at the University of the Pacific began using aligners to treat more complex cases—such as those involving the extraction of a mandibular incisor—to determine if the space could be closed in a manner parallel to that of fixed appliances, they discovered that both the technique and the material had to be altered to move the teeth bodily. They are now experimenting with premolar extraction cases. Based on those experiences, it was concluded that "the use of the Aligners is far more complicated than most people believe. It takes a knowledgeable clinician with considerable experience to use the appliance to its maximum."[3]

To determine just what that maximum might be with Invisalign in its current rendition of aligner materials, we must examine the biomechanics of tooth movement with Invisalign.

Biomechanics

For all practical purposes, the problems involved with extraction treatment can be broken down to controlling torque and root parallelism. To properly discuss these issues, a review of several definitions of biomechanical terms is in order.

The first of these is force. *Force* is a load applied to an object that tends to move the object to a different posi-

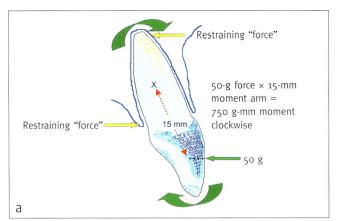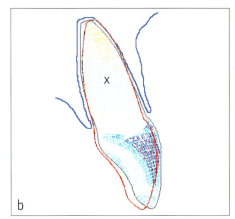

FIG 22-2 (a and b) Rotation around the center of resistance. The crown is displaced lingually and the apex facially. (X) Center of resistance and center of rotation are in the same location.

tion. Force, though defined in Newtons (mass times the acceleration of gravity), is usually measured in mass units of grams or ounces. Historically, the optimal amount of force required for most tooth movements has been considered to be 50 to 150 g (Table 22-1). Recent studies have suggested that given time, forces as low as 18 g are sufficient to produce bodily movement.[4] Because the force delivered with an aligner made from Align Technology's Ex30 polyurethane material is 200 g initially and decays to essentially a constant level of 40 g within hours, there should be no problem delivering adequate forces to the teeth to create desired movements. Controlling those forces then becomes the issue.

How the force is delivered and the reaction of the tooth to that force is a function of multiple factors. One of these factors is center of resistance. In engineering terms, *center of resistance* is a point at which resistance to movement can be concentrated for mathematical analysis. For an object in free space, the center of resistance is the same as the center of mass. If the object is partially restrained—as is the case for a pole or post embedded in the earth or a tooth root embedded in bone—the center of resistance is determined by the type of external constraints. The center of resistance for a tooth is roughly midway between the root apex and the crest of the alveolar bone.

If the point at which a force is applied to an object is not directly opposite the center of resistance, a moment is created. A *moment* is a force that acts at a distance and is defined as the product of the force times the distance to the center of resistance. It is measured in units of gram-millimeters or equivalent. If a force is applied at some distance to the center of rotation, not only will the force tend

to translate the object in space, it will also tend to rotate the object around the center of resistance. This effect, of course, is precisely the situation when a force is applied to the crown of a tooth. The tooth is not only displaced in the direction of the force, but it is also rotated around the center of resistance—thus, there is a tipping tooth movement (Fig 22-1).

When there are two forces acting on an object that are equal in magnitude and opposite in direction, the combination of the two forces is referred to as a *couple*. The result of applying two forces in this way is a pure moment, since the translatory effect of the forces cancels out. A couple produces pure rotation, spinning the object around its center of resistance. The combination of a force and a couple can change the way an object rotates while it is being moved.

The point around which rotation actually occurs when an object is being moved is referred to as the *center of rotation*. When a force is applied directly to the middle of the facial surface of the crown, the tooth rotates about the center of resistance. This results in a tipping movement with the crown being displaced lingually and the apex of the root displaced slightly in a facial direction (Figs 22-2a and 22-2b).

If a force and a couple are applied to an object, the center of rotation can be controlled and made to have any desired location. The application of a force and a couple to the crown of a tooth, in fact, is the mechanism by which bodily movement of a tooth, or even greater movement of root than the crown, can be produced.

By applying a secondary force on the lingual at the incisal edge, a couple is formed that moves the center of rotation apically. The net lingual force combined with a couple

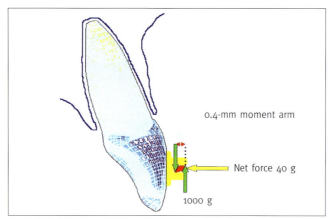

FIG 22-8 A moment-to-force ratio of 10 is needed for bodily movement. With a retraction force of 40 g and a moment arm of only 0.4 mm on a typical bracket, to avoid tipping the required moment is 400 g-mm, meaning a 1,000-g force at each corner of the archwire.

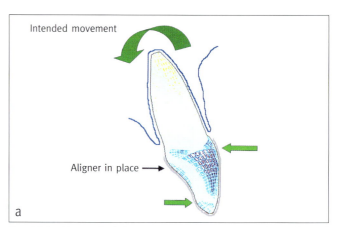

FIG 22-9a Theoretical force-moment system to achieve lingual root movement with an aligner.

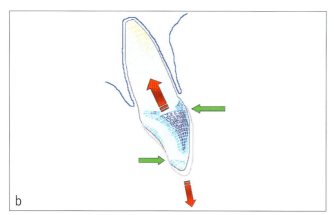

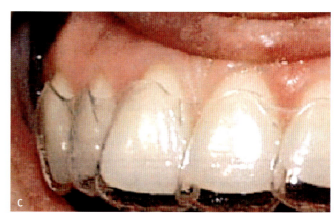

FIG 22-9 (b and c) Clinical expression of this force-moment system to achieve lingual root movement or bodily movement: The tooth is intruded or the aligner displaced as a result of lack of retention.

Torque control

To better understand the dynamics of root control with aligners, we will now examine the biomechanics of tooth movement with aligners and compare that with our understanding of movement with fixed appliances. Specifically, the design and placement of attachments and auxiliaries to accomplish controlled two-point force application will be examined.

One of the problems we see in attempts to move incisor roots with aligners is that the intended movement and the actual movement are often different. The reason for this is exactly what Proffit described for removable appliances in general: there is not enough retention to offset the force needed to generate the movement (Figs 22-8 and 22-9a to 22-9c).

The solution to aligner displacement is the proper design and placement of attachments. Figure 22-10 illustrates the evolution of attachments used to help eliminate

this problem. The key is to provide a ledge for the aligner to grip that is perpendicular to the direction of displacement and of sufficient size to provide enough surface area to offset the force delivered. Another simple rule of thumb is to place the attachment far enough away from the gingival margin that the aligner will not spread or stretch and slip off the attachment.

Proper attachment design allows clinical expression of this force-moment system to achieve lingual root movement or bodily movement—that is, torque control. The moment arm is measured from the most incisal aspect of the attachment that extends to the effective gingival point of contact of the aligner. The effective point of contact near the gingival margin is approximately 1 to 2 mm from the gingival edge of the aligner as a result of stretch of the aligner in this area. Figures 22-11 to 22-14 illustrate the effect of attachment design and placement on torque control.

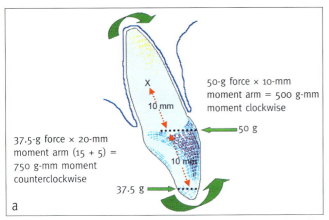
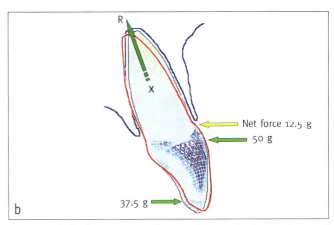

37.5-g force × 20-mm moment arm (15 + 5) = 750 g-mm moment counterclockwise

50-g force × 10-mm moment arm = 500 g-mm moment clockwise

50 g

37.5 g

a

Net force 12.5 g

50 g

37.5 g

b

FIG 22-6 (a and b) Greater force on facial than on lingual surface. Net counterclockwise moment of 250 g-mm results in rotation, and net force produces lingual movement (lingual crown torque). (X) Center of resistance; (R) center of rotation.

By applying a smaller force to the facial closer to the apex and an equal secondary force on the lingual at the incisal edge, a similar couple is formed that also moves the center of rotation apically. The net lingual force in this case is also zero. The net counterclockwise moment results in a rotational movement of the tooth with the apex moving slightly lingually and the crown moving facially (Figs 22-5a and 22-5b).

Applying a slightly greater force to the facial and maintaining the secondary force on the lingual at the incisal edge forms a similar couple that also moves the center of rotation apically. In this case, however, the net lingual force is greater than zero. The net counterclockwise moment results in a rotational movement of the tooth with the apex moving lingually and the crown moving slightly facially (ie, lingual crown torque) (Figs 22-6a and 22-6b).

The goal is to control root position during movement to achieve the desired results with the least possible complexity. This can be achieved through control of the moment-to-force ratio. The ratio between the force applied to move a tooth and the counterbalancing moment used to control root position determines the type of tooth movement. If the ratio between the counterbalancing moment and the retraction force is less than 1, the tooth will tip just apically to its center of resistance. As the moment-to-force ratio increases, the center of rotation is displaced farther away from the center of resistance, producing controlled tipping. With a moment-to-force ratio of 8 to 10, bodily movement occurs. If the moment-to-force ratio is greater than 10, the root apex will be retracted more than the crown, producing lingual root torque (Fig 22-7).

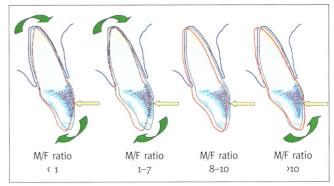

M/F ratio < 1

M/F ratio 1-7

M/F ratio 8-10

M/F ratio >10

FIG 22-7 Moment-to-force (M/F) ratios used to control root position during movement.

Tooth-Aligner Biomechanics

Proffit stated in his textbook that removable appliances are

"rarely satisfactory for adjunctive (or comprehensive) treatment. Removable appliances by their very nature produce simple tipping movements of teeth, making control of tooth position extremely difficult. In addition, removable appliances are by definition removable, and the adult patient's concept of continuous appliance wear does not always coincide with that of the dentist. Intermittent forces, though capable of producing tooth movement, are not as efficient as continuous forces, particularly in the presence of occlusal interferences."[1 p236]

He went on to say, "As a practical matter, it can be difficult to maintain removable appliances in place against the displacing effects of a pair of springs with heavy activation. The usual orthodontic solution is a fixed attachment on the tooth, constructed so that forces can be applied at two points".[1 p236]

199

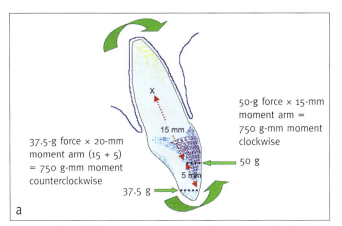
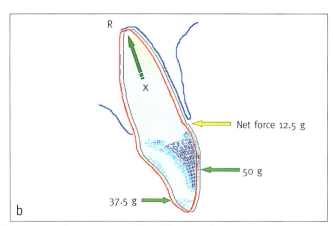

FIG 22-3 (a and b) Opposing moments form a couple that moves the center of rotation apically with a net force to the lingual that moves the tooth bodily. (X) Center of resistance; (R) center of rotation.

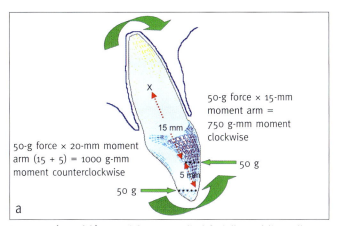
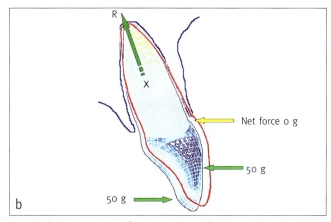

FIG 22-4 (a and b) Equal forces applied facially and lingually. Net counterclockwise moment of 250 g-mm results in rotation. The facial and lingual forces offset each other so there is no bodily movement. (X) Center of resistance; (R) center of rotation.

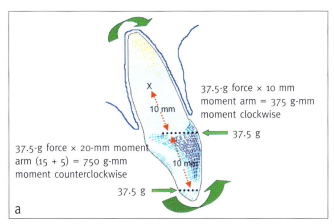
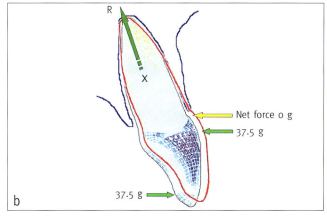

FIG 22-5 (a and b) Equal facial and lingual forces, with facial force applied more apically. Net counterclockwise moment (375 g-mm) results in rotation with no bodily movement. (X) Center of resistance; (R) center of rotation.

results in bodily movement of the tooth to the lingual. In this instance, forces applied to both facial and lingual surfaces produce the couple (Figs 22-3a and 22-3b).

By applying a secondary force on the lingual at the incisal edge equal to the force on the facial, a couple is

formed that moves the center of rotation farther apically. The net lingual force in this case is zero. The net counterclockwise moment results in a rotational movement of the tooth with the apex moving slightly lingually and the crown moving facially (Figs 22-4a and 22-4b).

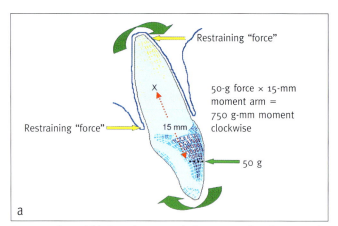 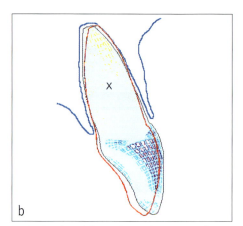

FIG 22-2 (a and b) Rotation around the center of resistance. The crown is displaced lingually and the apex facially. (X) Center of resistance and center of rotation are in the same location.

tion. Force, though defined in Newtons (mass times the acceleration of gravity), is usually measured in mass units of grams or ounces. Historically, the optimal amount of force required for most tooth movements has been considered to be 50 to 150 g (Table 22-1). Recent studies have suggested that given time, forces as low as 18 g are sufficient to produce bodily movement.[4] Because the force delivered with an aligner made from Align Technology's Ex30 polyurethane material is 200 g initially and decays to essentially a constant level of 40 g within hours, there should be no problem delivering adequate forces to the teeth to create desired movements. Controlling those forces then becomes the issue.

How the force is delivered and the reaction of the tooth to that force is a function of multiple factors. One of these factors is center of resistance. In engineering terms, *center of resistance* is a point at which resistance to movement can be concentrated for mathematical analysis. For an object in free space, the center of resistance is the same as the center of mass. If the object is partially restrained—as is the case for a pole or post embedded in the earth or a tooth root embedded in bone—the center of resistance is determined by the type of external constraints. The center of resistance for a tooth is roughly midway between the root apex and the crest of the alveolar bone.

If the point at which a force is applied to an object is not directly opposite the center of resistance, a moment is created. A *moment* is a force that acts at a distance and is defined as the product of the force times the distance to the center of resistance. It is measured in units of gram-millimeters or equivalent. If a force is applied at some distance to the center of rotation, not only will the force tend

to translate the object in space, it will also tend to rotate the object around the center of resistance. This effect, of course, is precisely the situation when a force is applied to the crown of a tooth. The tooth is not only displaced in the direction of the force, but it is also rotated around the center of resistance—thus, there is a tipping tooth movement (Fig 22-1).

When there are two forces acting on an object that are equal in magnitude and opposite in direction, the combination of the two forces is referred to as a *couple*. The result of applying two forces in this way is a pure moment, since the translatory effect of the forces cancels out. A couple produces pure rotation, spinning the object around its center of resistance. The combination of a force and a couple can change the way an object rotates while it is being moved.

The point around which rotation actually occurs when an object is being moved is referred to as the *center of rotation*. When a force is applied directly to the middle of the facial surface of the crown, the tooth rotates about the center of resistance. This results in a tipping movement with the crown being displaced lingually and the apex of the root displaced slightly in a facial direction (Figs 22-2a and 22-2b).

If a force and a couple are applied to an object, the center of rotation can be controlled and made to have any desired location. The application of a force and a couple to the crown of a tooth, in fact, is the mechanism by which bodily movement of a tooth, or even greater movement of root than the crown, can be produced.

By applying a secondary force on the lingual at the incisal edge, a couple is formed that moves the center of rotation apically. The net lingual force combined with a couple

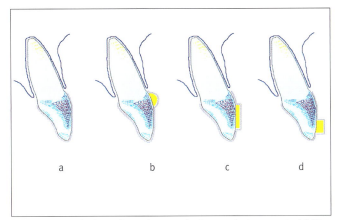

FIG 22-10 Evolution of attachment design and placement. (*a*) The aligner is easily displaced because there is no attachment or ledge to provide retention. (*b*) A ledge is created with an attachment, but it is placed too far gingivally and is inadequate for retention. (*c*) A ledge is created with an attachment, but it is placed too far gingivally and is too narrow for retention in this direction. (*d*) An attachment of proper design and placement, closer to the incisal edge and perpendicular to the direction of displacement, will provide sufficient retention.

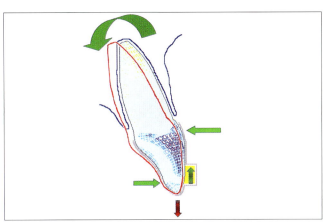

FIG 22-11 A 1 × 2 × 4–mm horizontal rectangular attachment placed near the incisal edge. The intrinsic, extrusive forces exerted on the aligner are now offset by the forces the attachment places on the "bubble" in the aligner. By providing a horizontal ledge 90 degrees to the force applied, retention of the aligner in its desired location is achieved, unwanted movements are reduced, and intended movements are enhanced.

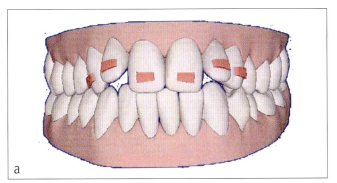

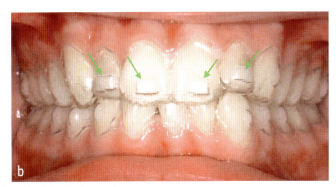

FIG 22-12 (a and b) Rectangular attachments as viewed in ClinCheck and clinically (*arrows*).

Figure 22-12a illustrates a typical set of attachments as viewed on ClinCheck. The clinical appearance of these attachments is seen in Fig 22-12b. The trapezoid appearance seen on the virtual image is an artifact of the manufacturing process.

Figures 22-13a and 22-13b illustrate a recent modification to the horizontal rectangular attachment that produces a beveled appearance. The beveled attachment accomplishes two things: it allows easier aligner insertion and is esthetically superior in that it is less noticeable because of the lack of shadow along the incisal aspect of the attachment.

A net force of 40 g intended to move the tooth lingually would require a moment of 320 to 400 g-mm (F/M ratio, 8 to 10) for bodily movement or greater than 400 g-mm (F/M ratio, < 10) for lingual root movement (Figs 22-14a and 22-14b). Improper attachment design or placement

allows the delivery of only 280 g-mm moment in conjunction with 40 g force, which results in controlled lingual crown tipping (Fig 22-14c).

Root parallelism

The other biomechanical consideration pertinent to extraction treatment is the controlled tipping to achieve root parallelism in the extraction sites. When a force is applied in an attempt to move a canine distally, the tooth will rotate around the center of resistance. It requires a sufficient moment to oppose the tipping movement. This is a more problematic area because in a typical extraction scenario, the aligner contacts the tooth in the buccal segments on a surface that is parallel to the direction of force. The result, of course, is that there is little, if any, moment arm created without the use of substantial attachments, auxiliaries, or both (Figs 22-15 to 22-17).

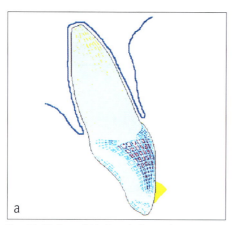
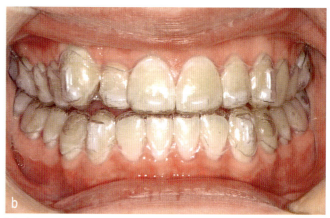

FIG 22-13 (a and b) Beveled attachments accomplish the goals of retention and resistance to unwanted movement, are discreet, and facilitate insertion and removal of aligners.

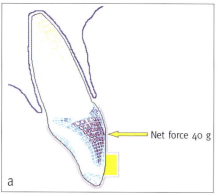
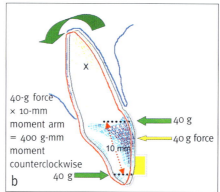
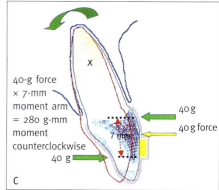

FIG 22-14 (a to c) Depending on attachment design and placement, a net force of 40 g on the facial surface (*a*) can create bodily movement (*b*) or lingual crown tipping (*c*). (X) Center of resistance.

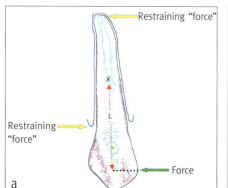
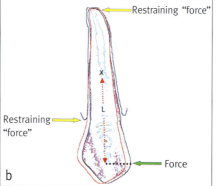
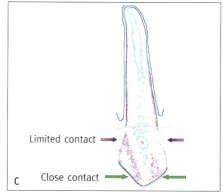

FIG 22-15 (*a and b*) The tooth rotates clockwise around the center of resistance. (*c*) Controlling movement of buccal segments can be difficult because of limited aligner contact in the direction of force application. To enhance force application requires placement of attachments and/or auxiliaries. (X) Center of resistance; (L) moment arm.

An idea dating back to the 1920s was to place an attachment on the gingival aspect of a bracket extending toward the center of resistance in an attempt to decrease the amount of tipping that occurs when teeth are moved mesiodistally. These gingival extensions are often described as *power arms*. A power arm can be added to the force system with Invisalign. The addition of a power arm auxiliary accomplishes two things. First, it moves the application of force closer to the center of resistance. Second, it creates a secondary moment as a result of pressure against the distal of the aligner. With the combined power arm and "T" attachment, it should be possible to control the distal root tip during retraction. This attachment design has been successful with some patients (Figs 22-18 to 22-23).

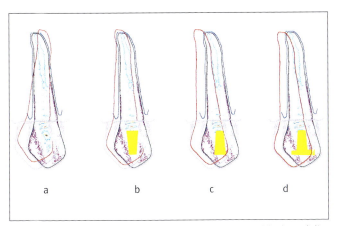

FIG 22-16 Attachment design and placement are critical to delivery of adequate couple to control root position but may still not be enough. Auxiliaries must be considered. (*a*) No attachment; tooth does not track with aligner. (*b*) Long vertical attachment helps provide couple but has intrusive vector and minimal retention. (*c*) Inverted long vertical attachment to provide couple has extrusive vector but still minimal retention. (*d*) "T" attachment design provides couple and added retention.

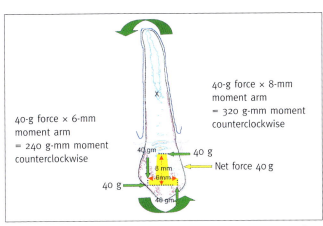

FIG 22-17 Combined 240-g-mm and 320-g-mm moments produce a 560-g-mm moment, assuming a full 40-g force at each corner.

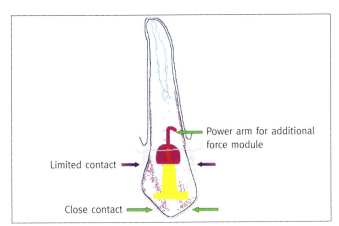

FIG 22-18 Addition of a power arm auxiliary and "T" attachment increases the likelihood of a proper force-moment system to control root movement during retraction.

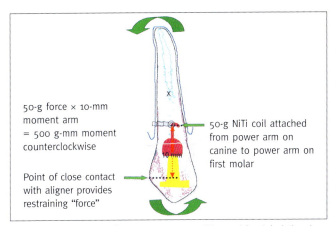

FIG 22-19 Addition of a power arm auxiliary with nickel-titanium coil adds additional retraction force.

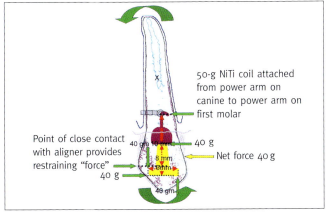

FIG 22-20 Force-moment system when attachments and auxiliaries are used. Combined 240-g-mm, 320-g-mm, and 500-g-mm moments produce a 1,060-g-mm moment with a 90-g distalizing force. (X) Center of resistance.

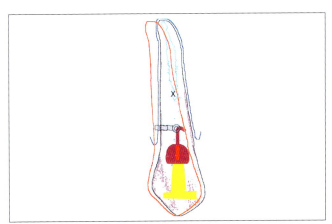

FIG 22-21 Proper planning and addition of a power arm auxiliary should allow the ability to effectively parallel roots.

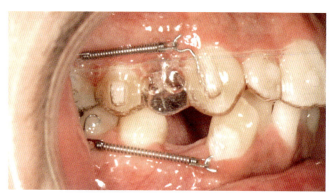

FIG 22-22 Power arms fabricated out of .020 SS round wire bonded with composite. NiTi coil springs are attached to apply force to the power arm.

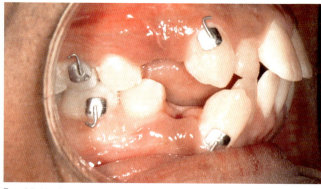

FIG 22-23 Attempt at manufactured power arms on orthodontic bonding bases. This was ineffective because the length of the power arm was insufficient to move the point of force application adequately to achieve the desired results.

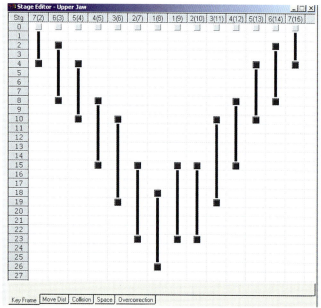

FIG 22-24 Staging diagram. The numbers across the top represent different teeth, and the vertical axis represents the aligner number. The vertical black bars in the diagram indicate the timing and rate of tooth movement. Each aligner number represents one stage.

Staging

Another aspect of proper control of tooth movement is staging. Staging is the sequence and speed that teeth are moved with aligners (Fig 22-24). Although most movements have default staging plans, the orthodontist can request custom staging when necessary. For more complex movements like extraction cases, a custom staging request is almost always required.

Planned rate of tooth motion per stage or aligner must not exceed the ability of the roots to keep up with desired movement. Proper staging is critical to effective space clo-

sure with aligners. It is usually necessary to reduce the rate of space closure with aligners to approximately one half that possible with fixed appliances. Even that rate may exceed the aligner's ability to provide the proper force system needed for root parallelism.

Clinical Issues

It should be obvious after reviewing the biomechanics of space closure with aligners that several variables combine to either produce acceptable desired results or unacceptable, undesired, and aberrant tooth movements. These are reviewed with reference to space closure and control of root position.

Foremost is the clinical crown length. The longer the clinical crown, the more likely it is that a sufficient couple can be created. Patients with very short clinical crowns are not good candidates to attempt extraction treatment with Invisalign. Single mandibular central incisor extraction tends to be successful because of the length of the clinical crowns relative to the forces applied (Figs 22-25a and 22-25b). Although root position of canines has been successfully maintained during retraction, the molars, especially maxillary molars, tend to tip mesially. This is frequently referred to as "dumping" (Figs 22-26a to 22-26c). Dumping occurs even when the molars are simply being used as anchorage for anterior retraction; this may be caused by the disadvantageous crown-to-root ratio combined with the large root surface area over which forces are distributed. Work is currently being done with various accentuated attachment designs, but as yet the ability to predictably avoid molar dumping has not been demonstrated.

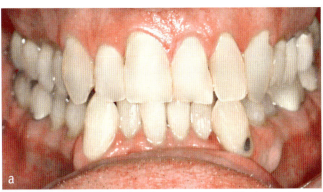
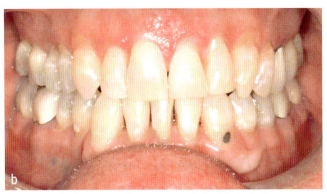

FIG 22-25 Pretreatment (*a*) and posttreatment (*b*) views of a mandibular central incisor extraction case treated with Invisalign.

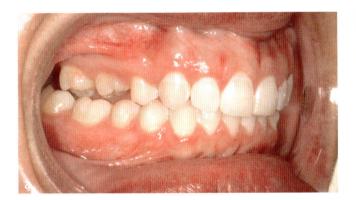
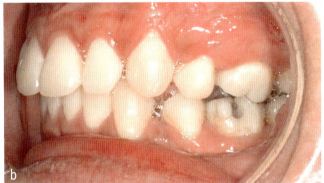

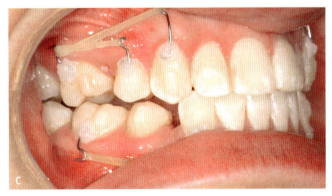

FIG 22-26 (a to c) Mesial tipping of maxillary molars sometimes occurs during Invisalign treatment.

Conclusion

With aligners, it is still difficult to achieve extraction treatment and subsequent space closure with proper tip and torque to produce root parallelism and esthetic crown inclination. Understanding the biomechanics of tooth movement with aligners and applying that knowledge to treatment planning and clinical execution should result in breakthroughs in the near future that will make such treatments more predictable and routine.

References

1. Proffit W, Fields HJ (eds). Contemporary Orthodontics, ed 1. St Louis: Mosby, 1986.
2. Sims MR. Brackets, epitopes and flash memory cards: A futuristic view of clinical orthodontics. Aust Orthod J 1999;15:260–268.
3. Dugoni AA. What price progress? Am J Orthod Dentofacial Orthop 2002;122(2):16A–18A.
4. Iwasaki LR, Haack JE, Nickel JC, Morton J. Human tooth movement in response to continuous stress of low magnitude. Am J Orthod Dentofacial Orthop 2000;117:175–183.

chapter 23

FORCE APPLICATION WITH INVISALIGN: CONSTANCY AND COMPLIANCE

by
Trang Duong, DDS and Robert Tricca, PhD

Duration of Force and Force Magnitude

Force duration and magnitude are important factors in tooth movement. Traditionally, it was believed that light, continuous forces applied 24 hours per day produce the most efficient tooth movement. It has been shown, however, that teeth can be successfully moved with shorter durations of force application; reportedly, the effective force application threshold is approximately 6 hours (Fig 23-1).[1]

Interrupted forces have been shown to produce tooth movement similar to that achieved with continuous force application, but with less damage to the structures of the periodontal ligament (PDL).[2] The response of periodontal tissues to orthodontic forces is discussed in detail in chapter 19. It will suffice to review here concepts of force magnitude and duration.

It is generally known that force magnitude, as well as force duration, plays an important role in producing optimal tooth movement. The ideal force magnitude is one that remains constant regardless of how the tooth moves in response. Unfortunately, force decay is inevitable after the tooth has moved a short distance (Fig 23-2). Even with the new nickel titanium and copper nitinol wires, forces decay as the teeth move.

Orthodontic force duration may be classified into three categories. The first is *continuous force*, which is a force maintained, at some fraction of the original, over time. The second category of orthodontic force duration is *interrupted force*, which describes a force level that falls to zero between activations (Fig 23-3). *Intermittent* force levels fall to zero when the appliance is removed or when a fixed appliance is temporarily deactivated.[1] The aligners worn by patients produce intermittent forces because the force is removed once the appliance is removed. Recent studies have shown that light, short-term or cyclic force applications can produce tooth movement that is comparable to that produced by light, continuous forces. Events associated with tooth movement, such as bone turnover, have been shown to continue for an indeterminate period after force decay or appliance removal. Theoretically, if a patient wears the aligners for 16 to 20 hours per day, clinically effective tooth movement will occur.

Oppenheim suggested that intermittent force was suitable for optimal tooth movement of monkey incisors, because the rest period allowed for reconstruction of the periodontal tissues (Fig 23-4).[3] In theory, light, continuous forces produce the most efficient tooth movement. Despite the best efforts to keep forces light enough to produce only frontal resorption, however, undermining resorption probably occurs in every patient.

Clinical experience with fixed appliances has shown that a 4- to 6-week appointment cycle is usually sufficient to track the length of activation. With the newest generation of memory archwires and self-ligating brackets, 8-week activations have been used. An appliance activated too frequently can inhibit the biologic repair process of the tooth and cause damage to the teeth.

Wear Time with Invisalign

When Invisalign was introduced, the optimum reactivation schedule (ie, the amount of time each aligner should be worn before advancing to the next aligner) was unknown. It was assumed, however, that over time as the aligners were worn, the magnitude of applied force would diminish (see Fig 23-4). This could be a consequence of material fatigue and the distance the teeth had moved. To understand the outcomes of forces applied to teeth under varying conditions, a randomized clinical trial was conducted at the University of Washington.[4] The objective was to specifically determine the activation time and optimal frequency of appliance change with Invisalign. This study also examined the optimal material stiffness.

The inclusion criteria for this study were that the patient must be over 18 years of age and have the ability to attend weekly appointments. Patients requiring orthognathic surgery were excluded from the study. After enrollment, consent, and collection of orthodontic records, four clinical investigators independently planned treatment for each patient. At least three of the four orthodontists had to agree on a particular plan before it was chosen.

Based on the severity of the malocclusion and the treatment plan, patients were placed in the extraction or nonextraction and high versus low peer-assessment rating (PAR) stratification. The extraction group consisted of either mandibular incisor or premolar extractions. Patients were then randomly assigned to one of four groups: hard or soft plastic, and 1- or 2-week schedule for appliance change. The hard material was twice as stiff as the commercial material; the soft material was one-tenth as stiff as the commercial material. The sample consisted of 51 patients with a mean age of 34 years (range: 19 to 55 years). There were no significant differences among the four groups in terms of age, gender, or race.

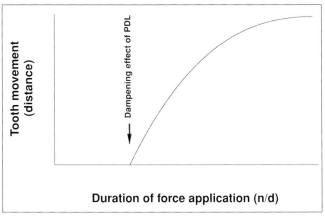

FIG 23-1 Theoretical plot of tooth movement efficiency versus duration of force. Successful tooth movement can be produced by shorter durations, with a threshold (periodontal ligament [PDL] dampening) at about 6 hours.

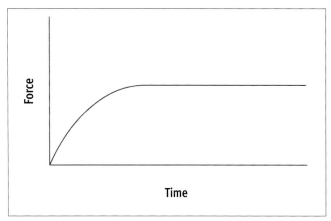

FIG 23-2 Diagram of force decay in an ideal spring situation. An ideal spring would maintain the same amount of force regardless of the distance a tooth moved. With any type of wire (or spring or aligner material), however, force decays as the tooth moves.

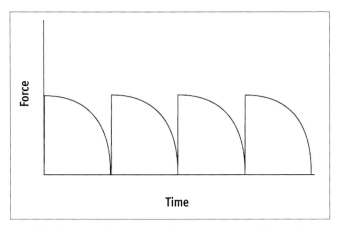

FIG 23-3 Diagram of interrupted forces. Interrupted forces drop to zero between activations.

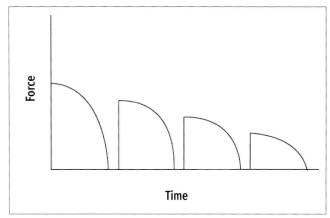

FIG 23-4 Diagram of intermittent force. This occurs in removable appliances when the force drops to zero when the appliance is taken out. The force resumes when the appliance is replaced. Forces with Invisalign would most resemble this type of diagram.

Although there were no statistically significant findings, some trends were observed. The patients who wore their aligners for 2-week intervals had a greater tendency to have completed the initial series of aligners than did patients in the 1-week groups (21% versus 37%, $P < .20$).[4] Of the four treatment protocols, the 2-week hard material group showed the best results in all measurements of occlusal and alignment improvement. This trend was seen for every index. It is possible that the lack of statistical significance is attributable to a lack of power in the study due to its small sample size. The difference between the 1- and 2-week groups might have been much larger and found to be statistically significant if the sample size were doubled.

This clinical trial concluded that the 2-week activation times achieved a higher degree of success than 1-week activation times. Subjects with a 2-week activation regimen, no extractions, and a low PAR score were more likely to complete their initial series of aligners. This study supports Align Technology's current recommendation of a 2-week wear time for each aligner.

Based on the results of this study, the optimal wear time per aligner is 2 weeks for approximately 16 to 20 hours per day. Tooth movement, however, is a complex phenomenon. Individual responses vary from patient to patient, tooth to tooth, and depending on the type of tooth movement. It is recommended, therefore, that each aligner be completely passive prior to progressing to the next aligner. Patients have been recommended to wear their aligners for 3 weeks if the teeth have not moved to the desired position after 2 weeks. For optimal progress and results, the clinician must monitor individual tooth movements and refer back to the ClinCheck at each appointment to ensure that the actual movements of the teeth match those from the programmed treatment.

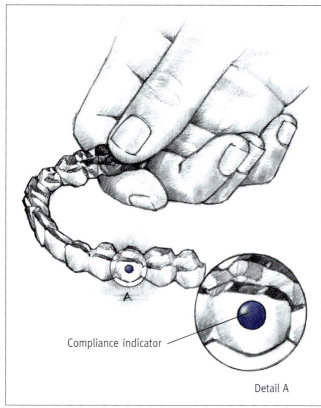

Compliance indicator

A

Detail A

FIG 23-5 Compliance indicator (A) on a posterior surface of an aligner.

The Invisalign System is most effective when the patient wears the aligners as prescribed by the orthodontist. In fact, just about any orthodontist would freely state, "Give me a good cooperator, and I'll treat anything." Clearly, patient cooperation is vitally important for a successful outcome—not only with fixed appliances, but also with the Invisalign System. Extended removal of the aligner for

any reason beyond what is recommended interrupts the treatment plan and lengthens the overall period of treatment. If the distance between each interval were to be increased, the expected outcome would be very little and unpredictable tooth movement.

Compliance with aligner wear during the course of Invisalign treatment is solely the responsibility of the patient. Reminders are a helpful method to aid patient cooperation. The orthodontist can objectively assess patient cooperation through the use of compliance indicators. Compliance indicators are mounted on each aligner (Fig 23-5) and are designed to give a visual indication as to how long a patient has been wearing the aligner. Some advantages of compliance indicators include the following:

- Better data for communicating aligner compliance with patients, including increased patient knowledge and recall of usage, increased compliance in wearing the dental appliance, and increased patient satisfaction as a result.
- A means of self-monitoring for the patient.
- Reduction of the patient's anxiety levels without requiring oral or written instructions. Because appliance usage is self-evident, there are no instructions to read or clocks to watch on the part of the patient.
- Better information for the orthodontist on patient progress during the treatment.

A compliance indicator with a layered-disk technology is shown in Fig 23-6. Interaction with oral fluids such as saliva causes a visual change (eg, color, mass, shape) in the indicator. Changes in an indicator occur as aligner wear time increases. The layered disk is composed of an active

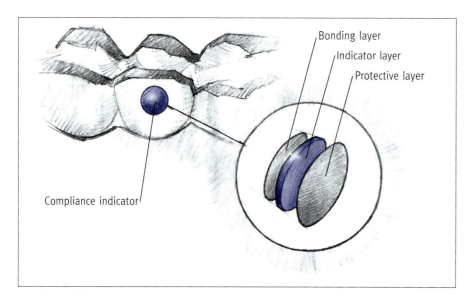

Bonding layer
Indicator layer
Protective layer
Compliance indicator

FIG 23-6 Compliance indicator with layered-disk technology.

FIG 23-7 Compliance indicator over time corresponding with good aligner wear.

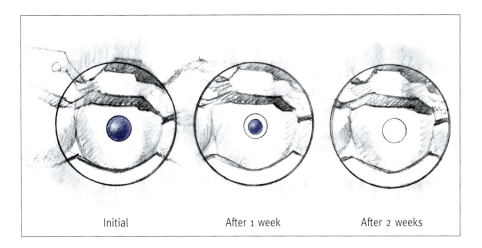

| Initial | After 1 week | After 2 weeks |

indicator layer, a protective layer, and a bonding layer. The protective layer is a thin, transparent film that protects the indicator layer from toothbrushing, buccal or lingual contact, and other external forces. The indicator layer can be composed of a water-soluble polymer and a pigment. Interaction with saliva and other oral fluids slowly dissolves the polymer and reduces the size of the indicator layer. For example, after 1 week with good compliance, the indicator may lose half its mass. After 2 weeks of good compliance, the indicator layer may be completely dissolved (Fig 23-7). The third layer of the compliance indicator is a bonding layer that is used to adhere the indicator layer to the aligner surface. The bonding layer can be composed of a biocompatible pressure-sensitive adhesive.

A compliance indicator on aligners provides a better understanding of patient compliance and aids in improving the clinical outcome for patients treated with the Invisalign System. It is best that the clinician prescribe 300 to 400 hours of aligner wear time. No harm can be done by wearing the aligners too long, but many problems are possible if the aligners are not worn constantly and long enough.

References

1. Stark T, Sinclair P. Effect of pulsed electromagnetic fields on orthodontic tooth movement. Am J Orthod Dentofacial Orthop 1987;91:91–104.
2. Gibson J, King G, Keeling S. Long-term orthodontic tooth movement response to short-term force in the rat. Angle Orthod 1992;62:211–215.
3. Oppenheim A. A possibility for physiologic orthodontic movement. J Dent Res 1944;30:277–328.
4. Bollen A, Huang G, King G, Hujoel P, Ma T. Activation time and material stiffness of sequential removable orthodontic appliances. Part 1: Ability to complete treatment. Am J Orthod Dentofacial Orthop 2003;124:496–501.

CLINICAL CONSIDERATIONS IN USING THE INVISALIGN SYSTEM

chapter 24

ADVANTAGES OF THE INVISALIGN SYSTEM

by
Trang Duong, DDS and Mitra Derakhshan, DDS

The First Appliances

Edward Angle is not only the father of modern orthodontics, he was also known to be a prolific inventor of orthodontic appliances. His first appliance was the E-arch. The E-arch was developed in the late 1800s and consisted of bands placed on the teeth with ligatures to the heavy archwire (Fig 24-1a). The pin and tube, which permitted precise torque and tip control to be accomplished by using a vertical tube on each tooth with a soldered pin on the base archwire, came next (Fig 24-1b). This appliance was impractical because of the time and effort required to activate it. The next appliance Angle developed was the ribbon arch. It incorporated a vertical rectangular slot behind the tube (Fig 24-1c). A ribbon arch consisted of gold wire and was placed into the slot and held in with pins. This appliance, unfortunately, could not torque the roots. The slot was then rotat-

ed 90 degrees and termed "edgewise" (Fig 24-1d). By changing the orientation, Angle was able to control crown and root position in all three planes of space. Just about all fixed appliances used today are based on Angle's designs.

Appliances Used Today

The appliances used today have evolved since Angle's edgewise appliance in the early 20th century. Numerous advances in cements, materials, techniques, and technology have allowed orthodontics to become more efficient, comfortable, and esthetically pleasing for the patient. In 1970, fewer than 5% of all orthodontic patients were age 18 years or older. Most of the growth of orthodontics in the 1980s was in the adult patient group. By 1990, adults consisted of approximately 25% of all orthodontic

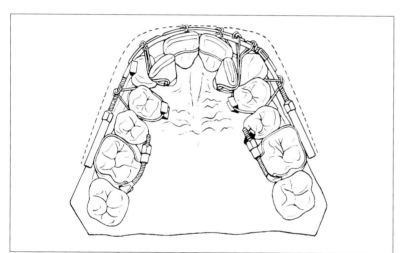

FIG 24-1a E-arch appliance.

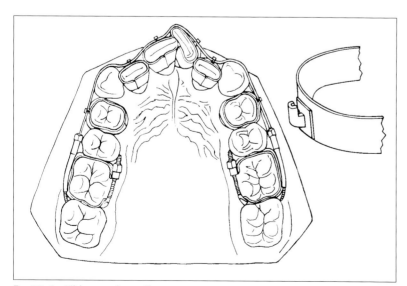

FIG 24-1c Ribbon arch appliance.

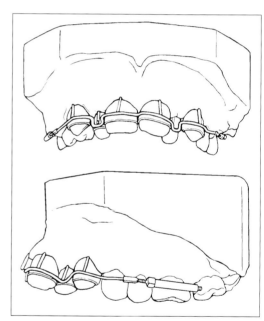

FIG 24-1b Pin and tube appliance.

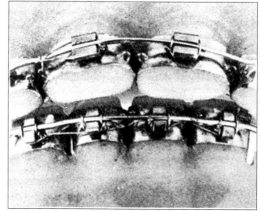

FIG 24-1d Edgewise appliance.

patients. This trend is related to the increase in the number of orthodontic patients aged 40 and older.[1]

Most adults express some concern about the appearance of orthodontic appliances. Today, there is a high demand for an esthetic orthodontic appliance. With the introduction of bonding in the 1970s, it was possible to place fixed attachments on the lingual surface of the teeth and produce an invisible fixed appliance. The small inter-bracket distance and the access, unfortunately, makes the use of lingual appliances difficult and time-consuming. In addition, the discomfort level on the tongue was significant and often intolerable. With the development of ceramic brackets in the late 1980s, another esthetic option for patients seeking orthodontic treatment became available. The ceramic bracket, however, still involved a bracket bonded onto the tooth and a metal archwire. Although esthetics was greatly improved over that of metal brackets, the orthodontic wire was still visible. Invisalign offers the advantages of superior esthetics and comfort as compared to all other appliances currently available.

Esthetics

There are numerous advantages of the Invisalign System. The main benefits are that the Invisalign aligners are clear, comfortable, and removable. Because aligners are clear, they are undetectable from a distance of at least 2 feet. Many adults and teenagers want their teeth straightened but are unwilling to wear a full set of conventional fixed appliances because of esthetic concerns. Like ceramic and plastic brackets, Invisalign is an esthetic alternative for straightening teeth: the difference is that aligners are removable. And because they are undetectable, patients can wear them during important personal or business matters. Invisalign is the most esthetic option (Figs 24-2a to 24-2e).

Removability

Aligners are removable. This allows patients to maintain their current oral hygiene practices. Patients can brush and floss normally, unfettered by brackets or wires. Also, patients do not need to change their diet or eating habits; they can eat or drink whatever they please with no fear of food sticking to or breaking their appliances. Patients can also remove their aligners for special occasions such as dinner parties.

Comfort

Aligners are comfortable and do not cause irritation to the cheeks or surrounding tissues, as can happen with wires or brackets. There is no need to dispense wax or provide patients with plastic sleeves to place over the appliances because there are no bulky brackets or wires.

Bonding to Enamel Defects

Invisalign can be used with patients for whom conventional fixed appliances are contraindicated because of metal or nickel allergies or the inability to bond appliances to teeth (as in cases of amelogenesis imperfecta). These types of cases present with hypocalcified enamel, which makes bonding to the teeth difficult (Figs 24-3a and 24-3b).

No Reported Root Resorption

There have been no reported cases in which a patient treated with Invisalign showed evidence of root resorption. Invisalign offers precisely controlled movements that can be specified by the treating clinician. Tooth movements can be reduced per aligner as requested by the clinician. Studies conducted at the University of the Pacific and the University of Florida have not shown any evidence of root resorption with the Invisalign appliance.[2] Based on the current University of Florida attachment study, which has 99 patients enrolled, there has been no incidence of root resorption.[2]

Less Discomfort and Pain

Adults who have had fixed appliances as adolescents and Invisalign treatment as adults have reported that treatment with Invisalign is more comfortable and induces less pain. Invisalign treatment is unique in that the treating clinician can specify to slow down movements programmed into each aligner in patients who have a lower pain threshold. The University of Florida conducted a study in which the treatment effects of Invisalign and fixed appliance therapy were compared during the initial week of treatment. The patients were asked to complete a questionnaire for the first 7 days. Patients treated with

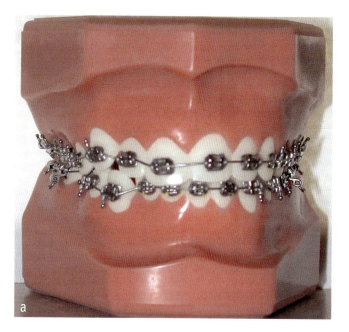

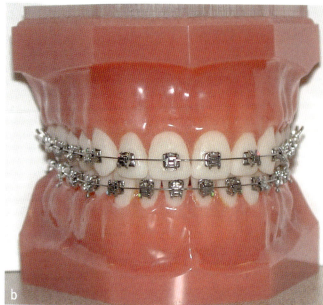

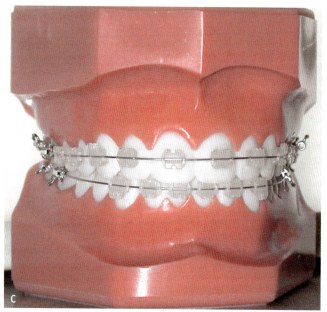

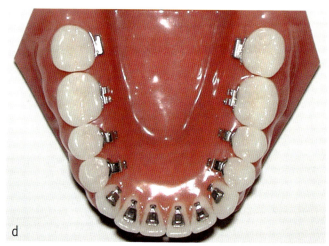

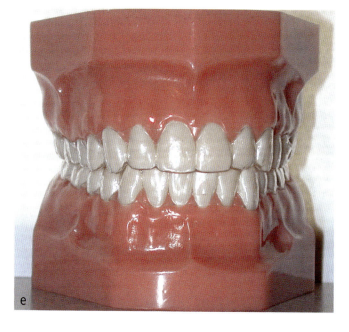

FIG 24-2 Comparison of the esthetics of orthodontic appliances: (*a*) metal brackets, (*b*) self-ligating brackets, (*c*) clear brackets, (*d*) lingual brackets, (*e*) Invisalign.

Invisalign reported less negative effects on their overall quality of life during the initial week. They also reported less pain from day 2 through day 7.[2]

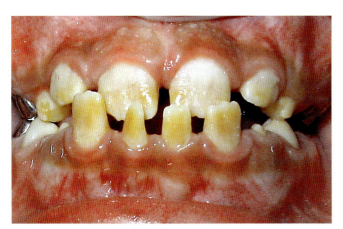

FIG 24-3a Amelogenesis imperfecta.

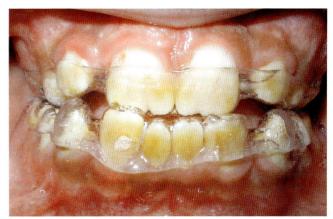

FIG 24-3b Amelogenesis treatment progress with Invisalign aligners in place.

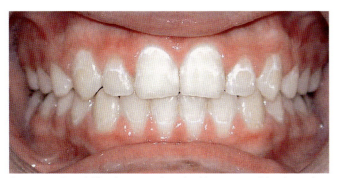

FIG 24-4a Decalcification associated with poor oral hygiene during fixed appliance therapy.

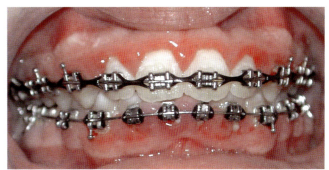

FIG 24-4b Poor oral hygiene during fixed appliance therapy causing gingivitis.

Hygiene

Oral hygiene is easier and better to maintain during Invisalign treatment than with fixed appliances. Because the Invisalign appliance is removable, it presents no obstacle to good oral hygiene, and thus poor hygiene with Invisalign is minimal. Brushing tools such as proxy brushes and floss threaders are not necessary. Adults who have had previous periodontal disease but are in good periodontal health have more difficulty maintaining good hygiene habits, especially during fixed appliance treatment. With Invisalign, these patients do well. A study has shown that there is an improvement in gingival health during treatment with Invisalign.[3] It is commonly known that decalcification (permanent markings), decay, or periodontal disease can occur if patients do not brush their teeth properly and thoroughly during fixed appliance treatment (Figs 24-4a and 24-4b). Patients treated with Invisalign have shown to have a lower incidence of decalcification or decay compared with those treated with fixed appliances.

Numerous Restorations or Crowns

Bonding brackets onto teeth that have crowns and restorations can be challenging. Although products such as hydrofluoric acid and porcelain primer can be used to bond onto crowns, the technique requires an extra step and is not predictable. In addition, using hydrofluoric acid requires the use of a rubber dam for safety because of its highly caustic effect on tissues. Treatment with Invisalign in these types of cases is ideal because the treating clinician can specify which teeth will not have attachments and therefore reduce or eliminate this challenge (Figs 24-5a and 24-5b).

Speech

The Invisalign appliance, since it does not cover the palate, does not affect speech. In contrast, Hawley retainers or quad-helix appliances are obtrusive and can affect speech and irritate the tongue (Figs 24-6a and 24-6b).

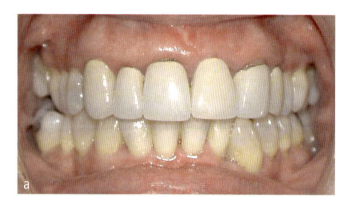

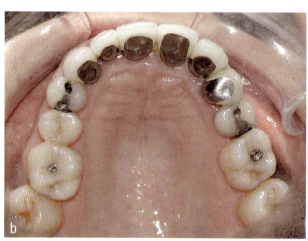

FIG 24-5 (a and b) Bonding is not an issue with patients who have numerous crown restorations.

Chair Time

With Invisalign, more of the clinician's time is invested up front for treatment planning with the use of ClinCheck. The advantage is that this time does not directly affect patient chair time. The chair time needed to monitor Invisalign patients is reduced. Treatment with Invisalign involves fewer instruments and inventory than treatment with fixed appliances (Figs 24-7a and 24-7b). There is no need for bands, wires, or brackets. Valuable chair time spent untying and tying A-lastics or C-chains is eliminated. All of the instruments and setup required for fixed appliances is eliminated. Office visits for patients undergoing Invisalign treatment involve the next set of aligners, a mirror, floss, and stripping instruments if interproximal reduction is part of the treatment plan. More staff time is spent on building patient relationships, which adds value to the practice. There is less armamentarium needed for each appointment. No large inventory of pliers is required, unless IPR is needed at the appointment.

Vertical Control

Invisalign has proved to be effective in controlling anterior open bite or shallow overbite. Unlike conventional fixed appliances, with which open bites can easily occur during the initial leveling stages, Invisalign treatment has been found to reduce this tendency. Because aligners cover the entire occlusal surface of the posterior teeth, they have a posterior bite block effect and as a result are excellent at controlling anterior open bites and open-bite tendencies (Figs 24-8a to 24-8c).

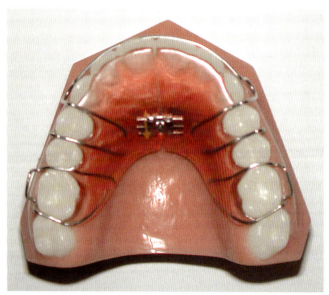

FIG 24-6a Hawley appliance covering palate.

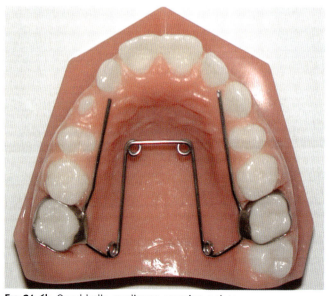

FIG 24-6b Quad-helix appliance covering palate.

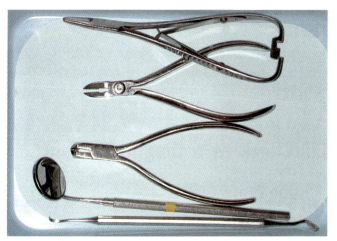

Fig 24-7a Basic instrument setup with fixed appliances.

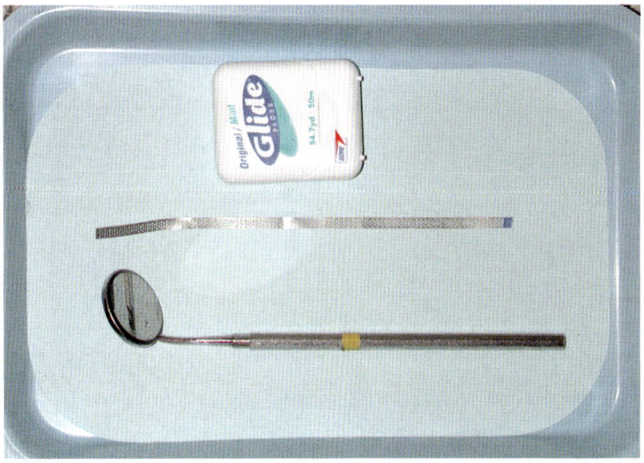

Fig 24-7b Basic instrument setup with Invisalign.

Treatment in Deep Bite Cases

Malocclusions with a deep overbite can be treated immediately in both arches and do not require bite planes or posterior bite blocks.

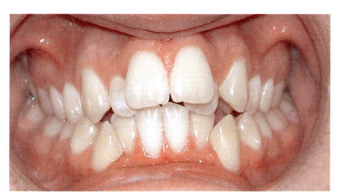

Fig 24-8a Initial photograph of an anterior open bite.

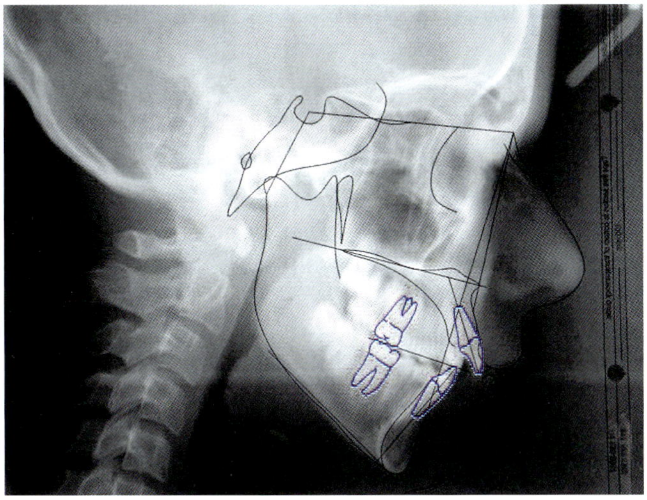

Fewer Emergencies

Emergencies with Invisalign treatment are fewer than with fixed appliances. There is no potential for broken brackets or protruding wires. Occasionally, there are instances where the patient loses an aligner or an aligner breaks, but neither situation requires immediate attention. For these situations, the patient can be seen the following day to arrange for a replacement aligner to be sent. More practically, depending on the timing, the patient may be able to simply advance to the next aligner. If this is not possible, the patient is usually advised to wear the previous aligner until the replacement arrives, which typically takes a few days. In some instances, the aligners may go off track, ie, they may no longer fit and the teeth are not moving to the desired positions. When this happens, the patient can call the doctor to schedule an appointment—this, too, is not an emergency.

Fig 24-8b Initial cephalogram.

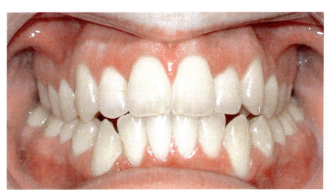

Fig 24-8c Progress: control of overbite.

Control of Individual Tooth Movements

Invisalign is unique in that the clinician can specify exactly which teeth are to be moved and which are to remain stable during treatment. With this option, for example, teeth with preexisting root resorption or fixed partial dentures can be programmed to remain stable during treatment.

Phase 2 Treatment

Invisalign treatment is recommended for patients that have a fully erupted dentition from second molar to second molar. A study of Invisalign treatment in adolescents showed that treatment in patients 12 to 18 years of age with a fully erupted dentition was effective (see chapter 29). When a patient has had phase 1 treatment during the mixed dentition to correct either habits, jaw discrepancies, or major alignment, by phase 2, he or she is usually tired of fixed appliance therapy. Invisalign can be used during phase 2 treatment once the permanent dentition is fully erupted. This provides a good change for the patient, as well as a great esthetic treatment at a time when physical appearance and social acceptance are of heightened importance.

Control of Bruxism

One advantage of aligner use in patients who suffer from bruxism or clenching habits is that the occlusal coverage acts as a protective barrier on the teeth. Therefore, during orthodontic treatment, there can be a reduction of wear facets that may occur from bruxism habits.

Special Patient Populations

Because of the removability and comfort of the aligner, Invisalign is the treatment of choice for athletes and patients who play instruments. The treatment does not interfere with the daily routine of an athlete or musician: they can always remove their aligners, when necessary, to compete or perform. Especially for athletes, the safety aspect of not having to worry about brackets breaking or irritation during sports is crucial. If an aligner is left in during sports, in a sense it acts as a mouth guard.

Bleaching During Treatment

An additional benefit is that, concurrent with Invisalign treatment, tooth bleaching can be administered. Thus, Invisalign can offer a full package of esthetic treatments.

ClinCheck as a Diagnostic Tool

One significant advantage of Invisalign treatment is the three-dimensional visualization of the treatment plan provided through ClinCheck. ClinCheck provides the first opportunity for the clinician to view the treatment from beginning to end before initiating treatment (see chapter 11).

Conclusion

Invisalign treatment offers patients a wide variety of advantages. Not only is Invisalign the most esthetically pleasing appliance available today, but it also can make orthodontic treatment more comfortable and convenient. Today, with the increasing development and use of digital and computer technology, a new generation of orthodontists is being developed. These orthodontists have the knowledge of the concepts and use of traditional fixed appliances, but are also schooled in the new technological tools that are available today. Those who can incorporate their scientific knowledge with technology and learn how to properly use them will have a distinct advantage in orthodontics today and in the future.

References

1. Patient census survey results. Bull Am Assoc Orthod 1997;15(4).
2. Miller K, Dolan T, Dolce C, McGorray S, Taylor M, Wheeler TT. A comparison of treatment impacts between Invisalign and fixed appliance therapy during the first seven days of treatment [poster presentation]. Presented at the Southern Association of Orthodontists Annual Meeting, New Orleans, October 2004.
3. Taylor MG, McGorray SP, Durrett S, et al. Effect of Invisalign aligners on periodontal tissues. Presented at the 32nd Annual Meeting and Exhibition of the American Association for Dental Research, San Antonio, March 2003.

chapter 25

REVIEW OF THE DIAGNOSTIC PROCESS

by
Robert L. Boyd, DDS

Just about all potential Invisalign patients require detailed explanation. They have seen the advertisements, talked to their dentists, or thoroughly explored the Invisalign website. But because orthodontic treatment has traditionally been associated with fixed appliances, patients may still believe that it is painful and that they have to come for appointments every month; most significantly, they may have the mindset that Invisalign treatment is faster.

Also, it is wrong to think that patients with certain malocclusions are better candidates for Invisalign treatment; but then, there are patients who can only be treated using fixed appliances. The importance of patient education cannot be overemphasized. Initially, it is best to have the treatment coordinator talk to the patient and explain what the Invisalign System is, how it works, and how important cooperation and compliance are for a successful outcome. This session with the patient, therefore, serves as an opportunity for the clinician to address mistaken impressions and to provide realistic expectations and understanding about orthodontic treatment. Specifically, it must be emphasized that Invisalign trays are not magical instruments that can correct everything. The patient has to realize that the process is painless, but that all the elements of the biology of tooth movement are still in effect.

The most important person in the patient-education process is the clinician. A focused question-and-answer conversation with the patient is critical. Obviously, the clinician must be well informed about Invisalign System appliance characteristics. This chapter provides an overview of a system that can be used to examine a patient and formulate a tentative treatment plan. A series of case reports is also presented to illustrate the potential of Invisalign treatment.

Initial Consultation

All prospective patients should be provided information about Invisalign treatment prior to their initial visit. This can be done by sending information about Invisalign with the initial health history (brochures are available from Align Technology), having the patient visit the Invisalign website, or developing your own website with this information.

Any staff member who comes in contact with the patient needs to be knowledgeable about the Invisalign System and ready to answer questions. This requires training that focuses on Invisalign treatment. The treatment coordinator should convey pertinent information about this patient and his or her concerns to the clinician before the clinician meets the patient.

Patients should be seated fully upright when introduced to the clinician. When initially speaking with the patient, the clinician should try to discover areas of mutual interest by asking patients about their own interests. The clinician should listen to the patient carefully rather than immediately respond or express opinions. A question-and-answer conversational style generally yields more meaningful information.

Clinical Examination

The following suggestions do not differ substantially from the general format followed for clinical examinations. After listening carefully to the patient's concerns, the clinician should determine the patient's true hopes and expectations for the treatment. The clinician should also determine if there are medical contraindications to treatment by carefully examining the medical history and asking follow-up questions where needed for additional information.

Then the clinician should ask the patient if it is agreeable to begin the initial clinical examination. The first thing to do is determine the patient's chief concern (eg, "crooked front teeth") in relation to his or her overall esthetic appearance. A good question to ask is, "What would you like to change about the way your teeth look?" and a follow-up question, "Are you satisfied with the color and shapes of your teeth?" Then the clinical exam starts with recording all relevant findings, preferably with an assistant taking notes as the clinician examines the patient. Things to note are:

The skeletal pattern (Class I, II, or III): This should be specific for explaining what skeletal proportion is not ideal. For example, a patient could have a retrognathic mandible or a protrusive maxilla.

Degree of lip competence: Lip length and thickness, and the way the lips relate to the nose and chin should be noted.

Symmetry: Are the dental midlines on? The middle of the philtrum should be used as a reference for the midline. The direction and amount (in millimeters) of deviation, if any, should be documented for both the maxillary and mandibular arch. If it is more than 2 mm, ask the patient if they have ever noticed this.

Analysis of the smile: The percentage of tooth display in speaking and full smile should be recorded. Does the lower lip follow the contour of the maxillary arch? Is the smile symmetric? Do the buccal corridors display excess space? Are the teeth as white as the patient wishes?

Analysis of the profile: Is the smile straight, convex, or concave from the side view? Are facial proportions balanced?

Frontal analysis: Deviation of the nose, alar base width, and chin deviation (which side and how many millimeters) should be noted. If noticeable asymmetries of the chin or nose are present, ask the patient, "Is there anything you would want to change about the way you look?" Avoid referring to any specific anatomic variation unless the patient brings this up as something he or she wants to change.

Analysis of the occlusion: Angle's classification of the molars and canines, overbite, overjet, presence of a cant of the occlusal plane, missing teeth, large restorations, and crossbites (anterior or posterior) should all be recorded. The clinician should also note whether centric relation is coincident with centric occlusion. If they are different, the degree (in millimeters) and direction of the mandibular movement should be recorded.

TMJ status: At the very least, maximum opening, jaw opening deviations, clicking and creptitus, muscle soreness on palpation, and history of pain must be established.

Periodontal status: The patient's ability to remove plaque and areas of poor plaque removal should be noted. Color variations, including red, edematous gingiva, should be recorded. The clinician should look for areas of thin gingiva (minimal attached gingiva) and gingival recession (especially in relation to labially prominent teeth), high frenum attachments, or gingival discolorations from amalgam or pigment. If all tissues appear healthy, at least all molars should be probed for increased pocket depth (greater than 3 mm) or bleeding upon gentle probing. All other areas of red or inflamed gingiva should be spot probed.

Decision About Treatment Feasibility

The primary conclusion that needs to be determined after this initial examination is whether the patient can be effectively treated with Invisalign. As with any other orthodontic appliance, it is very important that this decision take into consideration the level of the clinician's expertise using Invisalign. Many times the clinician will have to tell the patient that additional diagnostic records (panoramic or periapical radiographs, intraoral and extraoral photographs, cephalometric evaluation, periodontal evaluation, radiographs of the temporomandibular joint, etc) are necessary to make the final diagnosis and treatment plan. The clinician may wish to e-mail the digital photographs to Align Technology for an answer about the feasibility of treatment. A response can be provided at no charge within 48 hours.

Invisalign can provide predictable treatment in the following situations:

Patients who do not want fixed appliances. Patients who had orthodontic treatment before as adolescents frequently do not want fixed appliances again. They may also be extremely focused on esthetic issues, perhaps if they have a high public visibility. Fear of pain is another reason why many patients do not want fixed appliances. Many times high-school-age (ie, 15- to 18-year-old) adolescents are strongly motivated for improved esthetics of their smile but are not interested in having fixed appliances.

Functional posterior occlusion. A patient whose only complaint is the appearance of the teeth themselves is usually a good candidate for treatment, especially if there is a stable posterior occlusion.

Patients who do not require extensive restoration of anterior teeth. Patients who need extensive restoration of anterior teeth should be presented alternatives, such as restoration of the anterior teeth, that may be able to solve their esthetic concerns without orthodontic treatment. Many times, Invisalign treatment to improve tooth positions will create a situation in which less invasive restorative dentistry can be done. The improved tooth positions will necessitate lesser amounts of tooth reduction for placement of laminate veneers.

Patients who require primarily tipping movements. If the malocclusion can be solved primarily by mild amounts of proclination or expansion, the patient is usually a very good candidate for Invisalign.

Patients who are periodontally compromised or have high caries rates. Two published studies have found that there is less plaque and gingivitis during Invisalign treatment than before treatment.[1-3] This is in contrast to other studies that show an increase in plaque and gingivitis with fixed appliances.[4,5] Patients with a high caries rate can be better managed with Invisalign than with fixed appliances because of the decreased plaque retention and increased access to interproximal areas.

Patients who require prosthetic treatment. Coordination of prosthetic treatment is facilitated with Invisalign. The numerous trial treatments done on the ClinCheck images allow for testing the prosthetic result before the treatment actually starts. The restorative dentist can show patients virtual treatments with tooth replacements, and the patients will better understand the proposed treatment.

Patients with short roots or increased susceptibility to root resorption. A recent study showed that root resorption is not measurable with Invisalign treatment (Wheeler T, unpublished data, 2006). This is in contrast to fixed appliances, with which 10% of patients generally show clinically significant root resorption of 3 mm or more.[6]

Patients with shallow overbite or slight open bite. Because of the intrusive effect on the posterior teeth during aligner wear, overbite is usually improved by 1 to 2 mm during treatment. In contrast, fixed appliances generally have a small degree of bite opening effect on patients with edge-to-edge or slightly open bite malocclusions.[5]

Patients who have excessive wear on their teeth. Patients who grind or brux their teeth have no way to stop this problem during orthodontic treatment with fixed appliances unless they wear an appliance such as a nightguard during treatment, which is difficult for the patient to do. Invisalign creates a layer of plastic material between the teeth to prevent additional wear.

Patients with myofacial pain. Numerous studies have shown that single or double splints placed between the teeth disarticulate the teeth and decrease the effects of muscle soreness.[7] A recent study by Nedwed and Miethke[8] showed no increase in myofacial pain during Invisalign treatment.

Patients with mild Class II (end-on) malocclusion with acceptable facial esthetics and mild crowding. Use of Class II elastics and/or molar distalization of 2 to 3 mm is a predictable movement with Invisalign without opening the bite as fixed appliances frequently do. This is because molar distalization is usually associated with molar extrusion and loss of anchorage with flaring of the anterior teeth.

Patients with extensive porcelain, gold, or other restorations. Bonding and debonding procedures pose certain risk factors for these restorations and can be avoided with Invisalign.

Deep overbite. Generally with fixed appliances, a progression through initial archwires to a larger-diameter wire is necessary before significant bite opening can occur. This treatment may require 6 to 12 months, depending on the severity of the deep bite. In addition, fixed or removable bite-separating appliances may also be necessary to hold the teeth apart to prevent the occlusion from loosening fixed appliances. Wheeler (unpublished data, 2006) has shown that intrusion is one of the most predictable movements that can be achieved with Invisalign.

Anterior and posterior crossbites. For the same reason as in the case of deep overbite (clearance of tooth interferences), anterior and posterior crossbites can be more easily managed with Invisalign than fixed appliances because aligners provide disarticulation for the teeth and smooth surfaces for teeth to slide over each other without the need for bite-opening appliances.

Problem List and Treatment Goals

The next step is to formulate a problem list, which will help the clinician focus on the best solutions. This should include all of the issues that the patient presented with and the problems identified by the clinician at the initial exam.

Specific solutions to each of the problems are needed to be sure all of the problems are taken into account with the proposed treatment plan. The problem list and solutions will then serve as the basis of the treatment goals and objectives.

Treatment Plan

A sequenced step-by-step treatment plan is required to create the desired tooth movement that will fulfill the goals and objectives. This should include all other treatments such as periodontal, endodontic, restorative, and retention. Referring back to this list throughout treatment will ensure that the correct order of treatment priorities was maintained.

Treated Cases

The cases illustrated in Figs 25-1 to 25-28 show types of treatment possible with Invisalign. They are arranged in order of increasing difficulty. It is especially important to carefully analyze the face initially to determine the degree of lip support, midlines, overjet/overbite relationships, arch form, esthetics of the smile, and the areas mentioned in the beginning of this chapter. Each case includes still

Figs 25-1 to 25-4 Patient 1.

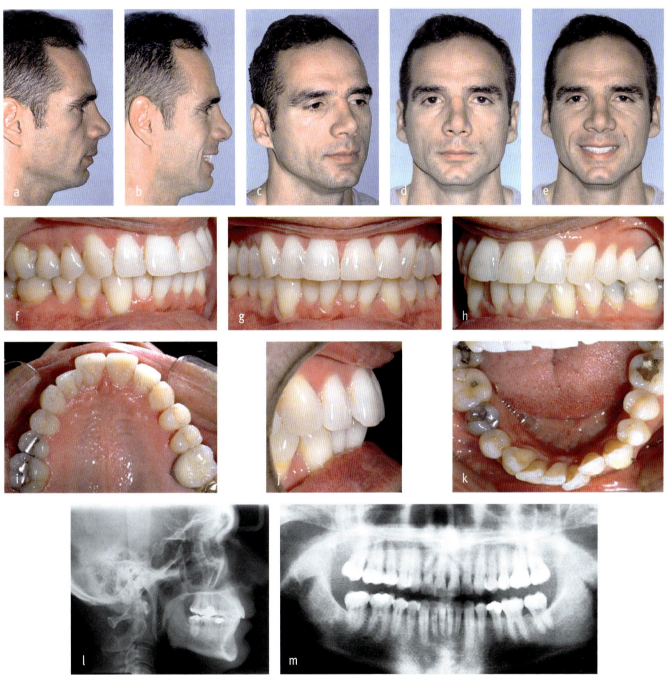

Fig 25-1 (a to m) This patient presented with the chief complaint of crowded teeth. The patient was very particular about his appearance. He liked his facial appearance and balance. The dimple in his chin was important. Radiographically, there were no findings of concern. After an attentive interview session with the patient and review of records, the decision was made to procline the incisors, perform interproximal reduction, and expand the dental arches.

photos of the beginning and final stage ClinChecks that were approved for the patient. It is important to analyze each of these ClinChecks to determine how close the actual results are to the final occlusion. Unfortunately, it is not possible to show the actual movement of the teeth in this printed form. However, the actual paths of movement and staging need to be carefully analyzed for correctness of biomechanics of movement, anchorage, and final tooth position using the Superimposition tool (see chapter 14).

An informed consent form such as the one shown in Fig 25-29 will be helpful to ensure good patient cooperation and uneventful progress of treatment.

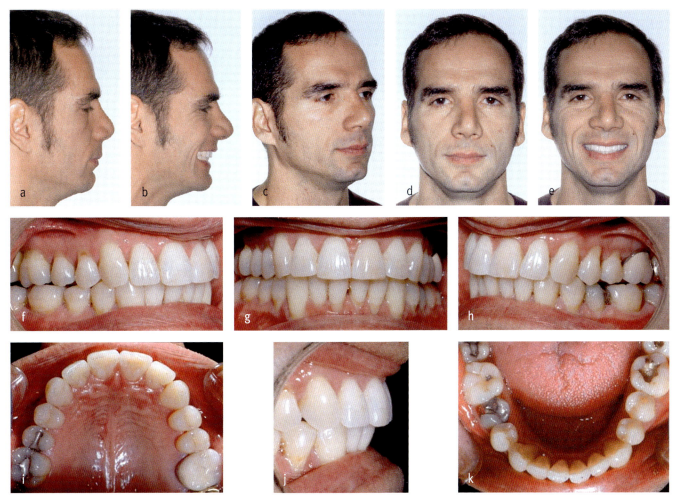

FIG 25-3 (a to k) The final result images display the characteristic posterior open bite. Despite this opening, however, the deep bite was improved. Note the disappearance of the canine tip and conservation of tooth morphology especially in the anterior segments. Teeth were slightly reduced mesiodistally, which helped reduce the presence of dark, open spaces interproximally (commonly referred to as "black triangles"). Also note the correction of the crossbite of the right second molars. The usual retention plan is to have the patient wear retainers full time for 4 to 6 months and then during sleep indefinitely. Patients are told retainer wear reduces tooth wear from nighttime bruxing and can also be used for periodic home bleaching. Once retainers are worn during sleep only, the slight posterior open bite closes within 4 to 6 weeks.

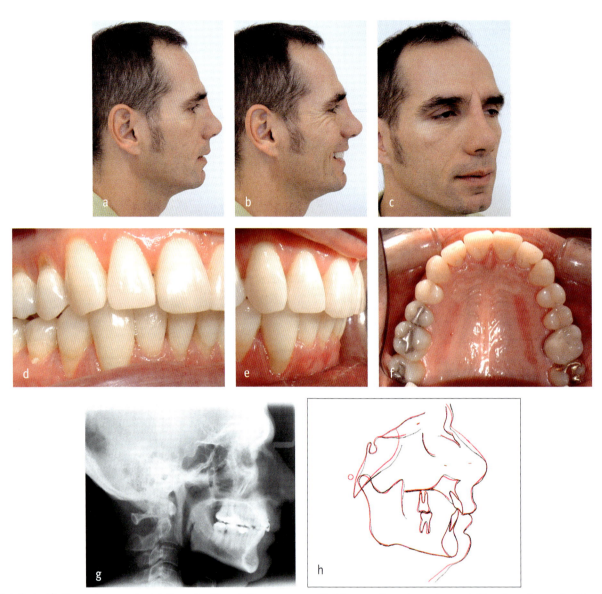

FIG 25-4 (a to h) These images depict the retention at the 3-year recall. All corrections have been stable since the end of treatment. The patient has been compliant with his retainers. Clearly, as in all cases, this patient's cooperation made a significant difference. The superimposed cephalometric tracings reveal the conservative nature of this particular treatment plan.

FIGS 25-5 TO 25-7 Patient 2.

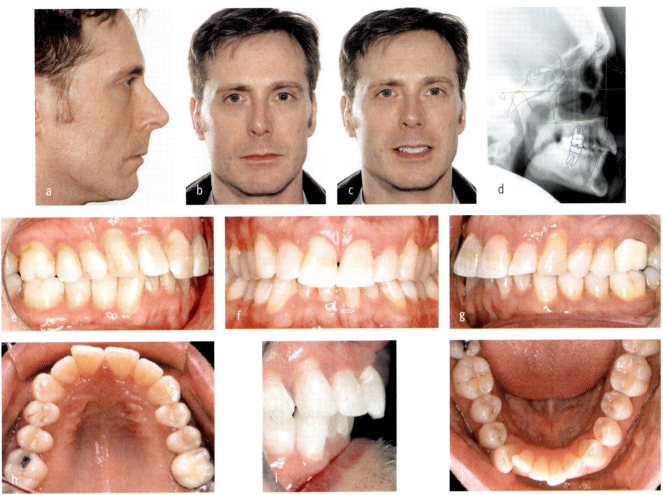

FIG 25-5 (a to j) This patient's chief complaint was that his teeth were "shifting" and "overlapped." The angular nature of his chin disguised the retrognathism, and the lips were competent. The position of the maxillary incisors was within esthetic norms, but his canine and molar occlusion was end-on. After working with the ClinCheck images (see Figs 25-6a to 25-6j), the decision was made not to disturb the posterior and canine occlusion, but rather open the bite, slightly expand the arches to gain more space, and eliminate the "black triangles" through interproximal reduction.

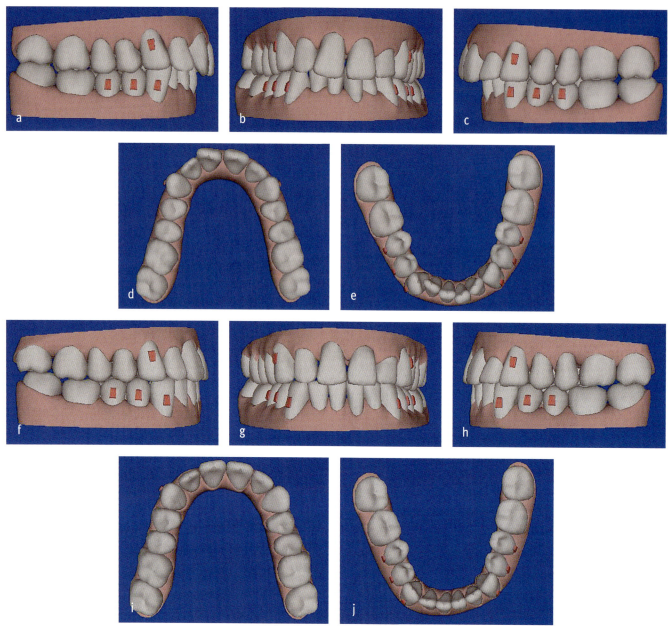

Fig 25-6 Comparison of these ClinCheck images (*a to e*, preoperative; *f to j*, treatment goal) and the end-of-treatment records show that the goals of treatment were achievable.

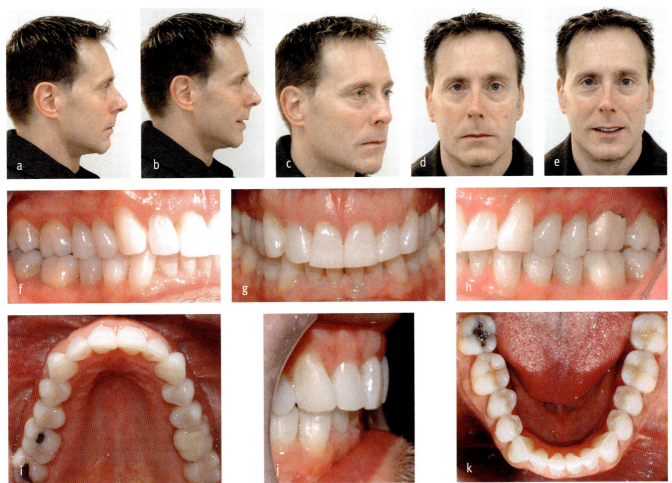

FIG 25-7 (a to k) Three years after the end of active treatment, the result is stable. Note the improved tooth morphology and profile appearance. The patient also bleached his teeth with a 30% carbamide peroxide gel, using his aligners as bleaching trays. His excellent cooperation during active treatment was essential to the results and their retention.

FIGS 25-8 TO 25-11 Patient 3.

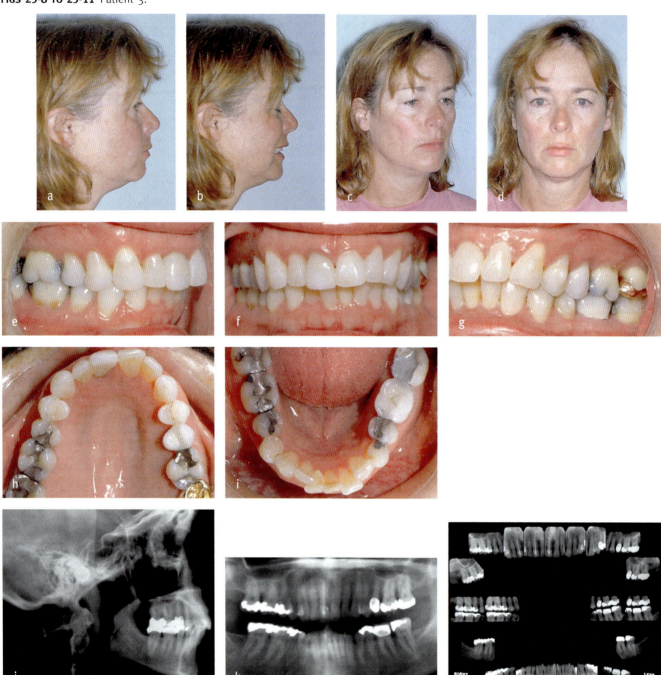

FIG 25-8 (a to l) The chief complaint of this 53-year-old patient was the overlap of her anterior teeth. She reported a history of trauma and endodontic treatment (at age 13) on the maxillary right central incisor. She had orthodontic treatment as a teenager, and her orthodontist had informed her that this tooth was ankylosed. Facial esthetics were good, and occlusion was Class I with a moderate overbite. Radiographic examination showed extensive restorative work, but this did not contraindicate orthodontic treatment. After her previous fixed orthodontic treatment, which included extraction of the four first premolars, the patient was not compliant with her retainers and stopped wearing them shortly after receiving them. The return of crowding, however, was slow. Perhaps because it was ankylosed, the maxillary right central incisor was in an acceptable position. The patient did not want fixed appliances again and decided to have Invisalign treatment. The treatment plan was to keep the maxillary right central incisor in its current position and resolve the crowding. This approach necessitated significant interproximal reduction (IPR) and slight expansion. IPR was further necessary to eliminate the black triangles between her anterior teeth.

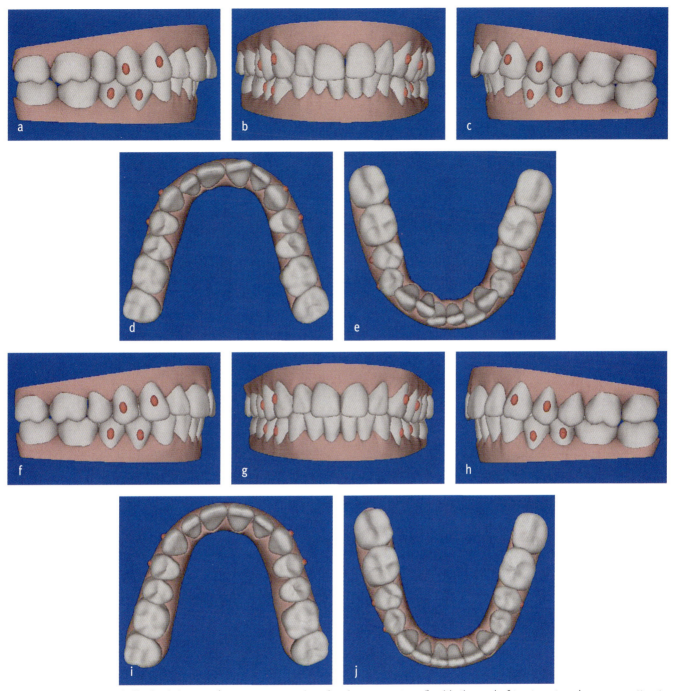

FIG 25-9 Comparison of ClinCheck images (*a to e*, preoperative; *f to j*, treatment goal) with the end-of-treatment and 3-year posttreatment images shows that the goals of treatment were achievable.

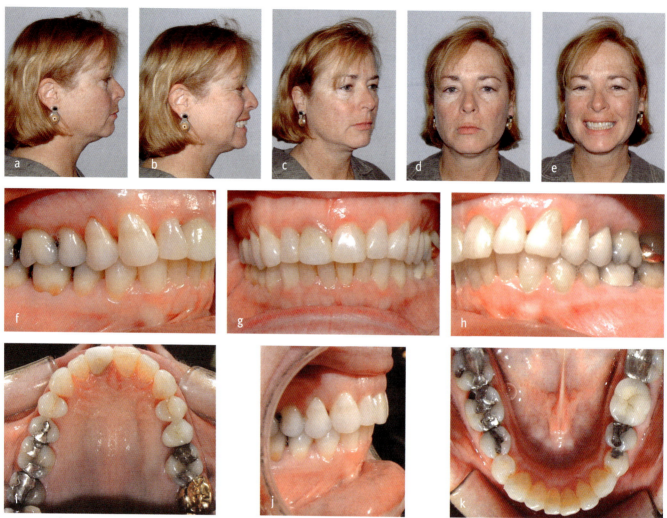

FIG 25-10 (a to k) Posttreatment success. ClinCheck predictions have been accomplished. An esthetically pleasing smile is present. Fourteen months of Invisalign treatment, including one series of case-refinement aligners, was required to correct the crowding.

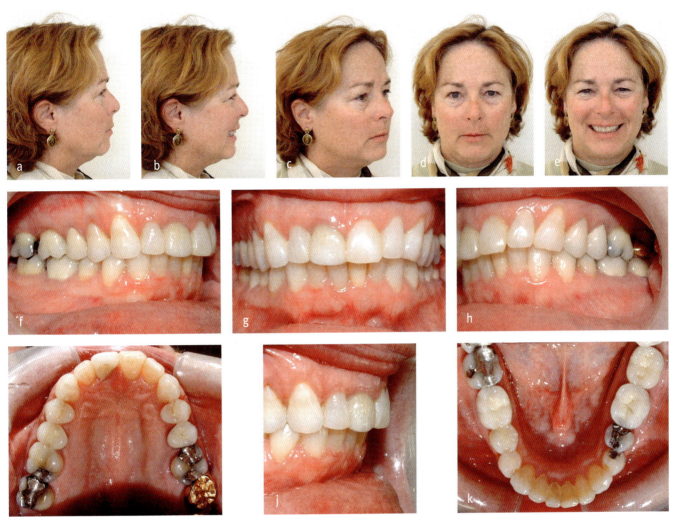

FIG 25-11 (a to k) The 3-year posttreatment images reveal that the end result was maintained successfully. These photos indicate stability of the orthodontic treatment with nighttime wear of retainers. Note that the improvement of the gingival recession of the mandibular left central incisor was maintained without the need for an epithelial graft as initially planned.

FIGS 25-12 TO 25-15 Patient 4.

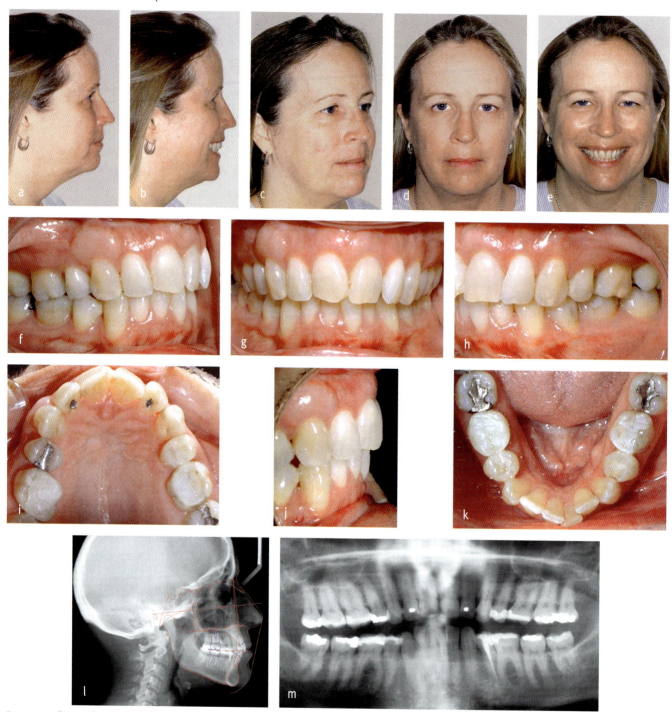

FIG 25-12 (a to m) The chief complaint of this patient was the mandibular incisor crowding and chipped maxillary incisors. She had orthodontic treatment with first premolar extractions as a teenager. She stopped wearing her retainers shortly after removal of the appliances. The patient preferred a broader smile, so the treatment plan was to expand her arches slightly and to improve the overjet, eliminate crowding, and establish better intercuspation. An epithelial graft had been previously placed on the maxillary right canine because of gingival recession, and another graft was planned for placement on the mandibular left central incisor, which was in labioversion. Space was created with posterior arch expansion and interproximal reduction in the mandibular arch. Care was taken not to move the mandibular left central incisor labially, and instructions were given to the Invisalign computer operator at the time of the ClinCheck to have this tooth's root moved lingually to encourage coronal movement of the gingival tissue. This was successful, and the posttreatment epithelial graft was not needed. It is also important to note that the chipped incisors were rounded off before the impressions were made so that the esthetic appearance was maintained throughout treatment.

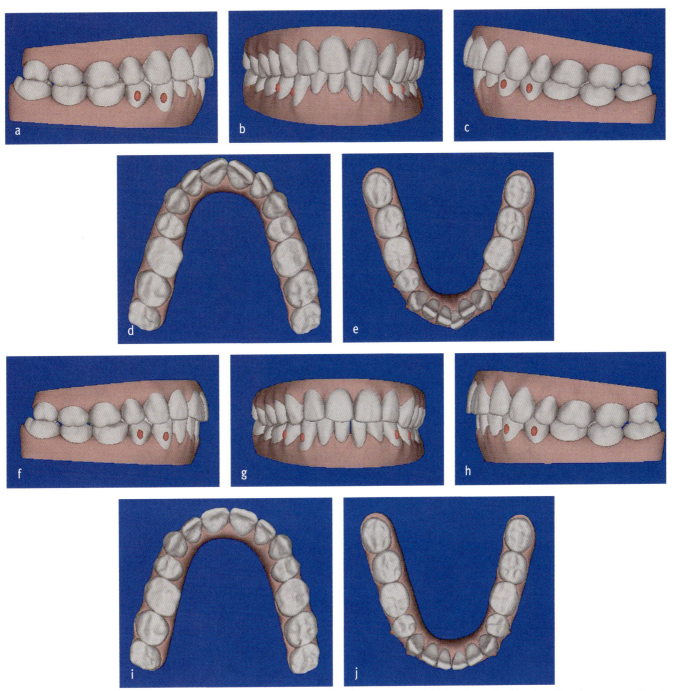

FIG 25-13 Comparison of ClinCheck images (*a to e*, preoperative; *f to j*, treatment goal) with the end-of-treatment and 3-year posttreatment images show that the goals of treatment were achievable.

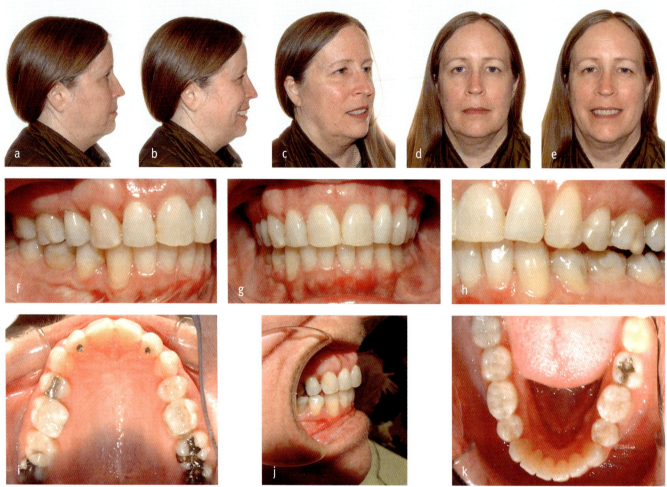

FIG 25-14 (a to k) The final result is as the ClinCheck images had predicted. Note improvement in the length of the clinical crown of the mandibular left central incisor due to the root being moved into the ridge. The maxillary midline was centered. The posterior occlusion was satisfactory, so no attempt was made to correct the mandibular midline, which was offset 1 mm to the right.

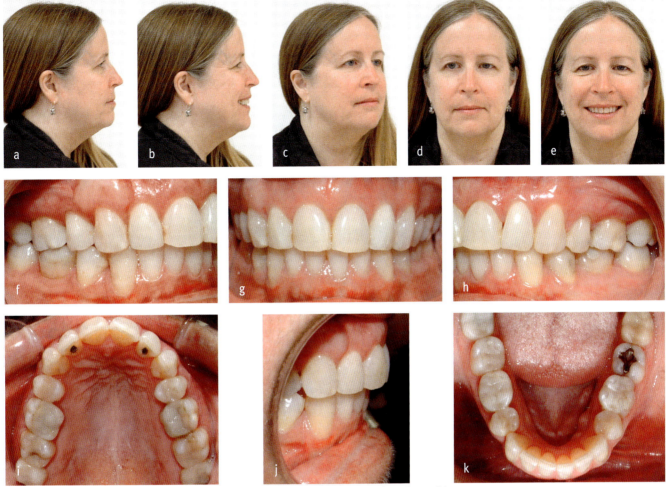

FIG 25-15 (a to k) The 3-year posttreatment photographs show the end result to be stable.

FIGS 25-16 TO 25-19 Patient 5.

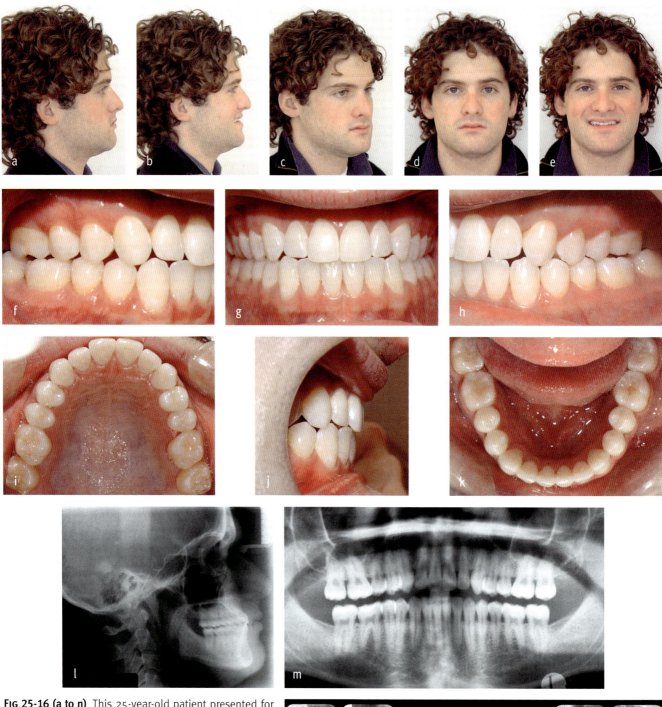

FIG 25-16 (a to n) This 25-year-old patient presented for an orthodontic evaluation complaining that his teeth had shifted since being treated with fixed appliances. Examination revealed that he had minor relapse of his occlusion, which had been corrected to a normal overbite/overjet and Class I posterior occlusion. He still wore his retainers. Further examination revealed that this patient most likely had later mandibular growth, which caused his well-aligned teeth to move into an edge-to-edge (Class III) anterior overjet relationship, with the midlines off by 1 mm. Radiographically, no concerns were noted. The patient wanted only Invisalign treatment if possible.

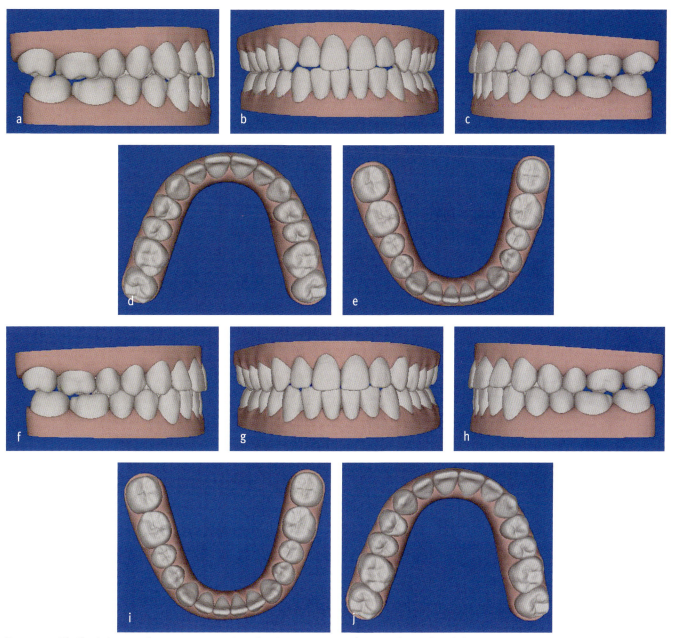

Fig 25-17 ClinCheck images (*a to e*, preoperative; *f to j*, treatment goal) correctly predicted the possible outcome.

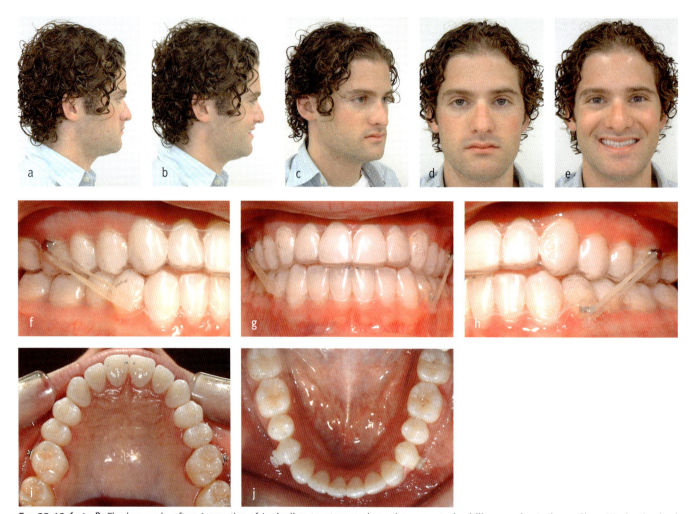

FIG 25-18 (a to j) Final records after 6 months of Invisalign treatment show the corrected midlines and rotations. Class III elastics had to be worn to correct the anteroposterior relationship. For this reason, clear buttons on the mandibular canines and metal buttons on the maxillary first molars were placed during treatment.

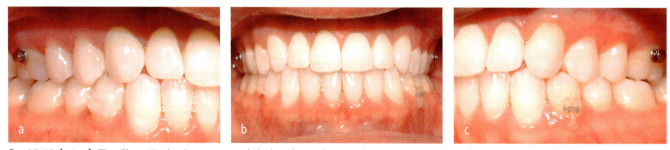

FIG 25-19 (a to c) The Class III elastics were used during the early retention stages. Retainer aligners were cut back 2 to 3 mm on the buccal to create space to place these buttons. Four-ounce elastics were used for these interarch mechanics.

Figs 25-20 to 25-23 Patient 6.

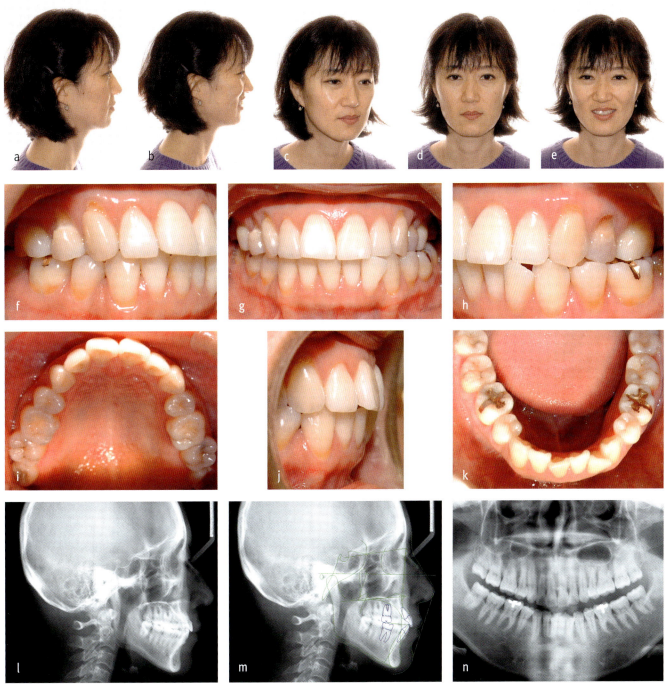

Fig 25-20 (a to n) This 33-year-old patient presented with a chief complaint of "crooked front teeth." She had excellent facial esthetics with competent lips and a Class I occlusion with a unilateral posterior crossbite on the left side. There was 3-mm maxillary and 5-mm mandibular arch crowding. Overbite and overjet were normal. The maxillary midline was centered, but the mandibular midline was deviated 2 mm to the left. Radiographic analysis indicated that her skeletal pattern was well balanced.

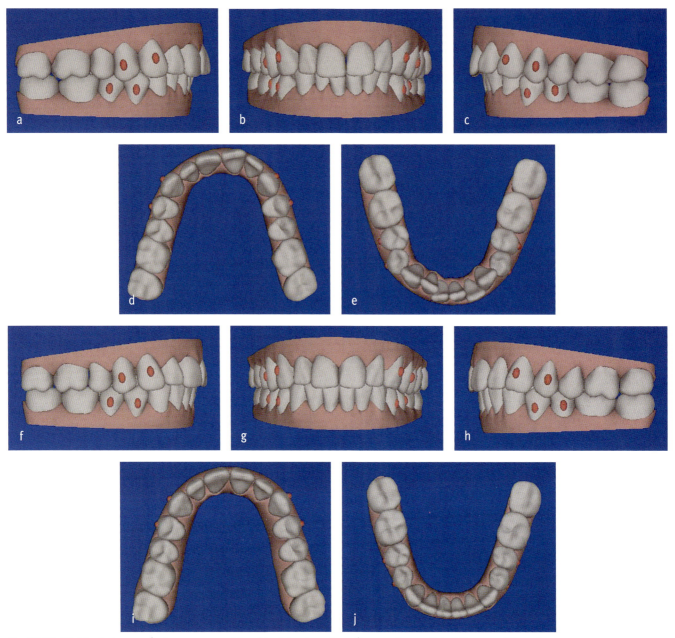

Fig 25-21 ClinCheck images (*a to e*, preoperative; *f to j*, treatment goal) correctly predicted the possible outcome.

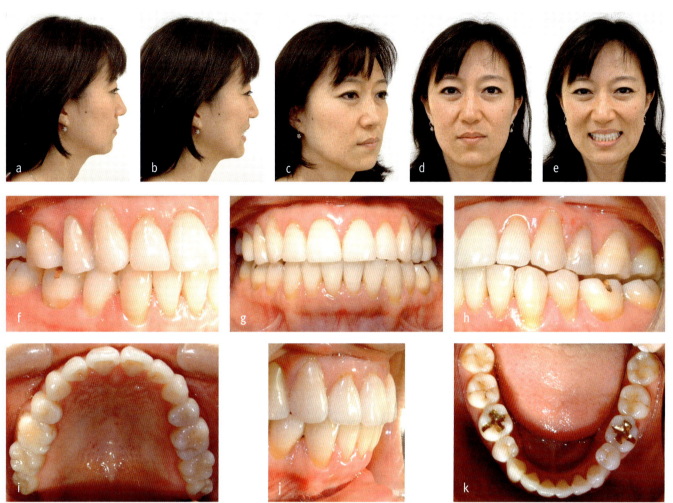

FIG 25-22 (a to k) Posttreatment photographs show correction of the posterior crossbite and alignment of the maxillary and mandibular anterior teeth. The maxillary crowding and posterior crossbite were corrected by expansion. Mandibular crowding was corrected by expansion and interproximal reduction.

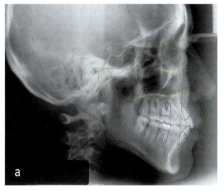

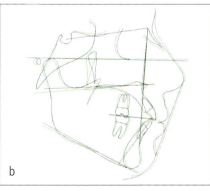

FIG 25-23 (a to c) Cephalometric radiograph and tracing reveal a well-executed Invisalign treatment for this patient. Note that the mandibular plane angle decreased 2 degrees, which reflects excellent vertical control during the posterior crossbite correction. (*c*) (tx) treatment; (S) sella; (N) nasion; (A) point A; (B) point B; (WITS) Wits analysis; (FMIA) Frankfort–mandibular incisor angle; (FMA) Frankfort–mandibular plane angle; (IMPA) incisor–mandibular plane angle; (Go) gonion; (Gn) gnathion; (U1) maxillary central incisor; (L1) mandibular central incisor; (IIA) interincisal angle; (Pog) pogonion. All measurements in degrees, unless otherwise noted.

Measures	Pre-tx	Post-tx	Normal
SNA	77	77	82
SNB	77	77	80
ANB	0	0	2
WITS (mm)	−3	−3	0
FMIA	58	57	65
FMA	29	28	22
IMPA	92	95	90
SN-GoGn	39	37	33
U1-SN	107	109	102
U1-NA (degrees/mm)	30/11	31/11	22/4
L1-NB	29/8	30/7	25/4
IIA	121	117	130
POG-NB (mm)	1.5	1.8	2

c

FIGS 25-24 TO 25-28 Patient 7.

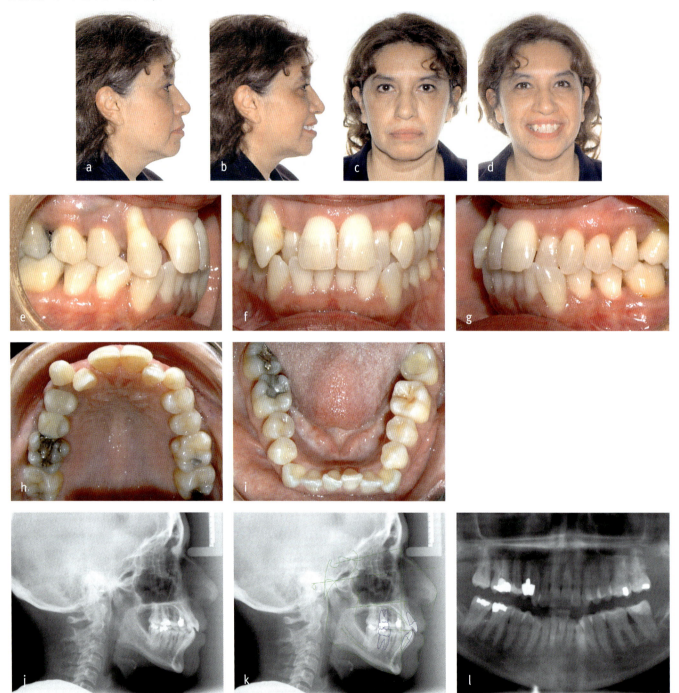

FIG 25-24 (a to l) This 46-year-old patient desired to have the moderate maxillary and mandibular crowding corrected specifically with Invisalign. She had previously declined a four-premolar-extraction treatment by another orthodontist. Mild protrusion was present, but the patient was satisfied with her facial appearance, and her lips were competent. She had a Class I posterior occlusion with anterior crossbite of both maxillary lateral incisors. The maxillary right canine had significant loss of clinical crown length as a result of previous periodontal disease. At initial presentation, she was in periodontal maintenance and had not lost additional bone in 4 years.

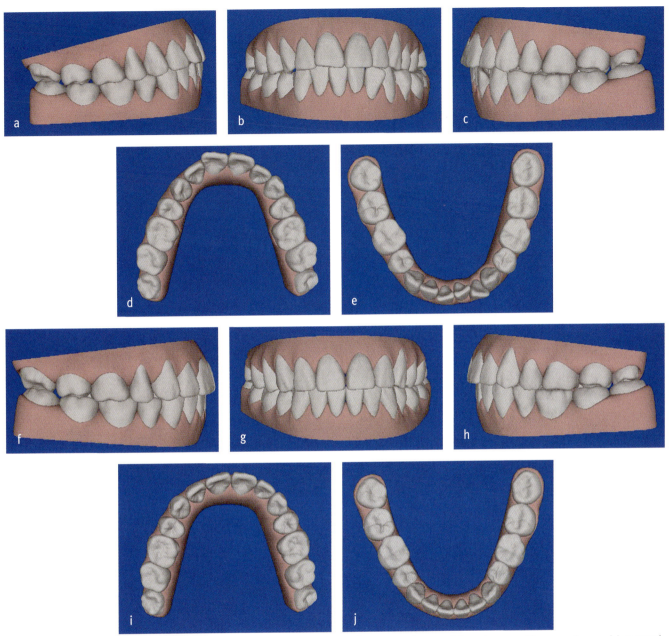

FIG 25-25 ClinCheck images (*a to e*, preoperative; *f to j*, treatment goal) suggested a possible outcome with expansion and interproximal reduction (IPR).

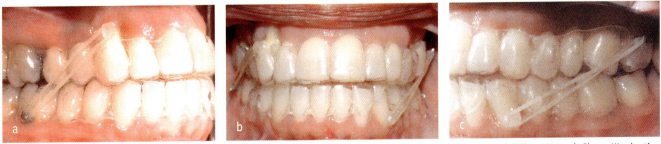

FIG 25-26 (a to c) Note the traditional use of midline elastics. Midlines were corrected by asymmetric Class II and Class III elastics attached to the teeth on clear buttons.

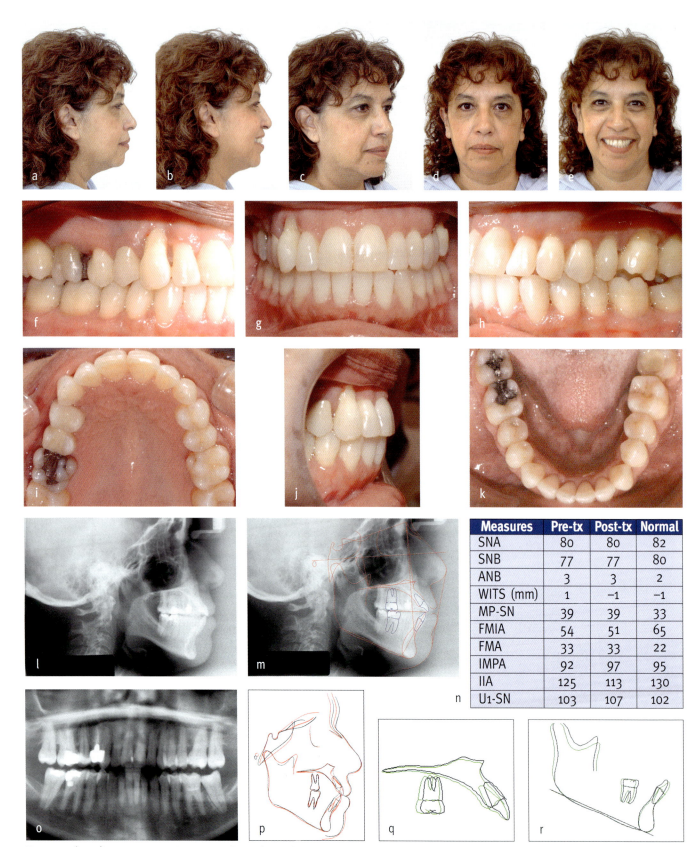

Measures	Pre-tx	Post-tx	Normal
SNA	80	80	82
SNB	77	77	80
ANB	3	3	2
WITS (mm)	1	−1	−1
MP-SN	39	39	33
FMIA	54	51	65
FMA	33	33	22
IMPA	92	97	95
IIA	125	113	130
U1-SN	103	107	102

Fig 25-27 (a to r) Posttreatment images. Radiographic evidence reveals a well-executed Invisalign treatment. Correction of crowding was accomplished by creating space by IPR, posterior expansion, and distal movement of posterior teeth into the space gained by IPR. The cephalometric superimposition does not show an increase in protrusion. (*n*) (tx) treatment; (S) sella; (N) nasion; (A) point A; (B) point B; (WITS) Wits analysis; (MP) mandibular plane; (FMIA) Frankfort–mandibular incisor angle; (FMA) Frankfort–mandibular plane angle; (IMPA) incisor–mandibular plane angle; (IIA) interincisal angle; (U1) maxillary central incisor. All measurements are in degrees unless otherwise noted.

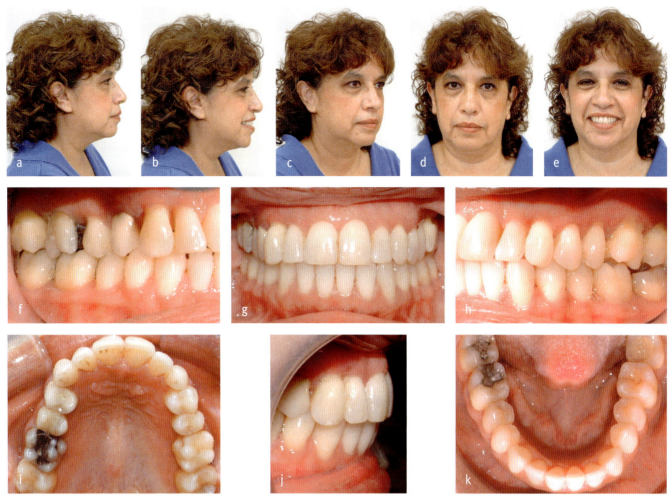

FIG 25-28 (a to k) Postretention figures. Note the improvement in the length of the clinical crown of the maxillary right canine, which was achieved because it was retracted lingually and the root was moved lingually into the ridge. Placement of a graft further improved the crown length. The corrected occlusion was stable with diligent nighttime wear of clear retainers.

Invisalign Patient Cooperation Acknowledgment
for Orthodontic Treatment with Dr _____

Your orthodontist is dedicated to providing you the best possible Invisalign treatment. To ensure that your Invisalign treatment progresses on schedule and as smoothly as possible, it is imperative that you understand the following procedures that are involved in your treatment.

- Make sure with your general dentist that **all cleanings, fillings, or other dental work is completed prior to starting your Invisalign treatment.**
- **Please maintain your usual frequency of appointments with your general dentist** during and after Invisalign treatment.
- **Aligners must be worn at least 22 hours a day.** The only exceptions are when eating, drinking, brushing, or flossing. Please remember that Invisalign only works while you are wearing your Aligners!
- **Small tooth-colored attachments are frequently attached to your teeth.** These attachments are nearly invisible and will aid the Aligners in moving your teeth properly.
- **Whenever possible, keep teeth together** (not clenching) especially for the first 3–4 days after changing Aligners, as this speeds up the fit and efficiency of treatment.
- **Many patients want to bleach their teeth** during treatment using their Aligners. Ask us about this benefit, as it is included in the cost of your Invisalign treatment.
- **It is critical that you follow the instructions covered in the use and care pamphlet in the Patient Starter Kit** regarding inserting and removing the Aligners, cleaning the Aligners, and proper brushing and flossing.
- **Always store your Aligners in their case** when they are not being worn to avoid loss. If you lose an Aligner, it will cost you $75.00 per Aligner to replace.
- **It is your responsibility to make sure you do not go to the next Aligner unless the Aligner fits completely with no space between the teeth and Aligner.** If you notice that the Aligner has space when due for a change in Aligners, you should keep that Aligner until it fits with no space.
- Because the Aligners are designed to sequentially move your teeth, it is very important to **wear each Aligner in the order prescribed by your orthodontist.** Usually you will wear each Aligner for about two weeks, but sometimes a few days to a week longer is required if wear is less than 22 hrs/day. Do not wear Aligners out of order.
- **Always keep at least the last 3 Aligners** in case of loss of a presently used Aligner or in case an Aligner does not fit. Your orthodontist may go back in sequence to catch up to have Aligners correctly fit.
- **Modifications to your Aligners or several additional Aligners or occasionally regular (clear) braces may be needed at the end of your treatment** in order to completely finish your treatment.
- After your treatment is complete, **clear** retainers are designed to maintain the smile you've invested in. Usually you will wear these for **6 months full time and then indefinitely at night while sleeping.**
- **Keep your scheduled appointments**—this is the only way we can be sure that your treatment is progressing as planned.
- I consent to the making of orthodontic records, including x-rays, photographs, prescriptions, and other information which may include personal identification, before, during, and after treatment, and to the orthodontic treatment prescribed by my doctor. I also consent to my doctor and/or Align Technology forwarding any of my orthodontic records to other licensed dentists and organizations employing licensed dentists for the purpose of consulting regarding my treatment.
- Finally, I consent to the use of my orthodontic records (eg, dental x-rays, photographs, and plaster models) for purposes of orthodontic consultations, educational and research purposes, publication in professional journals, or use in professional collateral materials, but not to use or disclosure of my specific name, address, or other personal identification information.
- Please don't hesitate to call our office if you should have any questions or problems with your Aligners.

I have read and understand these tips to my successful Invisalign treatment.

Patient Signature _____ Date _____

Parent/Guardian Signature _____ Date _____

Fig 25-29 *(left)* Informed consent form.

References

1. Bollen A, Huang G, King G, Hujoel P, Ma T. Activation time and material stiffness of sequential removable orthodontic appliances. Part 1: Ability to complete treatment. Am J Orthod Dentofacial Orthop 2003;124:496–501.
2. Clements KM, Bollen AM, Huang G, King G, Hujoel P, Ma T. Activation time and material stiffness of sequential removable orthodontic appliances. Part 2: Dental improvements. Am J Orthod Dentofacial Orthop 2003;124:502–508.
3. Taylor MG, McGorray SP, Durrett S, et al. Effect of Invisalign Aligners on periodontal tissues [abstract]. J Dent Res 2003;82(special issue A):1483.
4. Boyd RL. Longitudinal evaluation of a system for self-monitoring plaque control effectiveness in orthodontic patients. J Clin Periodontol 1983;10:380–388.
5. Boyd RL, Leggott PJ, Quinn RS, Eakle WS, Chambers D. Periodontal implications of orthodontic treatment in adults with reduced or normal periodontal tissues versus those of adolescents. Am J Orthod Dentofacial Orthop 1989;96:191–198.
6. Baumrind S, Korn EL, Boyd RL. Apical root resorption in orthodontically treated adults. Am J Orthod Dentofacial Orthop 1996;110:311–320.
7. Johnston LE. A systems analysis of occlusion. In: Carlson D, McNamara J, Ribbens K (eds). Developmental Aspects of Temporomandibular Disorders, monograph 16, Craniofacial Growth Series. Ann Arbor, MI: University of Michigan Press, 1985:191–205.
8. Nedwed R, Miethke RR. Motivation, acceptance and problems of Invisalign patients. J Orofac Orthop 2005;66:162–173.

chapter 26

INTERPROXIMAL ENAMEL REDUCTION

by
Rainer-Reginald Miethke, Prof Dr Med Dent and
Paul-Georg Jost-Brinkmann, Prof Dr Med Dent

Most patients seek orthodontic treatment because of crowding. According to a 2003 study by Meier et al,[1] 87% of randomly interviewed individuals interested in orthodontic treatment with the Invisalign System displayed various severities of crowding. Crowding problems may be eliminated by creating sufficient space. The traditional means to accomplish this are extraction of posterior teeth (mostly premolars) or incisors (mainly in the mandible), expansion (mainly in the sagittal plane, and to a limited degree also in the transverse plane), and interproximal enamel reduction (IPR). The appropriateness of these procedures for a given malocclusion depends on many factors.

IPR has several notable advantages, especially when patients are treated with the Invisalign System. In the course of treatment, it might become obvious that teeth collide, though this should have been noticed already in the ClinCheck images. At such times, IPR might be the most reasonable approach.

It is commonly accepted that IPR removes a certain amount of enamel from the proximal tooth surface. In orthodontic parlance, this is referred to as *stripping*. Alternatively, terms such as *slicing*, *slenderizing*, *trimming*, *mesiodistal (enamel) reduction*, *re(ap)proximation*, or *interproximal wear*, *selective grinding*, *reshaping*, *recontouring*, *coronoplasty*, and *Hollywood trim* are sometimes used.[2–4] The term *stripping* is ambiguous and should not be used. Other terms listed above downplay the seriousness of this procedure and thus are also inappropriate. *Interproximal enamel reduction* is the most neutral and accurate term and will be used in this chapter.

History of Interproximal Enamel Reduction

The first orthodontist to advocate IPR as a means to resolve asymmetry of tooth size was Ballard in 1944.[5] Later, Bolton concluded that this procedure was best to correct tooth-size discrepancies between the maxillary and mandibular dental arches.[6,7] In 1954, considerable attention was drawn to IPR by Begg, whose article on Stone Age man's dentition demonstrated that attrition can occur to a remarkable degree.[8] According to Begg, tooth wear helps to prevent impaction and crowding of third molars. The first clinician to describe how to perform IPR was Hudson in 1956.[9] According to Hudson—and others later—IPR is completed by polishing the teeth and applying topical fluoride.[2] This

suggests that IPR is not simply a procedure of grinding off enamel, but also that it has to be performed with the same care as any other invasive procedure. Hudson was also the first to give exact numbers about enamel thickness and the amount of safe IPR. Subsequently, other researchers reevaluated the question of enamel thickness.[10]

The first study on IPR was conducted by Rogers and Wagner, who investigated the effect of fluoridation after enamel reduction in vitro.[11] They showed that fluoride significantly lowered the rate of decalcification. This study provided the first scientific argument against critics who opposed IPR on the basis that irreplaceable material was removed and tooth damage inflicted. Opponents had argued that enamel injury induced through IPR could lead to caries and ultimately to loss of the entire tooth.

A new era in IPR began in 1985 when Sheridan first presented his concept of air-rotor stripping.[12] Sheridan was obviously heavily influenced by Begg. IPR, which had been mainly restricted to anterior teeth, was extended by Sheridan to include posterior tooth segments. According to Sheridan, this allowed for the removal of up to 8 mm of tooth material. Also, Sheridan realized that effective and sufficient IPR in the posterior segments of the dental arch could not be accomplished easily and safely with rotating disks. To overcome this problem, Sheridan propagated tungsten carbide burs at high speed.[12] He named his IPR method *air-rotor stripping* (ARS).[12,13]

Another person who had a strong impact on IPR was Zachrisson.[4] Although others had already mentioned the influence of IPR on the gingiva ("gingival improvement"),[14] Zachrisson was probably the first to emphasize the importance of enamel reduction to avoid unesthetic void interproximal spaces ("black triangles").

A new concept of IPR, in which mechanical enamel removal was combined with the application of a microabrasive chemical (37% phosphoric acid), was advocated in studies conducted by Joseph et al[14] and Rossouw and Tortorella.[15] These studies showed that this combination IPR method produces relatively smooth surfaces, which have a potential to "heal themselves" by crystal growth. These reports of in vitro studies had no clinical impact: nothing of substance was subsequently published about this combination IPR. In contrast, Piacentini and Sfondrini considered enamel surfaces treated by this approach "susceptible to decalcification," as the clinician is unable to check whether the patients use calcifying or fluoridating solutions.[3] Subsequent to these milestone articles, much has been published on IPR.[16–27]

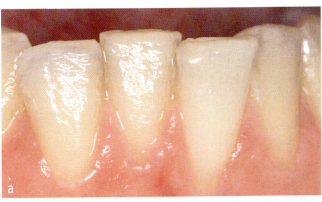 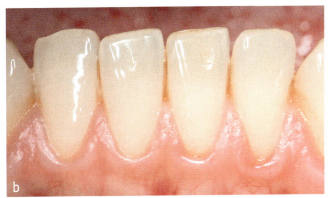

FIG 26-1 Teeth with a triangular crown shape (*a*) are better suited for IPR than are those with a square crown configuration (*b*).

Indications

The following indications for IPR are listed in the order of their presumed importance:

- Elimination of anterior and posterior crowding.
- Avoidance of open gingival embrasures.[4,28–30] This is of particular concern for patients with advanced periodontal disease and gingival recession.
- Correction of tooth-size discrepancies between the two dental arches. This problem could also be solved by widening the relatively smaller teeth through bonding or veneers, but IPR is more readily available and far less expensive.
- Establishment of congruent tooth morphology on both sides of the dental arch.
- Improvement of occlusion (ie, correction of improper interdigitation, overjet, and overbite). This procedure can sometimes help to correct a sagittal skeletal malocclusion by limiting the corrective movements to the dentoalveolar complex.
- Reduction of one-jaw or bimaxillary protrusions without extractions.
- Recontouring of abnormally shaped teeth toward a more ideal morphology.[4]
- Prevention of crowding.[31,32] This effect remains unsubstantiated.[33]

Contraindications

Contraindications are more difficult to list because they are seldom clearly stated. Some important considerations are as follows:

- IPR is not an option in patients with microdontia or an abnormal crown shape (ie, their widest extension is in the gingival, not the occlusal, area). The possible impact of IPR in teeth with abnormal crowns is not only poor esthetics, but also food impaction that can lead to further complications.
- Teeth with a square crown configuration—as opposed to teeth with a triangular crown shape (Fig 26-1)—are poor candidates for IPR.
- Hypersensitivity to hot or cold may be a reason to avoid IPR, as the hypersensitivity might increase after IPR.
- It has been argued that closeness of roots is a reason to avoid IPR.[34] Although not proven, the presumption prevails that the more the roots of adjacent teeth approach each other, the narrower the bone between the roots becomes, which in turn reduces the blood supply and ultimately makes the periodontium less resistant to bacterial invasion. This argument seems unreasonable because in many crowding situations the roots are closer to each other before alignment than they are after—even when IPR was performed.[35] Furthermore, a study by Årtun et al showed that root approximation caused by orthodontic treatment did not increase a patient's risk of developing periodontal problems.[36] Similarly, Crain and Sheridan did not see differences in the alveolar crest morphology when they compared areas with and without IPR.[37]
- Although poor oral hygiene is sometimes mentioned as a contraindication, this argument has no merit because (1) orthodontic treatment of any kind should not be undertaken in any patient with compromised oral hygiene; (2) if IPR is performed to resolve crowding, the accessibility to all interproximal tooth surfaces is improved after treatment, which makes interproximal hygiene (ie, salivary flushing or flossing) easier; and (3) not only is plaque removal easier after IPR, but even the retention of plaque may decrease if the correct polishing technique is used after IPR.

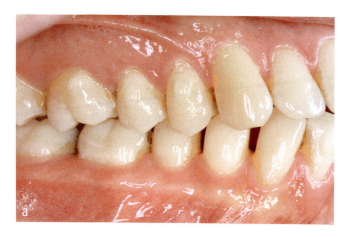
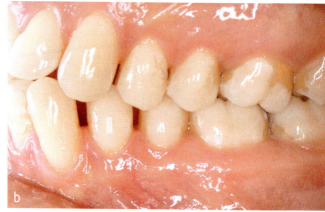
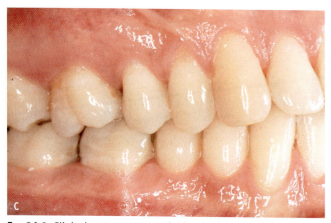
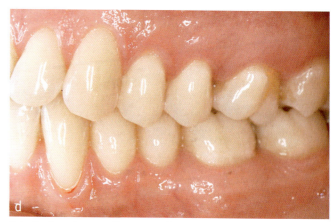

Fig 26-2 Clinical appearance at the beginning of (*a, b*) and after (*c, d*) Invisalign therapy. The space for aligning the crowded anterior teeth was achieved primarily by posterior IPR prior to taking impressions.

Preliminary Requirements

As stated initially, IPR is often indicated to correct crowding of dental arches. In these and similar situations (eg, protrusions) the question is: should enamel reduction take place before or during treatment?

During ClinCheck, the responsible laboratory technician will recognize the amount of space that needs to be created by IPR—if no other means are indicated. Still, every method has some inherent errors. This means that every treatment can be better staged if most of the enamel reduction is done before the polyvinyl siloxane (PVS) impressions are made (Figs 26-2a to 26-2d). To make sure that not too much enamel is removed, some IPR is left to be performed as prescribed in ClinCheck.

The question then arises: how much enamel must be removed? Orthodontic literature is replete with methods to evaluate crowding.[38–45] Unfortunately, none of these methods is sufficiently reliable. Thus, it is preferable to define the amount of space needed through a modified diagnostic setup (Fig 26-3). During this setup, one tooth is eliminated on both sides (or only a single tooth if all IPR is supposed to take place in the mandibular anterior segment only), and the remaining teeth are optimally aligned within the dental arch. This leaves a space whose size can be compared to the mesiodistal width of the tooth that originally occupied this area. In our view, the difference yields the most accurate amount of IPR that is needed.

Allocation of Interproximal Enamel Reduction

After the required amount of IPR is determined, the clinician must decide on which surfaces it should be carried out. The choice is generally between the anterior and the posterior teeth. Before the decision about the location of IPR is made, the following factors must be considered:

- IPR should take place close to the area where space is required. The advantage of this is that teeth require less movement, and thus the crowding is relieved more quickly. This fact favors IPR mainly in the anterior region.

FIG 26-3 (*a*) For this patient, crowding should be corrected primarily by IPR and only by a limited protrusion of the incisors on the right coupled with retrusion on the left. (*b*) Diagnostic setup defines the amount of IPR needed. After arbitrary removal of the two second premolars with a mesiodistal width of 6.8 mm, the remaining space amounts to 3.6 mm on the right and 5.7 mm on the left. Thus, IPR must extend to 3.2 mm on the right side and only to 1.1 mm on the contralateral side.

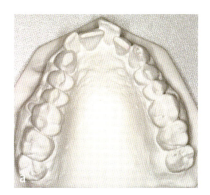
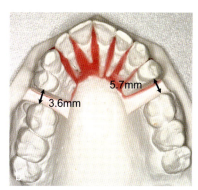

- IPR between anterior teeth has the added advantage of preventing open gingival embrasures or even eliminating them. It works best, however, if the distance between the contact point and the alveolar crest is less than 6 mm.[28,29,46]
- The main disadvantage to IPR in the anterior area is that it is limited because the enamel layer is relatively thin (Fig 26-4).
- IPR between anterior teeth of just one dental arch changes the Bolton ratio.[6,7] This would be favorable if a discrepancy existed before, but if this is not the case, overjet and overbite will be affected. Of course, the various compensation factors for the Bolton ratio have to be taken into account.[6,7] Given that, the overall Bolton ratio normally varies between 87.5% and 94.8%, considerable tooth-size discrepancies can be compensated by manipulations of angulation and inclination, and by finishing with a modicum of overbite. This means, for example, that for an average total maxillary tooth mass (first molar to first molar) of 96.4 mm,[47] every mandibular width first molar to first molar between 84.4 and 91.4 mm is acceptable. In other words, within this range IPR may be carried out but is not an absolute necessity.

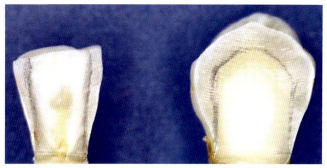

FIG 26-4 Vertical sections at the greatest mesiodistal width of a mandibular incisor (*left*) and a first premolar (*right*) demonstrate the thickness of the enamel layer. The border between enamel and dentin is marked with a pencil line.

- Table 26-1 reflects the amount of enamel that can be safely removed by IPR in the anterior area according to Fillion.[48]
- IPR in the posterior region is favorable because the enamel layer of the premolars and molars is much thicker than that of the anterior teeth (see Fig 26-4, Table 26-2). Thus, much more enamel can be removed without running the risk of mutilating the respective teeth.

TABLE 26-1 Minimum amount of enamel (mm) that can be removed with IPR in the anterior area*						
	Central incisor		**Lateral incisor**		**Canine**	
	Mesial	Distal	Mesial	Distal	Mesial	Distal
Maxillary	0.3	0.3	0.3	0.3	0.3	0.6
Mandibular	0.2	0.2	0.2	0.2	0.2	0.3

* Without additional diagnostic measures (eg, periapical radiographs).

TABLE 26-2 Minimum amount of enamel (mm) that can be removed with IPR in the posterior area*						
	First premolar		**Second premolar**		**First molar**	
	Mesial	Distal	Mesial	Distal	Mesial	Distal
Maxillary	0.6	0.6	0.6	0.6	0.6	0.6
Mandibular	0.6	0.6	0.6	0.6	0.6	0.6

* Without additional diagnostic measures (eg, periapical radiographs).

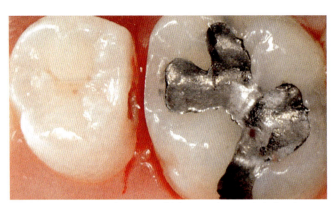

FIG 26-5 Interproximal caries, which was observed during inspection of the individual bitewings and was accessible after IPR for a minimally invasive restoration.

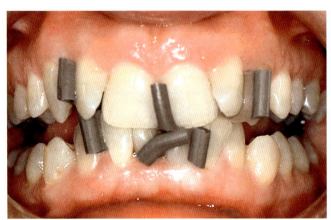

FIG 26-6 Multiple dumbbell separators were placed by the patient. Since the patient has a Class II, division 2 malocclusion with a 100% overbite, the separation effect is intensified when she bites down.

- IPR in posterior teeth has the disadvantage that more teeth have to be moved over a certain distance before the problem—usually crowding of anterior teeth—is solved. This leads to a prolonged treatment time—a fact any patient should be well informed about. Moreover, the intercuspation changes if IPR is executed only in one dental arch.

- IPR should never be routinely distributed evenly between teeth of any given dental arch region without previous consideration of individual tooth shape and size, with the final goal of a symmetric dentition in mind. Factors like midline deviations should be accounted for.

These arguments make the decision of where to perform the indicated IPR rather demanding. It is generally agreed that half of the normal enamel layer thickness can be removed without any harm. Thus, the question arises as to how thick the layer of enamel of all teeth is. There are respective tables by Hudson,[9] Shillingburg and Grace,[10] and Stroud et al.[49] However, these numbers are of limited use in an individual patient, since one looks at minimum values to be on the safe side (see Tables 26-1 and 26-2).

It might be asked whether periapical radiographs should be taken initially to define the individual enamel layer thickness, especially if more IPR in the anterior area is desirable. Although such an approach can be reasonable in individual situations, it is not generally advisable since all intraoral radiographs give an enlarged image and are of limited sharpness. If teeth are rotated or overlap each other because of existing crowding, radiographs are of no value. Nevertheless, the radiographic records should be carefully examined before IPR is performed to detect any existing abnormalities. Figure 26-5 shows a second premo-

lar with interproximal caries that was accessible after IPR and treated with only minimally invasive procedures. However, the patient was upset that he had not been informed earlier about the manifest caries.

To summarize, Tables 26-1 and 26-2 can help to allocate necessary IPR. If needed, the given amounts can be increased following evaluation of high-quality orthoradial periapical radiographs. Sheridan's rule of thumb that 0.5 mm of enamel can be reduced from practically all anterior interproximal spaces and 1.0 mm from all posterior proximal areas is a helpful guide. Overall, space that can be gained by IPR between the mesial aspects of the first molars amounts to at least 10 mm in the maxillary and almost 9 mm in the mandibular arch.

Preparatory Measures

In situations with severe crowding, it is sometimes difficult, if not impossible, to conduct a judicious IPR because the respective proximal surfaces overlap. This holds especially true for the anterior teeth. Therefore, one must either begin IPR with the usually uncrowded posterior teeth or overcome this problem by separation, as was described by Tuverson as early as 1980.[50] Such a separation could be performed immediately in the orthodontic office, or the patient can start this process at home. The latter is often preferable for both parties because it is less traumatic, since movements of the teeth occur over a longer period (at best, overnight). In such situations the authors use Maxian (dumbbell) separators, which are available in different sizes (Fig 26-6). They are cut into pieces and delivered to the patient, who is taught how to apply them (lending a pair of hemostats is advisable).

If the separators stay in the mouth overnight, there is sufficient space after their removal the following morning to start a qualified IPR. In patients with severe crowding, it might be necessary to repeat this procedure several times. Under these circumstances, separation starts at the most accessible (ie, the least crowded) area. After the first IPR, the crowding decreases spontaneously, which implies uncontrolled tooth movements. Still, this is a desirable landscape because such "unraveling" facilitates IPR at all proximal surfaces that are considered. Although it would be disadvantageous if the posterior teeth were to come forward and occupy the created space, it is not clinically practical or necessary to place a thermoformed retainer while IPR is still in progress. Therefore, IPR is carried out until sufficient space is created; at this point, the retainer is inserted. In the rare case, however, that separation of posterior teeth becomes necessary, standard O-rings or metal spring separators should be inserted.

If particular teeth are severely angulated, it might be difficult to perform a perfect IPR—especially if the clinician lacks experience. In this situation, it may be advisable to inspect the teeth in question beforehand and mark the area that is to be removed by IPR (Fig 26-7).

Enamel Removal

A plethora of instruments is advocated for IPR; single- or double-sided versions include manually driven abrasive strips of various materials,[30,51] motor-driven abrasive strips,[52-55] abrasive (diamond-coated) disks or oscillating disk segments,[55,56] tungsten carbide burs,[3,48,57] and diamond-coated burs.[3,58,59] Some of the above listed devices are either operated freehand or clamped into a type of holder to improve their effectiveness; others are operated using a contra-angle handpiece.

IPR roughens the enamel surface. The degree of roughness, however, depends primarily on the aggressiveness of the device used.[3] On the other hand, the abrasiveness determines the effectiveness of the procedure. A device that is less abrasive can only do the job when it operates for a much longer time or at a much higher speed. If this method takes an inordinate amount of time, then what is the point? And at times, IPR is so minuscule that the enamel removal cannot be well controlled if it occurs at high speed.

IPR can leave behind a plaque-retentive surface and an increased risk of caries.[59,60] It is crucial, therefore, to produce an enamel surface not rougher than natural, untreat-

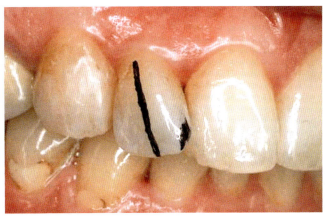

FIG 26-7 Patient with a mesially angulated right lateral incisor for which perfect IPR requires sound clinical experience. In such a situation it can be helpful, after separation, to mark the long axis of the tooth and, parallel to it, the enamel area that is to be removed.

ed enamel—preferably, even smoother. To achieve this, polishing of the surface is necessary after IPR.[4] Other criteria for selecting the best IPR protocol are safety and reliability, as perfect results must be achieved in every patient.

Our own studies and experiences have led to the protocols described below.[54,58]

IPR in posterior teeth (when more than 0.5 mm enamel is to be removed): A modified ARS technique seems to be most adequate. This is achieved through placement of a tungsten carbide bur (no. 699L) horizontally underneath the interproximal contact point of two adjacent teeth. The bur is then run at high speed (> 100.000 min⁻¹) and pulled with gentle force straight toward the occlusal surfaces. To achieve even surfaces, cutting should not be interrupted. This is done twice, once from the buccal side and once from the lingual side. Considerable heat is generated in this process; therefore, water cooling is highly recommended.

This vertical approach is preferable to a horizontal movement of the bur from the buccal or lingual side, as the bur has a conical shape such that horizontal movement would produce a triangular shape of the proximal area with the contact point far too gingival.

On the other hand, it might be traumatic to place the bur into the interproximal space if it is completely filled by a papilla. To protect the soft tissue, Sheridan has advocated placement of an "indicator wire"—a thick brass wire (0.5 to 0.7 mm) below the bur (on top of the papilla).[12] Unfortunately, the placement and presence of the indicator wire can be painful, and thus its use is not advisable.

IPR is a procedure well tolerated by the patient. In our experience, no patient has complained following the removal of 0.5 mm (or slightly more) enamel.

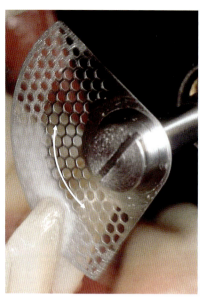

FIG 26-8 Perforated oscillating disk segment during IPR. It is obvious that the visibility through the segment is excellent, and no safeguard is needed.

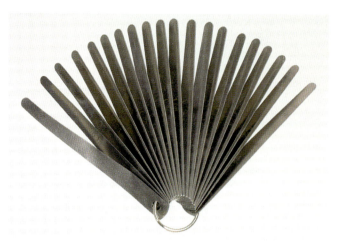

FIG 26-9 The authors' preferred device for measuring the amount of enamel reduction: a gauge for spark plugs. This gauge includes 20 blades and can measure spaces 0.05 to 1.00 mm wide.

IPR in anterior teeth: This can be accomplished most effectively with very thin (0.1 mm), flexible, diamond-coated perforated disks spinning at 10,000 min⁻¹ or by oscillating disk segments at 5,500 min⁻¹. Rotating disks must be operated with a safeguard. If the disk is perforated, the visibility of the working field is excellent. To prevent aspiration of airborne cooling water mixed with intraoral bacteria, staff members must wear face-masks and protective goggles. The patient should also be covered. In the event that separation was not sufficient or not performed, it may be prudent to start with lightening strips. After access is created, the remaining cutting can take place with the disk as described above.

Oscillating segmental disks are favored (Fig 26-8). These differ from conventional disks in that they oscillate 30 degrees at 5,500 min⁻¹. The oscillating disk segments have two major advantages: they are unlikely to cut the lip and tongue and, therefore, do not require safeguards, and they are much smaller than full disks and thus are unlikely to cut any antagonist teeth.

Independent of the region where IPR is to take place, three aspects need to be considered:

1. Whenever a natural and an artificial tooth surface neighbor each other, the restorative surface should be preferred for reduction—either entirely or at least to a greater extent.

2. If IPR is only indicated at one of two adjacent tooth surfaces, it is difficult to leave one completely untouched. In such a situation, it is advisable to place a steel matrix over the surface to be protected or use single-sided disks or disk segments.

3. Most important, however, is the question, should IPR be performed before the PVS impressions are made and before any treatment is started, or should it be performed during treatment as prescribed by ClinCheck? The answer depends on the amount of enamel that is to be removed. If the amount is relatively small (less than 1.5 mm), IPR could be performed during therapy. More extensive IPR should take place up front. In other words, the more accurately the tooth morphology is reflected in the impression, and thus in the virtual model, the more precise the treatment outcome prediction can be. If IPR is executed before PVS impressions are made, the following points should be considered:

- Stay about 0.3 mm short of the necessary IPR. This approach prevents overextended enamel removal as well as residual spacing between teeth at the end of treatment. In a case with minimally sufficient IPR, it is left to ClinCheck technicians to disclose any possible collisions between teeth. Naturally, at every visit, contacts between the moving teeth should be checked with dental floss and, if tight, minimal IPR may be performed.
- Once the preimpression IPR is done, a thermoformed retainer must be placed.
- Information should be given in the Special Instructions section of the treatment planning form so that the

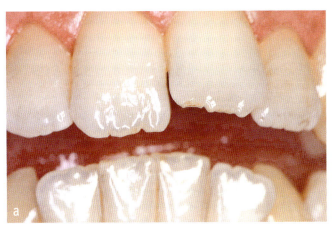 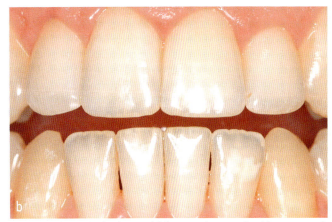

FIG 26-10 Incisors before (*a*) and after (*b*) treatment, including recontouring of the incisal edges, which were characterized by mammelons as a result of the existing open bite.

technician will not interpret the observed space for imperfections in the impression. Concurrently, it is crucial to submit intraoral photographs taken immediately after the IPR.

Measuring the Amount of Enamel Removal

To prevent excessive enamel removal, IPR should be initiated with a cutting device that is thinner than the amount of enamel to be removed. Thus, the amount of IPR and created space needs to be measured repeatedly. There is a multitude of measuring devices, from very simple sliding calipers to elaborate and costly ones, as presented by Sheridan and Hastings.[61] Each has its advantages. For a device to be practical for IPR, it should fulfill four conditions: simplicity of use (ie, applicable in all areas of the dental arch); measurement gradations from 0.1 mm to at least 1.2 mm, with all steps in between; sterilizability; and reasonable cost.

These requirements are fulfilled mainly by two devices. The first is a simple series of wires with various diameters. To distinguish them from one another, one end can be bent into the respective digit, or each is identified by a small numbered tag as suggested by Philippe,[62] or one end can be covered with a plastic tube that is inscribed with the diameter of the wire.

The second, even more practical, device is a measuring gauge used for spark plugs, which can be bought from any automotive supply store (Fig 26-9). Common gauges allow measurement of any gap between 0.1 and 2.0 mm, with

increments of 0.1 mm. If the individual gauge also contains a blade of 0.05 mm thickness, all measurements can be further refined. The main disadvantage of these gauges is that they are generally not made out of stainless steel but rather from an inferior alloy. Thus, if they are sterilized, they will corrode. This can be overcome by a thorough disinfection followed by wrapping the individual blades with fine plastic or metal foil.

Once the IPR procedure has started, the orthodontist should repeatedly insert the gauge into the created gap until it slides easily in and out. To avoid removing too much enamel, it is advisable to use a blade (combination) that is 0.1 mm smaller than the intended IPR value. The last 0.1 mm is removed by the recontouring and polishing process.[58]

Contouring of Teeth After Interproximal Enamel Reduction

After removal of interproximal enamel, the individual teeth are recontoured to give them a natural look. This is especially necessary for posterior teeth and maxillary incisors,[20] whereas for mandibular incisors this procedure can often be omitted. The contouring is best performed with fine (red ring) diamond-coated burs of various shapes, preferably ones that have a blank (not coated) tip. This guiding—polished, nonabrasive—tip, when moved buccolingually, helps level any surface irregularities, since it does not cut additional enamel. Sufficient water cooling is mandatory. The length of time needed for a perfect recontouring should not be underestimated.

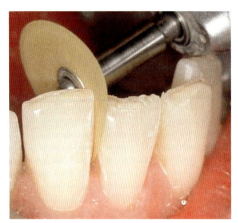

Fig 26-11 Enamel polishing with a Sof-Lex XT disk. Because of its flexibility, it can be directed into various areas to create a smooth transition from treated to untreated surfaces.

Polishing of Teeth After Interproximal Enamel Reduction

Polishing of all manipulated tooth surfaces is the next step. Irrespective of the devices used, the shaved surface will display furrows up to 40 µm wide and deep. Such rough surfaces accumulate plaque more readily and increase the risk for caries or periodontal disease.[60,63,64] To achieve perfectly polished enamel, it is crucial to avoid coarse instruments from the beginning.[3,51]

As with enamel cutting, a variety of polishing instruments and methods are described in the literature. Several studies[3,55,56,58,65] prove that with careful polishing the previously rough surface can be made very smooth (Fig 26-10). In an investigation by Zhong et al,[58] a minimum of 94% of all polished surfaces at the various heights of the interproximal space were smoother than untreated enamel in vivo. This was also true for the remaining 6%, where a few isolated furrows of up to 3 µm in depth could be observed. In commenting on this study, Zachrisson wrote, "The satisfactory result should relieve the orthodontist of any apprehension about inducing a carious environment in areas treated by enamel reduction."[4]

This was accomplished by using two extra-thin polishing disks with different surface coating (Sof-Lex XT fine and ultrafine, 3M), each attached to a handpiece, for 40 seconds with water cooling at 4,000 min⁻¹. Instead of water cooling, fluoride gel can be used. Many other techniques and variations were tested, but none produced results of a comparable quality within the same amount of time.

Even if polishing with the Sof-Lex disks produces a superior smoothness of the enamel surface, it has to be pointed out that because of the small size of the Sof-Lex disks (radius: approximately 6.5 mm), it can be difficult in large teeth to polish all treated surfaces. The disk must therefore be introduced from different angles. Such a maneuver does not present a problem because the extra-thin Sof-Lex disks are extremely flexible (Fig 26-11). This flexibility also helps to accomplish a smooth transition from the surfaces that have been worked on to the natural enamel. It should be mentioned that intensive use of a polishing disk leads to its rapid degradation. Thus, every disk has to be discarded after use on one patient.

Is it essential to use the micro motor of the dental unit for polishing, or can the same result be accomplished manually? The answer is that enamel smoothness is the result of the distance a polishing medium has traveled over a tooth surface. A simple test shows that an abrasive strip is moved an average of 10 mm. With full concentration, a clinician can jiggle such a strip 140 times/minute. Thus, after 40 seconds the polishing distance amounts to 1.87 m. On the other hand, considering the working range of a polishing disk is about 4.5 mm from its center (not at the outer edge, which would make the calculation even more stunning), it travels with one rotation ($2\pi r$) 28 mm. At a speed of 4,000 min⁻¹, the polishing surface has traveled 75.4 m after 40 seconds. Obviously, machine polishing is more than 40 times more effective than any manual method. Put differently, to produce a comparable surface texture, the manual polishing time must be extended to almost 27 minutes—not considering whether the polishing strip would last that long and whether it would need to be changed, or whether the manual speed could be maintained over this time. The answer, then, to whether manual polishing can achieve the same result as polishing with the micro motor is simply, no!

Another question relates to the fact that all teeth have a physiologic mobility: could the roughness after IPR reduce itself through a naturally induced polishing? Radlanski et al investigated this question and found that after 1 year only a very limited area of the previously reduced enamel achieved even a slight smoothness.[66] The answer to this second question, then, is also no: self-polishing after IPR cannot be expected.

Fluoridation

Even if polishing has been performed with all required care, some furrows might remain and enhance plaque accumulation. This remains a theoretical possibility[37,67] and should not be ignored—especially since the most fluoridated enamel layer is removed with IPR.[68–70] Removal by itself is not significant, as the fluoride concentration of the new outermost enamel layer is increased by saliva and can be further increased by fluoride-containing substances.[71–75] Incorporation of fluorine increases the microhardness of the enamel surface[76] and may actually result in an enamel structure that is more caries-resistant than the original surface layer.[77] Zachrisson recommends twice-daily mouth rinsing with a weak fluoride solution; he considers special topical fluoridation superfluous.[4] His opinion was substantiated by a long-term study[4] over more than 10 years that did not reveal any adverse effects of IPR in a group of 59 consecutive orthodontic patients. El-Mangoury et al even concluded that enamel after IPR remineralized spontaneously without an increased pathological caries risk.[78]

Although it is generally agreed that low-concentration fluoride preparations over longer time periods are ideal,[72,73,79] higher concentrations also achieve this goal, as more calcium fluoride is precipitated if higher fluoride concentrations are applied.[75,80,81] Furthermore, it is known that about 10% of patients do not comply with the instructions.[82] It is best to apply a higher-concentration fluoride topically[30] and advise the patient to use fluoride-impregnated floss, fluoridated toothpaste applied with a toothpick, fluoride-containing sugar-free chewing gum, or one of the following: daily fluoride tablets, fluoridated cooking salt, weak fluoride mouth rinses, or fluoride gel once a week.[83] Where available, amine fluoride has a better effect than other formulations.[74,84,85] For topical fluoridation, there are further alternatives: highly concentrated fluoride varnishes, less concentrated fluoride solutions and gels (eg, Elmex fluid and gel, GABA International), and fluoride- and thymol-containing varnish. In the future slow-release formulations[76] that enhance fluoride uptake in deeper enamel layers may also be considered.[86] Finally, it should be noted that aligners can be used as appropriate fluoride-preparation carriers.

Advantages and Disadvantages of Interproximal Enamel Reduction

The clinician may still wish to extract premolars in severe crowding cases, but IPR has its place. IPR transforms a crowded dentition into one with spacing that is thus easier to treat. Careful IPR never produces more space than is necessary, in stark contrast to premolar extraction therapy. Further, if crowding is resolved without IPR, open gingival embrasures can hardly be avoided in adult patients with long clinical crowns, particularly if they suffer from gingival recession.[46,87]

Finally, IPR is patient friendly, as demonstrated in the study by Zhong et al, in which 32 consecutive patients with 296 treated surfaces completed an anonymous questionnaire.[58] On a discomfort scale ranging from 1 (no discomfort) to 10 (pain), 81% selected grades 1 to 3. The remaining patients mainly reported minor trauma of the interproximal papilla, which is often a side effect of IPR. None of the patients said they would choose local anesthesia for further IPR.

The main disadvantage of IPR is that, if performed with adequate precision, it consumes a good amount of the clinician's time. A time study showed that high-quality IPR takes approximately 2.2 minutes per tooth surface with the change of various instruments. This time may be reduced by clinical experience, but likely not by much. Other disadvantages include removal of the most-fluoridated enamel layer and the inevitable slight gingival traumas. Finally, it is sometimes a challenge to overcome a patient's concern regarding IPR. The rationale we use is mainly that IPR is the reproduction of a physiologic process that no longer occurs because of changed nutritional habits.

References

1. Meier B, Wiemer KB, Miethke RR. Invisalign—Patient profiling. Analysis of a prospective survey. J Orofac Orthop 2003;64:352–358.
2. Pinheiro MLRM. Interproximal enamel reduction. World J Orthod 2002;3:223–232.
3. Piacentini C, Sfondrini G. A scanning electron microscopy comparison of enamel polishing methods after air-rotor stripping. Am J Orthod Dentofacial Orthop 1996;109:57–63.
4. Zachrisson BU. Actual damage to teeth and periodontal tissues with mesiodistal enamel reduction ("stripping"). World J Orthod 2004;5:178–183.
5. Ballard ML. Asymmetry in tooth size: A factor in the etiology, diagnosis, and treatment of malocclusion. Angle Orthod 1944;14:67–71.

6. Bolton WA. Disharmony of tooth size and its relation to the analysis and treatment of malocclusion. Angle Orthod 1958;28:113−130.

7. Bolton WA. The clinical application of a tooth-size analysis. J Dent Res 1962;48:504−529.

8. Begg PR. Stone Age man's dentition. J Dent Res 1954;40:298−312, 373−383, 462−475, 517−531.

9. Hudson AL. A study of the effects of mesiodistal reduction of mandibular anterior teeth. J Dent Res 1956;42:615−624.

10. Shillingburg HT Jr, Grace CS. Thickness of enamel and dentin. J South Calif Dent Assoc 1973;41(1):33−36.

11. Rogers GA, Wagner MJ. Protection of stripped enamel surfaces with topical fluoride applications. J Dent Res 1969;56:551−559.

12. Sheridan JJ. Air-rotor stripping. J Clin Orthod 1985;19:43−59.

13. Sheridan JJ. Air-rotor stripping update. J Clin Orthod 1987;21:781−788.

14. Joseph VP, Rossouw PE, Basson NJ. Orthodontic microabrasive reproximation. Am J Orthod Dentofacial Orthop 1992;102:351−359.

15. Rossouw PE, Tortorella A. A pilot investigation of enamel reduction procedures. J Can Dent Assoc 2003;69:384−388.

16. Kelsten LB. A technique for realignment and stripping of crowded lower incisors. J Pract Orthod 1969;3(2):82−84.

17. Paskow H. Self-alignment following interproximal stripping. J Dent Res 1970;58:240−249.

18. Peck H, Peck S. An index for assessing tooth shape deviations as applied to the mandibular incisors. J Dent Res 1972;61:384−401.

19. Peck H, Peck S. Crown dimensions and mandibular alignment. Angle Orthod 1972;42:148−153.

20. Tuverson DL. Anterior interocclusal relations. Part II. J Dent Res 1980;78:371−393.

21. Lusterman EA. Treatment of a Class II Division 2 malocclusion involving mesiodistal reduction of mandibular anterior teeth. J Dent Res 1954;40:44−50.

22. Ley M, Muller-Hartwick R, Jost-Brinkmann PG. Approximale Schmelzreduktion. Wann und wie? Inf Orthod Kieferorthop 2005;37:2−4.

23. Begg PR, Kesling PC. Begg Orthodontic Theory and Practice, ed 3. Philadelphia: Saunders, 1977.

24. Boese LR. Fiberotomy and reproximation without lower retention 9 years in retrospect: Part II. Angle Orthod 1980;50:169−178.

25. Alexander RG, Sinclair PM, Goates LJ. Differential diagnosis and treatment planning for the adult nonsurgical orthodontic patient. J Dent Res 1986;89:95−112.

26. DiPaolo RJ, Boruchov MJ. Thoughts on stripping of anterior teeth. J Clin Orthod 1971;5:510−511.

27. Sheridan JJ, Ledoux PM. Air-rotor stripping and proximal sealants. An SEM evaluation. J Clin Orthod 1989;23:790−794.

28. Kurth JR, Kokich VG. Open gingival embrasures after orthodontic treatment in adults: Prevalence and etiology. Am J Orthod Dentofacial Orthop 2001;120:116−123.

29. Atherton JD. The gingival response to orthodontic tooth movement. J Dent Res 1970;58:179−186.

30. de Harfin JF. Interproximal stripping for the treatment of adult crowding. J Clin Orthod 2000;34:424−433.

31. Lashar MC. A consideration of the principles of mechanical arches as applied to the dental arch. Angle Orthod 1943;4:248−268.

32. Williams R. Eliminating lower retention. J Clin Orthod 1985;19:342−349.

33. Betteridge MA. The effects of interdental stripping on the labial segments evaluated one year out of retention. Br J Orthod 1981;8:193−197.

34. Kramer GM. A consideration of root proximity. Int J Periodontics Restorative Dent 1987;7(6):8−33.

35. Philippe J. De l'harmonie entre la taille des dents et celle des arcades. Rev Orthop Dento Faciale 2004;38:37−51.

36. Årtun J, Kokich VG, Osterberg SK. Long-term effect of root proximity on periodontal health after orthodontic treatment. Am J Orthod Dentofacial Orthop 1987;91:125−130.

37. Crain G, Sheridan JJ. Susceptibility to caries and periodontal disease after posterior air-rotor stripping. J Clin Orthod 1990;24:84−85.

38. Musich DR, Ackerman JL. The catenometer: A reliable device for estimating dental arch perimeter. J Dent Res 1973;63:366−375.

39. Beazley WW. Assessment of mandibular arch length discrepancy utilizing an individualized arch form. Angle Orthod 1971;41(1):45−54.

40. Kinast H. Herstellungstechnische Grundlagen des Arcumeters und sein Gebrauch. J Orofac Orthop 2000;61:297−304.

41. Nance HN. The limitations of orthodontic treatment. I. Mixed dentition diagnosis and treatment. Am J Orthod Oral Surg 1947;33:177−223.

42. Nance HN. The limitations of orthodontic treatment. II. Diagnosis and treatment in the permanent dentition. Am J Orthod Oral Surg 1947;33: 253−301.

43. Carey CW. Treatment planning and the technical program in the four fundamental treatment forms. J Dent Res 1958;44:887−898.

44. Moorrees CFA. The dentition of the growing child. A longitudinal study of the dental development between 3 and 18 years of age. Cambridge: Harvard University Press, 1959.

45. Lundström A. The significance of early loss of deciduous teeth in the etiology of malocclusion. J Dent Res 1955;41:819−826.

46. Wu YJ, Tu YK, Huang SM, Chan CP. The influence of the distance from the contact point to the crest of bone on the presence of the interproximal dental papilla. Chang Gung Med J 2003;26: 822−828.

47. Miethke RR. Zahnbreiten und Zahnbreitenkorrelationen [thesis]. Berlin, 1972.

48. Fillion D. Vor- und Nachteile der approximalen Schmelzreduktion. Teil II. Inf Orthod Kieferorthop 1995;27:64−90.

49. Stroud JL, English J, Buschang PH. Enamel thickness of the posterior dentition: Its implications for nonextraction treatment. Angle Orthod 1998;68:141−146.

50. Tuverson DL. Anterior interocclusal relations. Part I. J Dent Res 1980;78:361−370.

51. Lundgren T, Milleding P, Mohlin B, Nannmark U. Restitution of enamel after interdental stripping. Swed Dent J 1993;17:217−224.

52. Hugo B, Lussi A, Gygax M. Anwendungen des EVA-Systems (II). Schweiz Monatsschr Zahnmed 1991;101:1587−1592.

53. Gygax M, Lussi A, Hugo B. Anwendungen des EVA-Systems (I). Schweiz Monatsschr Zahnmed 1991;101:1429−1434.

54. Hugo B, Lussi A, Hotz P. The preparation of enamel margin beveling in proximal cavities [in German]. Schweiz Monatsschr Zahnmed 1992;102:1181−1188.

55. Hein C, Jost-Brinkmann PG, Schillai G. The enamel surface quality after interproximal stripping—A scanning electron microscopic assessment of different polishing procedures [in German]. Fortschr Kieferorthop 1990;51:327−335.

56. Zhong M, Jost-Brinkmann PG, Radlanski RJ, Miethke RR. SEM evaluation of a new technique for interdental stripping. J Clin Orthod 1999;33:286−392.

57. Lucchese A, Porcu F, Dolci F. Effects of various stripping techniques on surface enamel. J Clin Orthod 2001;35:691−695.

58. Zhong M, Jost-Brinkmann PG, Zellmann M, Zellmann S, Radlanski RJ. Clinical evaluation of a new technique for interdental enamel reduction. J Orofac Orthop 2000;61:432−439.

59. Leclerc JF. Etat de la surface de l'email apres remodelage amelaire proximal? Etude au microscope electronique. J l'Edgewise 1992;25:25–33.

60. Radlanski RJ, Jäger A, Schwestka R, Bertzbach F. Plaque accumulations caused by interdental stripping. Am J Orthod Dentofacial Orthop 1988;94:416–420.

61. Sheridan JJ, Hastings J. Air-rotor stripping and lower incisor extraction treatment. J Clin Orthod 1992;26:18–22.

62. Philippe J. A method of enamel reduction for correction of adult arch-length discrepancy. J Clin Orthod 1991;25:484–489.

63. Swartz ML, Phillips RW. Comparison of bacterial accumulation on rough and smooth enamel surfaces. J Periodontol 1967;28:304–307.

64. Arends J, Christofferson J. The nature of early carious lesions in enamel. J Dent Res 1986;65:2–11.

65. Jost-Brinkmann PG, Otani H, Nakata M. Surface condition of primary teeth after approximal grinding and polishing. J Clin Pediatr Dent 1991;16:41–45.

66. Radlanski RJ, Jäger A, Zimmer B. Morphology of interdentally stripped enamel one year after treatment. J Clin Orthod 1989;23:748–750.

67. Kapur K, Fischer EE, Manly RS. Effect of surface alteration of permeability of enamel to a lactate buffer. J Dent Res 1961;40:1174–1182.

68. Joseph VP, Rossouw PE, Harris AM, Adams L. Stereometric evaluation of the enamel-stripping effect of hydrochloric acid. J Clin Orthod 1992;26:761–764.

69. Keene HJ, Mellberg JR, Pederson ED. Relationship between dental caries experience and surface enamel fluoride concentration in young men from three optimally fluoridated cities. J Dent Res 1980;59:1941–1945.

70. Konttinen ML, Hanhijarjvi H. Fluoride concentrations of the surface enamel of children living in an optimally fluoridated community. Scand J Dent Res 1986;94:427–435.

71. Amaechi BT, Higham SM. In vitro remineralisation of eroded enamel lesions by saliva. J Dent 2001;29:371–376.

72. Inaba D, Kawasaki K, Iijima Y, et al. Enamel fluoride uptake from mouthrinse solutions with different NaF concentrations. Community Dent Oral Epidemiol 2002;30:248–253.

73. Kashani H, Birkhed D, Petersson LG. Fluoride concentration in the approximal area after using toothpicks and other fluoride-containing products. Eur J Oral Sci 1998;106:564–570.

74. Mok Y, Hill FJ, Newman HN. Enamel fluoride uptake affected by site of application: Comparing sodium and amine fluorides. Caries Res 1990;24:11–17.

75. Lagerweij MD, ten Cate JM. Remineralisation of enamel lesions with daily applications of a high-concentration fluoride gel and a fluoridated toothpaste: An in situ study. Caries Res 2002;36:270–274.

76. Bottenberg P, Cleymaet R, Rohrkasten K, Lampert F. Microhardness changes in surface enamel after application of bioadhesive fluoride tablets in situ. Clin Oral Investig 2000;4:153–156.

77. Iijima Y, Koulourides T. Fluoride incorporation into and retention in remineralized enamel. J Dent Res 1989;68:1289–1292.

78. el-Mangoury NH, Moussa MM, Mostafa YA, Girgis AS. In-vivo remineralization after air-rotor stripping. J Clin Orthod 1991;25:75–78.

79. Featherstone JD, Glena R, Shariati M, Shields CP. Dependence of in vitro demineralization of apatite and remineralization of dental enamel on fluoride concentration. J Dent Res 1990;69(special issue):620–625.

80. Hellwig E, Lussi A. What is the optimum fluoride concentration needed for the remineralization process? Caries Res 2001;35(suppl 1):57–59.

81. Øgaard B. CaF_2 formation: Cariostatic properties and factors enhancing the effect. Caries Res 2001;35:40–44.

82. Geiger AM, Gorelick L, Gwinnett AJ, Benson BJ. Reducing white spot lesions in orthodontic populations with fluoride rinsing. Am J Orthod Dentofacial Orthop 1992;101:403–407.

83. Heintze SD, Jost-Brinkmann P-G, Finke C, Miethke R-R. Oral Health for the Orthodontic Patient. Chicago: Quintessence, 1998.

84. Chan JC, Hill FJ, Newman HN. Uptake of fluoride by sound and artificially carious enamel in vitro following application of topical sodium and amine fluorides. J Dent 1991;19:110–115.

85. Petzold M. The influence of different fluoride compounds and treatment conditions on dental enamel: A descriptive in vitro study of the CaF_2 precipitation and microstructure. Caries Res 2001;35(suppl 1):45–51.

86. Capilouto ML, DePaola PF, Gron P. In vivo study of slow-release fluoride resin and enamel uptake. Caries Res 1990;24:441–445.

87. Burke S, Burch JG, Tetz JA. Incidence and size of pretreatment overlap and posttreatment gingival embrasure space between maxillary central incisors. Am J Orthod Dentofacial Orthop 1994;105:506–511.

chapter 27

FACIAL ESTHETHIC EXAMINATION AND ANALYSIS

by
Marc B. Ackerman, DMD

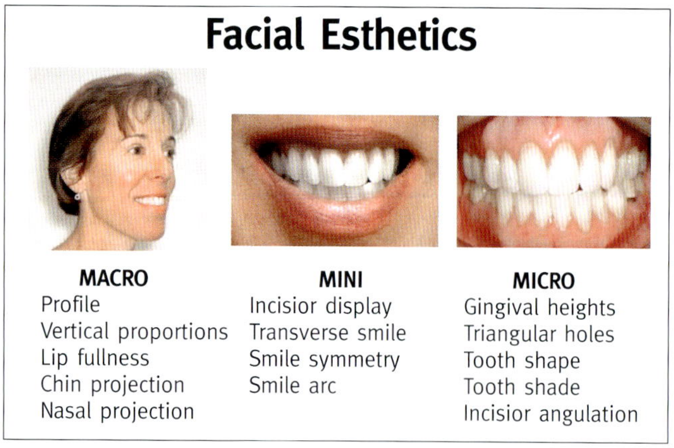

Facial Esthetics

MACRO	**MINI**	**MICRO**
Profile	Incisor display	Gingival heights
Vertical proportions	Transverse smile	Triangular holes
Lip fullness	Smile symmetry	Tooth shape
Chin projection	Smile arc	Tooth shade
Nasal projection		Incisior angulation

FIG 27-1 Facial esthetic classification.

The first 100 years of treatment planning in orthodontics were based on measurements taken from a system of static records, with the primary goal of treatment aimed at the attainment of a tooth-centered, occlusal model. A significant shortcoming of this focus on measurements from hard tissue anatomic elements from the lateral cephalogram and plaster study casts was that clinicians did not take into account the esthetics of resting and dynamic soft tissue relationships, which is regarded by patients as the most critical aspect in treatment planning. Orthodontics in the 21st century utilizes enhancement technologies with a range of techniques aimed not only at correcting the patient's functional deficiencies or treating his or her "disease," but also at improving the esthetic appearance of the face and in particular the smile.[1,2] Systematized patient examination and esthetic treatment planning with the Invisalign System are the focus of this chapter.

Contemporary Facial Esthetic Treatment Planning

Problem-oriented treatment planning, with its focus on the identification of problems and their possible solutions, has served orthodontists very well in the last several decades. Problem-oriented treatment planning should now include the identification of favorable attributes as well as the identification of problems. The sole emphasis on patient problems and their solutions may result in a treatment plan that has a potentially negative effect on the esthetic elements of that patient. A classic example is the extraction of maxillary premolars in the correction of a skeletal Class II malocclusion, which, while satisfying functional and occlusal issues, may produce an unfortunate effect on nasal and lip esthetics in profile. The goal of orthodontic treatment is minimization of a patient's negative attributes and preservation of attributes that are esthetically favorable.

Facial esthetics can be divided into three subcategories: macroesthetics, miniesthetics, and microesthetics (Fig 27-1). The specific concerns of the patient can be elucidated through open-ended clinician-patient communication and then integrated into the diagnostic decision tree. The physical burden of treatment is borne by the patient and must be weighed in determining the extent of intervention. A systematic approach to clinical examination of the patient is essential for the development of an optimization-oriented database.

Data Collection

Primary data collection begins at the clinical examination and is supplemented with static and dynamic recordings of the patient in three spatial dimensions. Record taking should replicate the functional and esthetic presentation of the patient. Findings from the clinical examination should either be confirmed or challenged by data obtained from the records. Analysis of the clinical database generates a diagnostic summary and optimized problem list. An emerging soft tissue paradigm[3] in orthodontic treatment planning has refocused analysis on facial proportionality and balance versus reliance on normative data derived from cephalometrics. The art of esthetic treatment planning in orthodontics lies in the clinician's ability to envisage the patient's desired three-dimensional (3-D) soft tissue outcome and then to engineer the dental and skeletal hard tissues to produce such a change.

In today's clinical environment there are three methods of data collection. The first and most commonly used method includes still photography, study casts, and cephalometric radiographs. The second is the use of data-basing programs to document direct clinical measurement of the patient's resting and dynamic relationships. The third involves the use of digital video to record the dynamics of facial movement.

Conventional records

Standard orthodontic records have not changed significantly in many years. In clinical practice, standard records include film or digital photographs, radiographs, and study casts (whether plaster, mounted or unmounted, or

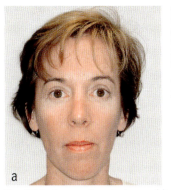
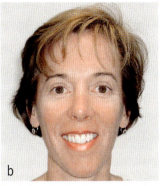
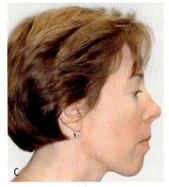
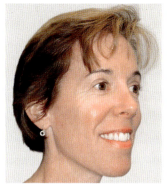

FIG 27-2 Conventional views: (*a*) frontal portrait photograph at rest, closed lips; (*b*) frontal portrait photograph on smile; (*c*) profile portrait photograph, closed lips.

FIG 27-3 Supplemental view: oblique (45-degree) portrait photograph on smile.

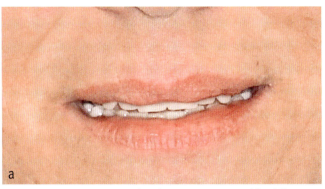
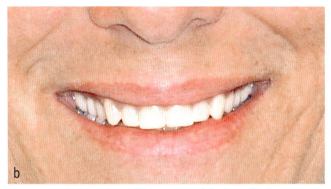

FIG 27-4 Views for direct facial measurements: (*a*) philtrum and commissure height, interlabial gap, and incisor display at rest; (*b*) philtrum and commissure height, interlabial gap, and incisor/gingival display on social smile.

electronic models). The facial images, which are universally considered standard records, include frontal at rest, frontal smile, and profile-at-rest images (Figs 27-2a to 27-2c). While these orientations do provide an adequate amount of diagnostic information, they do not contain all of the information needed for 3-D visualization and quantification. Ideally, supplemental images should be taken in the oblique or three-quarter view (Fig 27-3).

Direct facial measurement

The goal of the clinical examination is to quantitatively assess soft and hard tissue attributes of the dentofacial complex and record what elements are satisfactory and which are in need of optimization. Measurement should be thorough, systematic, and consistent—and should minimize the chance that something of importance will be overlooked.

Contemporary clinical examination uses a computer-databasing program to facilitate data entry. These data are then merged into reports and treatment planning screens or forms.[4] By using a computer database, the orthodontist saves valuable time both in the clinical examination and

in the diagnostic and treatment planning workup. The information is stored for recall and analysis and can even have predefined parameters that identify problematic measurements automatically.

The following frontal measurements should be performed systematically in evaluation of anterior dental display, both at rest and on smile (Figs 27-4a and 27-4b): philtrum height, commissure height, interlabial gap, amount of incisor display at rest, amount of incisor display on smile, crown height, gingival display, and smile arc.

The philtrum height is measured in millimeters from the subnasale (the base of the nose at the midline) to the most inferior portion of the upper lip on the vermilion tip beneath the philtral columns. In the adolescent, it is common to find the philtrum height to be shorter than the commissure height, and the difference can be explained in the differential in lip growth with maturation.

The commissure height is measured from a line constructed from the alar base through the subspinale, then from the commissures perpendicular to this line.

The interlabial gap is the distance in millimeters between the upper and lower lips.

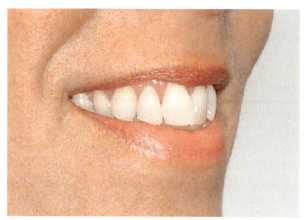

FIG 27-5 The smile arc is best visualized in the oblique view.

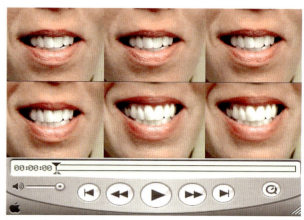

FIG 27-6 Digital videography affords the clinician multiple frames for evaluation of lip-tooth relationships during speech and smiling.

The amount of maxillary incisor display at rest is a critical esthetic parameter because one of the inevitable characteristics of an aging tooth-lip relationship is diminished maxillary incisor display at rest and on smile. For example, an adult patient with 3 mm of gingival display on smile and 3 mm of maxillary incisor display at rest should only carefully consider maxillary incisor intrusion to reduce gingival display, since reduction in gingival display also results in diminished incisor show at rest and during conversation (a characteristic of the aging face). When smiling, patients will either show the entire maxillary incisor or only a percentage of the incisor. Measurement of the percentage of incisor display, when combined with the crown height, helps the clinician decide how much tooth movement is required to attain the appropriate smile for that patient.

The vertical (crown) height of the maxillary central incisors in the adult is normally between 9 and 12 mm, with an average of 10.6 mm in men and 9.6 mm in women. The age of the patient is a factor in crown height because of the rate of gingival apical migration in the adolescent.

The amount of gingival display on smile varies in terms of what is acceptable esthetically, but it is important to always remember the relationship between gingival display and the amount of incisor shown at rest. In broad terms, it is better for a patient to be treated less aggressively in reducing gingival display during a smile when considering that the aging process results in a natural diminishment of this characteristic. A gummy smile is more often esthetically pleasing than a smile with diminished tooth display.

The smile arc should be defined as the relationship of the curvature of the incisal edges of the maxillary incisors and canines to the curvature of the lower lip in the posed social smile.[5] The ideal smile arc has the maxillary incisal edge curvature parallel to the curvature of the lower lip upon smile: the term *consonant* is used to describe this parallel relationship. A *nonconsonant*, or flat, smile arc is characterized by a maxillary incisal curvature that is flatter than the curvature of the lower lip on smile. The smile arc relationship is not as quantifiable as the other attributes, so the qualitative observation of consonant, flat, or reverse smile arcs is generally cited (Fig 27-5).

Digital videography

Dynamic recording of a patient's facial motion is accomplished with the use of digital videography.[6] This technology may be used to document and evaluate such characteristics as range of mandibular motion on opening and laterotrusive movements and deviations upon opening, smile, and speech. Digital video and computer technology has primarily been used to record anterior tooth display during speech and smiling. Digital videos can be recorded in a standardized fashion with the camera at a fixed distance from the subject. These images should be taken in a standard format with emphasis on natural head position, so that future analysis and research possibilities may be maximized. Video should be taken in the frontal, oblique, and lateral dimensions. Clinically, this technology is most relevant in the patient with an asymmetric smile. The question that arises is, does the patient have a dental asymmetry, skeletal asymmetry, or asymmetric movement of the lip curtain during animation? The single-smile photograph cannot corroborate the clinical impression gained during the data collection process. The video clip may be reviewed and evaluated during all planning phases of treatment as well as for comparison of the treatment effects (Fig 27-6).

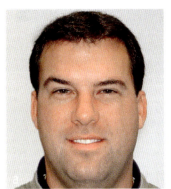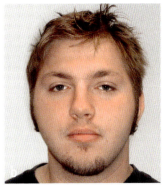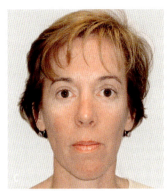

FIG 27-7 Common facial types: (*a*) mesocephalic, (*b*) brachycephalic, and (*c*) dolichocephalic.

Systematic Clinical Examination of Facial and Smile Esthetics

Macroesthetics

Frontal perspective

The starting point for the macroesthetic examination is the frontal view. Transverse and vertical relationships comprise the major components of the frontal examination and analysis. The proportional relationship of height and width is far more important than absolute values in establishing overall facial type. Faces can be broadly categorized as mesocephalic, brachycephalic, or dolichocephalic[7] (Figs 27-7a to 27-7c). The differentiation between these facial types has to do with the general proportionality of facial breadth to facial height, with brachycephalic faces being broader and shorter. Generally, the most attractive faces tend to have common proportions and relationships that differ from normative values.[8]

Vertical facial proportions

The ideal face is vertically divided into equal thirds by horizontal lines adjacent to the hairline, eyebrows, the nasal base, and menton (Fig 27-8). Orthodontic treatment is to a large extent limited to the lower facial third. Measurement of the upper face is often hindered by the variability in identification of such broad landmarks as location of the hairline and radix.

Clinical examination begins with the evaluation of lower facial height. In the ideal lower third of the face, the upper lip makes up the upper third, and the lower lip and chin compose the lower two thirds (Fig 27-9). Disproportion of the vertical facial thirds may be a result of many dental and skeletal factors, and these proportional relationships may help define the contributing factors related to vertical discrepancies.

Transverse facial proportions

The assessment of the transverse components of facial width is best described by the rule of fifths.[4] This method describes the ideal transverse relationships of the face. The face is divided sagittally into five equal parts from helix to helix of the outer ears (Fig 27-10). Each of the segments should approximate the width of one eye. Transverse fifths should be individually examined and then assessed as a complete group.

The middle fifth of the face is delineated by the inner canthi of the eyes. A vertical line from the inner canthus should be coincident with the alar base of the nose. Variation in this facial third could be due to transverse deficiencies or excesses in either the inner canthi or alar base. A vertical line from the outer canthi of the eyes frames the medial three fifths of the face, which should be coincident with the gonial angles of the mandible. Although disproportion may be very subtle, it is worth noting since treatments can positively change the shape or relative proportion of the gonial angles. The outer two fifths of the face are measured from the lateral canthus of the eye to the lateral helix of the ear, which represents the width of the ears. Another significant frontal relationship is the midpupillary distance, which should be transversely aligned with the commissures of the mouth.

Nasal anatomy in the transverse plane should also be assessed through proportionality. The width of the alar base should be approximately the same as the intercanthal distance, which should be the same as the width of an eye. If the intercanthal distance is smaller than an eye width, it is better to keep the nose slightly wider than the intercanthal distance. The width of the alar base is heavily influenced by inherited ethnic characteristics.

Asymmetry of the face is a somewhat natural occurrence. Systematic examination of the patient's facial symmetry should be directly measured in the frontal plane.

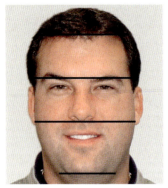

Fig 27-8 Vertical proportions in the frontal view: delineation of the vertical facial thirds.

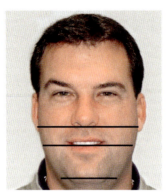

Fig 27-9 In the ideal lower third of the face, the upper lip makes up the upper third and the lower lip and chin compose the lower two thirds.

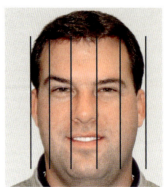

Fig 27-10 Transverse proportions in the frontal view: delineation of the transverse facial fifths.

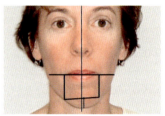

Fig 27-11 Measurement of the midsymphysis to the midsagittal plane is a logical indicator of chin asymmetry, but the parasymphyseal heights should also be measured when chin asymmetry is suspected.

The following measurements make up this portion of the clinical exam: nasal tip to midsagittal plane, maxillary dental midline to midsagittal plane, mandibular dental midline to midsymphysis, mandibular asymmetry with or without functional shift, chin asymmetry, maxillomandibular asymmetry, oblique perspective, and profile perspective.

To measure nasal tip to midsagittal plane, the clinician has the patient elevate his or her head slightly and then visualizes the nasal tip in relation to the midsagittal plane to best view the position of the nasal tip. Any deviation of the nasal tip should be noted in relation to the maxillary midline. The clinician should not make the mistake of treating the maxillary midline according to a distorted nose. An attempt to obtain the etiology of nasal tip asymmetry is recommended. The patient should be questioned as to any previous history of nasal trauma or nasal surgery for deviated septum. The patient may then be advised appropriately as to whether this deviation is severe enough to consider correction.

The maxillary dental midline should be recorded relative to the midsagittal plane. A discrepancy could be due to either dental factors or skeletal maxillary rotation. Maxillary rotation is a rare clinical finding and is usually accompanied by posterior dental crossbite (Sarver DM, personal communication, 2001).

The mandibular dental midline to midsymphysis relationship is best visualized by standing behind the patient and viewing the mandibular arch from above. The patient should open his or her mouth for the clinician to view the mandibular arch and its relationship to the body of the mandible and symphysis. Mandibular dental midline discrepancies are usually due to tooth-related issues such as dental crowding with

shifted incisors, premature exfoliation of primary teeth and subsequent space closure in preadolescents, congenitally missing teeth, or an extracted unilateral tooth. If the mandibular dental midline is not coincident with the midsymphysis, it usually indicates a dental shift. However, chin asymmetry should also be considered.

Mandibular asymmetry is suspected when the midsymphysis is not coincident with the midsagittal plane. An important diagnostic factor is whether a lateral functional shift is present secondary to a functional shift of the mandible as a result of crossbite. When the patient's jaw is manipulated into centric relation, a bilateral, end-to-end crossbite is usually present, and as the patient moves his or her teeth into full occlusion, he or she must choose a side to move the mandible into maximum intercuspation. This lateral shift is not indicative of true mandibular symmetry but of transverse maxillary deficiency and a resultant functional shift of the mandible. True mandibular asymmetry is suspected when, in closure into centric relation, no lateral functional shift occurs. The truly asymmetric mandible may be due to an inherited asymmetric facial growth pattern or as a result of localized or systemic factors. A thorough history of traumatic injuries and a review of the patient's medical history will help ascertain potential etiologies of true mandibular asymmetry.

Facial asymmetry may in some cases be limited to the chin only. If the systematic evaluation of facial symmetry determines dental and skeletal midlines and vertical relations of the maxilla to be normal and lower facial asymmetry is noted, then the asymmetry may be isolated to the chin. Measurement of the midsymphysis to the midsagittal plane is a logical indicator of chin asymmetry, but the parasymphyseal heights should also be measured when chin asymmetry is suspected (Fig 27-11). The frontal view is recommended, but a view from the superior facial aspect (much like for the evaluation of the mandibular dental midline) with the mouth closed also affords the clinician excellent visualization of the chin in relation to the body of the mandible and the midsymphysis.

Mandibular asymmetry is often accompanied by maxillary compensation, which is reflected clinically by a transverse cant of the maxilla. This means that evaluation of mandibular deformity should include the possibility of maxillomandibular deformity. Transverse tilting of the maxilla may be detectable cephalometrically but is most evident during the macroesthetic examination. The transverse cant of the maxilla is often determined by the relative difference in gingival display at the level of the canine moving posterior on smile.

Oblique perspective

The oblique view in the macroesthetic examination affords the orthodontist another perspective for evaluating the facial thirds. With regard to the upper face, the clinician may view the relative projection of the orbital rim and malar eminence. Orbital and malar retrusion are often seen in craniofacial syndromes. Cheek projection is evaluated in the area of the zygomatic and malar scaffold. Skin laxity and atrophy of the malar fat pad in this area may actually be a characteristic of aging and therefore seen in the older patient population.[9] This area can be described as deficient, balanced, or prominent. Nasal anatomy, which was described in the frontal examination, may also be characterized in this dimension (Fig 27-12). Lip anatomy is also viewed in the oblique and lateral view. The philtral area and vermilion of the maxillary lip should be clearly demarcated. The height of the philtrum should be noted as short, balanced, or excessive. Vermilion display should be termed as excessive, balanced, or thin. The relative projection of the maxilla and mandible can be assessed in the oblique view. Midface deficiency can result in increased nasolabial folding, relaxed upper lip support, and altered columellar and nasal tip support.

One of the other values of the oblique view is visualization of the body and gonial angle of the mandible as well as the cervicomental area. Mandibular deficiency with associated dental compensation may produce lower lip eversion, excessive vermilion display, and a pronounced labiomental sulcus. A characterization of mandibular form is also very important. The oblique view also demonstrates the effects of animation on the appearance of lip and chin projection.

Profile perspective

The last view in the macroesthetic examination is the profile or sagittal perspective. Natural head position is essential for accurate evaluation of profile characteristics. The patient should be instructed to look straight ahead and if possible into his or her own image in an appropriately placed mirror. The visual axis is what determines "natural head position." This axis very often, but not always, approximates the Frankfort horizontal plane. The classic vertical facial thirds should also be applied in profile view (Fig 27-13). An assessment of lower facial deficiency or excess should be noted.

The nasolabial angle describes the inclination of the columella in relation to the upper lip and should be in the range of 90 to 120 degrees.[10] The nasolabial angle is determined by several factors: (1) anteroposterior position of the maxilla, (2) anteroposterior position of the maxillary incisors, (3) vertical position or rotation of the nasal tip, and (4) soft tissue thickness of the maxillary lip, which contributes to the nasolabial angle, where a thin upper lip favors a flatter angle and a thicker lip favors an acute angle.

The characterization of the lower face in profile is measured by the relative degree of lip projection, the labiomental sulcus, the chin-neck length, and the chin-neck angle. Maxillary and mandibular sagittal position can be described by means of facial divergence. The lower third of the face is evaluated in reference to the anterior soft tissue point at glabella. Based on the position of the maxilla and mandible relative to this point, a patient's profile will be described as straight, convex, or concave and either anteriorly or posteriorly divergent.

Lip projection is a function of maxillomandibular protrusion or retrusion, dental protrusion or retrusion, or lip thickness. The description of lip projection should include pertinent information from any of the above sources. For example, a patient with lower lip protrusion may be maxillary (midface) deficient with dentoalveolar compensation including flared incisors and a thin maxillary vermilion display, or may simply have a thick lower lip that appears protrusive.

The labiomental sulcus is defined as the fold of soft tissue between the lower lip and the chin and may vary greatly in form and depth (Fig 27-14). The clinical variables that can affect the labiomental sulcus are mandibular incisor position (upright mandibular incisors tend to result in a shallow labiomental sulcus because of a lack of lower lip projection, whereas excessive mandibular incisor proclination deepens the labiomental sulcus) and vertical height of the lower facial third, which has a direct bearing on chin

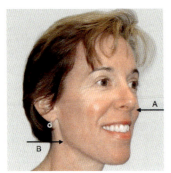

FIG 27-12 The oblique view provides visualization of the nasal anatomy and form (A) and the mandibular form and gonial angle (B).

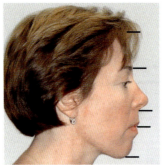

FIG 27-13 Delineation of the vertical facial thirds in the profile view. This patient has a longer lower facial third with excess height from the lower lip to menton.

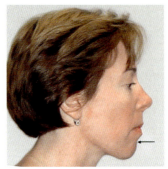

FIG 27-14 The labiomental sulcus is defined as the fold of soft tissue between the lower lip and the chin and may vary greatly in form and depth.

position and the labiomental sulcus. Diminished lower facial height usually results in a deeper labiomental sulcus (as in the patient with a complete denture who has an overclosed bite, whereas a patient with a long lower facial third has a tendency toward a flat labiomental sulcus.

Chin projection is determined by the amount of anteroposterior bony projection of the anterior, inferior border of the mandible and the amount of soft tissue that overlays that bony projection. The amount of profile chin projection is measured by the distance from pogonion (the most anterior point on the bony chin) to soft tissue pogonion (the most anterior point on the soft tissue profile of the chin) and is not generally alterable by surgical means. In the adolescent, the amount of chin is directly correlated to the amount of mandibular growth that occurs, because the chin point itself is borne on the mandible as it grows anteriorly.

Miniesthetics
Frontal perspective
Vertical characteristics/lip-tooth-gingival relationships
Key features of vertical facial miniesthetic characteristics is the relationship of the incisal edges of the maxillary incisors relative to the lower lip as well as the relationship of the gingival margins of the maxillary incisors relative to the upper lip. The gingival margins of the canines should be coincident with the upper lip and the lateral incisors positioned slightly inferior to the adjacent teeth (Fig 27-15). It is generally accepted that the gingival margins should be coincident with the upper lip in the social smile. However, this is very much a function of the age of the patient, since children show more teeth at rest and gingival display on smile than do adults.[11]

The vertical characteristics of facial miniesthetics impact the relative amount of gingival display at rest and animation. Gingival display is the amount of "gumminess" of the smile. Measuring the amount of gingival display on smile easily quantitates a gummy smile. The decision whether the amount of gingival display is an esthetic problem, in which treatment is desirable, is a personal choice. Orthodontists tend to see the gummy smile as an unesthetic characteristic, whereas laypersons attach importance only in the more extreme cases. The use of computerized graphic simulation of the frontal view of the smile is useful in counseling a patient and showing potential treatment changes. The individual is then able to guide the clinician and express opinions about what should and should not be corrected. Computer imaging not only provides the patient with a visual template for treatment, but also provides the clinician with a testing ground for treatment options.

Transverse characteristics
The three transverse characteristics of facial miniesthetics in the frontal dimension are arch form, buccal corridor, and transverse cant of the maxillary occlusal plane (Fig 27-16). Arch form plays a pivotal role in the transverse dimension. In cases in which the arch forms are narrow or collapsed, the smile may also appear narrow and therefore present inadequate transverse smile characteristics. An important consideration in widening a narrow arch form, particularly in adults, is the axial inclination of the buccal segments. Cases in which the posterior teeth are already flared laterally are not good candidates for dental expansion. Patients in whom the premolars and molars are upright have more capacity for transverse expansion—certainly in the adolescent, but it is particularly important in the adult, where

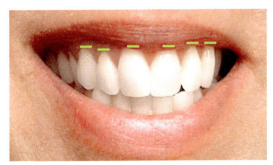

FIG 27-15 It is generally accepted that the gingival margins should be coincident with the upper lip in the social smile. However, this is very much a function of the age of the patient, since children show more teeth at rest and gingival display on smile than do adults. In this adult patient, there is asymmetrical lip curtain with greater elevation on the patient's right side. Thus, the asymmetric gingival heights are further highlighted because of the asymmetry of the dynamic lip.

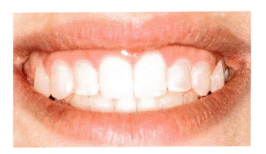

FIG 27-16 The three transverse characteristics of facial miniesthetics in the frontal dimension are arch form, buccal corridor, and transverse cant of the maxillary occlusal plane. This patient's maxillary arch has been overexpanded with conventional orthodontic treatment. The arch form is exceedingly broad, the buccal corridor has been completely obliterated, and there is a flat smile arc.

sutural expansion is less likely. Orthodontic expansion and widening of collapsed arch form can dramatically improve the appearance of facial esthetics and smile by decreasing the size of the buccal corridors and improving the transverse smile dimension. The transverse smile dimension (and the buccal corridor) is related to the lateral projection of the premolars and molars into the buccal corridors. The wider the arch form is in the premolar area, the greater the portion of the buccal corridor that is filled.

Arch expansion can have undesirable effects. Expansion of the arch form may fill out the transverse dimension of the smile, but two undesirable side effects may result. First, the buccal corridor can be obliterated and create a "denturelike" smile. Second, when the anterior sweep of the maxillary arch is broadened, the smile arc may be flattened. While it may not be possible to avoid these undesirable aspects of expansion, the clinician must make a judgment in concert with the patient as to what compromises are acceptable in the pursuit of the ideal facial esthetic outcome. Careful observation should be made to avoid these side effects if possible.

The last transverse characteristic of facial miniesthetics is the transverse cant of the maxillary occlusal plane. Transverse cant of the maxilla can be due to differential eruption and placement of the anterior teeth and to skeletal asymmetry of the skull base or mandible that results in a compensatory cant to the maxilla. Intraoral images or even mounted dental casts do not adequately reflect the relationship of the maxilla to the smile. Only frontal smile visualization permits the orthodontist to visualize any

tooth-related asymmetry transversely. Smile asymmetry may also be due to soft tissue considerations such as an asymmetric smile curtain. In the asymmetric smile curtain, there is a differential elevation of the upper lip during smile, which gives the illusion of transverse cant to the maxilla. This smile characteristic emphasizes the importance of direct clinical examination in treatment planning the smile, since this soft tissue animation is not visible in a frontal radiograph or reflected in study casts. It is not well documented in static photographic images, and is documented best in digital video clips.

Oblique perspective

The oblique view of the smile reveals characteristics not obtainable on the frontal view and certainly not obtainable through any cephalometric analysis. The palatal plane may be canted anteroposteriorly in a number of orientations. In the most desirable orientation, the occlusal plane is consonant with the curvature of the lower lip on smile. Deviations from this orientation include a downward cant of the posterior maxilla, upward cant of the anterior maxilla, or variations of both.[12] In the initial examination and diagnostic phase of treatment, it is important to visualize the occlusal plane in its relationship to the lower lip.

Early definitions of the smile arc were limited to the curvature of the canines and the incisors to the lower lip on smile because smile evaluation was made on direct frontal view. The visualization of the complete smile arc afforded by the oblique view expands the definition of the smile arc to include the molars and the premolars (Fig 27-17).

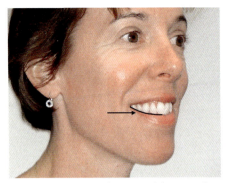

FIG 27-17 The visualization of the complete smile arc afforded by the oblique view expands the definition of the smile arc to include the molars and the premolars.

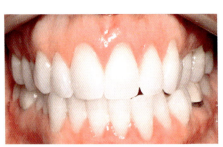

FIG 27-18 Microesthetic evaluation.

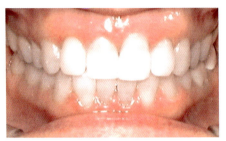

FIG 27-19 Obliterated gingival papillae or "dark triangles" in the anterior dentition should be noted. Note the small black triangles in between the maxillary and mandibular central incisors. This is due to mild horizontal bone loss over time as well as to a tooth shape issue. Reproximation of the contact points should be undertaken to broaden the area of contact and reposition the interdental papilla.

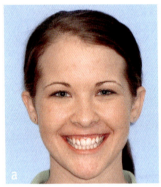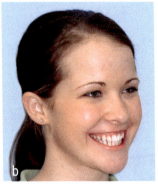

FIG 27-20 Patient case example: (*a*) frontal portrait photograph on smile; (*b*) oblique (45-degree) portrait photograph on smile.

Profile perspective

The two miniesthetic characteristics visualized in the profile view are overjet and incisor angulation. Excessively positive overjet is one of the most recognizable dental traits to the layperson. Excessive positive overjet is not as readily perceived in the frontal dimension as it is in the sagittal dimension. Many Class II patterns have very esthetic smiles frontally, but not when the patient's smile is observed from the side. In Class III patterns, the same phenomenon may be true: on frontal smile the smile looks esthetic, but on the oblique or sagittal view, the overall appearance reflects the underlying skeletal pattern and dental compensation. The patient and/or parents have to decide with the clinician whether this is an acceptable outcome.

The amount of maxillary anterior projection also has great influence on the transverse smile dimension in the frontal view. When the maxilla is retrusive, the wider portion of the dental arch is positioned more posteriorly relative to the anterior oral commissure. This creates the illusion of greater buccal corridor in the frontal dimension. Overall, the sagittal cant of the maxillary occlusal plane in natural head position can influence smile arc in the frontal dimension, affecting vertical characteristics. A negative cant of this plane will diminish the apposition of the incisal edges of the maxillary anterior teeth to the superior vermilion border of the lower lip at smile.

Microesthetics

The microesthetic portion of the clinical examination focuses on the morphology of tooth-to-tooth contacts and the surrounding intraoral tissues (Fig 27-18). As a structural unit, the dentogingival complex is defined by the relationship of the teeth to the alveolar bone and surrounding gingival and masticatory mucosa. The factors that influence the appearance of the dentogingival complex are the patient's periodontal status and past history of disease, the proximal and occlusal contacts of the teeth, the shape of the individual teeth, and the type of gingival architecture.

An assessment of the patient's current periodontal status is exceedingly important from an orthodontic point of view. The clinician should take an accurate dental history to ascertain whether the patient has had any periodontal disease and related treatment. Clinically, the teeth should be examined for plaque accumulation and supragingival calculus. Patients who cannot maintain a satisfactory

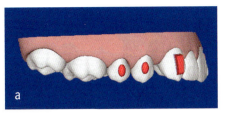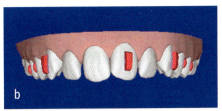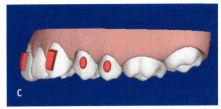

FIG 27-21 (a to c) ClinCheck images from the patient in Fig 27-20. Note the orientation of the maxillary arch.

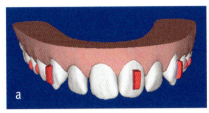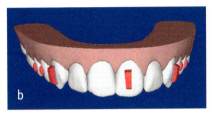

FIG 27-22 Reoriented ClinCheck images. A slight inferior cant of the anterior maxillary arch simulates the natural head position relationship. (a) Pretreatment; (b) simulated final result.

level of oral hygiene are at risk for gingival inflammation and caries during treatment. Periapical radiographs along with a panoramic radiograph will reveal alveolar architecture and any evidence of horizontal or vertical bone loss. Suspected periodontal defects should be probed and the depths recorded. The extent of attachment loss and degree of tooth mobility will influence tooth movement. "Black triangles" or obliterated interdental papillae should be noted (Fig 27-19).

Integration of Clinical Database with ClinCheck Images

The data obtained from the comprehensive clinical examination of the patient in the frontal, oblique, and profile perspectives should be correlated with the virtual case setup in the ClinCheck program. Esthetic treatment planning involves the integration of the patient's 3-D lip-tooth relationships with the virtual images of the teeth and gingival scaffold seen in ClinCheck. The clinician should, in his or her mind, reorient the virtual arches into their corrected positions within the framework of the patient's soft tissues at rest and during speech and smiling (Figs 27-20 and 27-21). Because the arches automatically appear in ClinCheck with the occlusal plane perpendicular to the computer screen, it should be noted that in reality there is a cant of the occlusal plane in natural head position (Figs 27-22a and 27-22b). This information becomes crucial when planning vertical maxillary incisor positioning relative to the preservation or creation of a consonant smile arc.

References

1. Ackerman MB. Orthodontics and its discontents. Orthod Craniofac Res 2004;7:187–188.
2. Ackerman JL, Keane ML, Ackerman MB. Orthodontics in the age of enhancement. Aust Orthod J 2004;20:3A–5A.
3. Sarver DM, Ackerman JL. About face: The re-emerging soft tissue paradigm. Am J Orthod Dentofacial Orthop 2000;117:575–576.
4. Sarver DM. Esthetic Orthodontics and Orthognathic Surgery. St Louis: Mosby, 1997.
5. Ackerman JL, Ackerman MB, Brensinger CM, Landis JR. A morphometric analysis of the posed smile. Clin Orthod Res 1998;1:2–11.
6. Ackerman MB. Digital video as a clinical tool in orthodontics: Dynamic smile design in diagnosis and treatment planning. In: McNamara JA, Ferrara AM (eds). Information Technology and Orthodontic Treatment, vol 40, Cranofacial Growth Series. Ann Arbor, MI: University of Michigan Press, 2003.
7. Farkas LG, Munro JR. Anthropometric Facial Proportions in Medicine. Springfield, IL: Charles C. Thomas, 1987.
8. Peck H, Peck S. A concept of facial esthetics. Angle Orthod 1970;40:284–318.
9. Pessa JE. The potential role of stereolithography in the study of facial aging. Am J Orthod Dentofacial Orthop 2001;119:117–120.
10. Krugman ME. Photoanalysis of the rhinoplasty patient. Ear Nose Throat J 1981;60:328–330.
11. Zachrisson BU. Esthetic factors involved in anterior tooth display and the smile: Vertical dimension. J Clin Orthod 1998;32:432–445.
12. Burstone CJ, Marcotte MR. Problem Solving in Orthodontics: Goal-Oriented Treatment Strategies. Chicago: Quintessence, 2000: 31–50.

chapter 28

SURGICAL TREATMENT AND INVISALIGN

by
Ross Miller, DDS and Trang Duong, DDS

The utilization of Invisalign in orthognathic surgery is an exciting prospect. Clear plastic appliances continue to be the esthetic standard in orthodontics and are thus a valuable part of the orthodontist's armamentarium. The goal of this chapter is to explain the value of Invisalign in orthognathic surgery cases, both as an appliance and as a diagnostic tool (ClinCheck) to help plan the patient's surgery and orthodontic treatment.

Most orthodontic records—photographs, casts, radiographs, and written records—are static in nature: there is no movement. ClinCheck offers movement, and movement offers a window into the future, revealing the patient's progress over a given series of aligners or time.

Treatment Planning

Sound goals are the foundation of orthodontic treatment, and this is especially true of surgery. The use of Invisalign as part of a treatment plan should not change or modify the goals set for the patient, unless one discovers that unrealistic goals have been set. The Invisalign System influences visualization of treatment and timing of Invisalign and fixed appliances. ClinCheck should be seen as a supplemental part of diagnosis and treatment planning, as it is extremely helpful in visualizing the treatment and can further help to clarify the relationships between vertical, transverse, and anteroposterior movements.

ClinCheck offers the orthodontist a new way of viewing treatment goals, even if fixed appliances are used for part of the treatment, and permits the orthodontist to visualize movement of not only the teeth but also the jaws, in three dimensions. Even though ClinCheck is model based—that is, created from an impression of the teeth without the reference of the skeletal base—it can provide simulations that will help with the diagnostic process. At the time of publication, skeletal changes that can be performed easily in ClinCheck are anteroposterior corrections of the maxillary and mandibular jaws.

ClinCheck can simulate the following movements: vertical movements (of teeth and jaws), dental or skeletal expansion, anteroposterior movements (of jaws), and asymmetric movements. Surgical movements that are difficult to describe or that require multiple-piece maxillary or mandibular surgery can also be performed. The actual visualization of bony segments on ClinCheck is not currently possible. That is to say, an orthodontist cannot ask Align Technology to move segments of bone on ClinCheck.

Align technicians can, however, move the maxillary or mandibular arches in any direction.

Timing

Timing refers to when and what appliances are to be applied. Some clinicians prefer to use fixed appliances before Invisalign, and others opt for Invisalign first. Our preference is to use Invisalign until 2 to 4 months before surgery and then fixed appliances until 6 months after surgery.

Realistically, the patient should understand that treatment will take more than 2 years. A well-planned treatment plan can be executed in 2 years, but we recommend a 6-month buffer for possible midcourse correction or patient noncompliance with the removable appliances. Timing is dependent on factors such as skill of the orthodontist and surgeon, patient compliance, case severity, treatment goals, and surgical plan. One timeline will not apply to all cases. The orthodontist planning the treatment should allow enough leeway to deal with unexpected developments and delays and build time into the treatment plan so the patient understands the timeline.

Communication

The first communication the orthodontist should have is with the patient and the oral surgeon. Everyone involved should understand that Invisalign, in combination with fixed appliances, is to be used in the treatment. There should be agreement about the treatment plan, especially on the part of the patient. It is critical to discuss with the patient the sequence of appliances (especially the fixed) before treatment. An orthodontist does not want to present fixed appliances to a patient who was not aware of and in agreement with the treatment plan.

Communication in ClinCheck is very important for accurate tooth and jaw setups. This is especially true for surgical treatment plans. The "Comments" section of the Virtual Invisalign Practice (VIP) treatment planning form (see chapter 15) is the correct place to log specific requests. In some instances, these comments are communicated directly to the technicians that set up the cases. Communication needs to be clear and concise and might include several ClinCheck iterations or possibly even a phone call to the clinical department. Following are some examples of instructions that might be included for surgical cases:

- *Mandibular advancement*: "This is a surgical treatment. Please move the mandible forward 4 mm and do the orthodontic setup in that position. Please use Class I canine as the guide to distance. As the mandible comes forward, please do dental expansion on the maxillary arch. Please move the mandible forward at stage 1 and do all orthodontic movement from that position."

- *Mandibular setback*: "This is a surgical treatment. Please move the mandible back 2 mm and do the orthodontic setup in that position. Please use Class I canine as the guide to distance. As the mandible moves back, please do dental expansion on the mandibular arch. Please move the mandible back at stage 1 and do all orthodontic movement from that position."

- *Maxillary advancement*: "This is a surgical treatment. Please move the maxilla forward 4 mm and do the orthodontic setup in that position. Please use Class I canine as the guide to distance. As the maxilla comes forward, please do dental expansion on the maxillary arch. Please move the maxillary jaw forward at stage 1 and do all orthodontic movement from that position."

- *Maxillary setback*: "This is a surgical treatment. Please move the maxilla back 2 mm and do the orthodontic setup in that position. Please use Class I canine as the guide to distance. As the maxilla moves back, please do dental expansion on the maxillary arch. Please move the maxillary jaw back at stage 1 and do all orthodontic movement from that position."

- *Vertical movements*: Vertical movements that are symmetric (in vertical movement) for both arches up or down do not generally require special instructions; however, those that include autorotation of the mandible will require special comments: "This is a surgical treatment. The surgical plan includes a 2-mm vertical movement of the maxillary arch in the upward direction. Please simulate a mandibular movement with 3 degrees of rotation of the mandible. Please perform the surgical movements at stage 1 and adjust the teeth at that point. Expand maxillary arch as needed."

- *Multiple-piece maxillary surgery*: At first glance, it may appear that this would be extremely difficult, and in fact, ClinCheck cannot provide for multiple cuts. This limitation of ClinCheck, however, does not mean that such a procedure cannot be planned; the instructions given would be identical to those given above for vertical movements.

These comments are not appropriate for every patient and are not intended as instructions for any given surgical treatment; they are meant as general comments for various types of surgical treatment. Note that the comments are written in clear, concise language.

ClinCheck visualization is not intended to be a final display of the diagnosis and treatment plan, but it can be part of the "database" that is used to develop the optimal treatment plan. As the clinician runs ClinCheck a number of times, he or she can get a feel for the validity of the treatment plan and make minor modifications as necessary. The clinician will most likely have to communicate directly with the clinical team to obtain exactly what is needed in the treatment plan. Basic advances and setbacks, of course, are much easier to simulate than vertical movements or multiple-piece surgeries.

ClinCheck and Surgical Cases

ClinChecks are made from four general parts: initial position, bite, final position, and movements from initial to final position. These components must flow smoothly and be well integrated into the treatment plan. The clinician must not ignore the last point and should be mindful of such questions as "What is the root doing?" and "Can a plastic appliance move the root like that?"

The clinician is advised to not just accept the ClinCheck but to review it thoroughly: laboratory technicians set up the ClinCheck files for the clinician to evaluate. In particular, the clinician should note all vertical movements. The treatment plan should not aim to obtain "socked in" first or second molars; this should be done with the fixed appliances. An assessment of the ClinCheck gives the clinician the opportunity to ask whether extrusion is needed or whether relative intrusion of neighboring teeth will achieve better results. It also provides the clinician the opportunity to get rid of unwanted root torques and tips. In assessing the ClinCheck, the clinician should keep in mind that extrusive movements do not work well with clear plastic appliances.

An evaluation of the initial bite and position should also be undertaken. When performing this evaluation, the clinician should have the patient's treatment form, casts, photographs, and charts available. The clinician should also be certain that stage 1 on ClinCheck matches the patient's bite and should check this from multiple views. If the initial bite is not correct, the clinician can determine what modifications are needed to make the setup work.

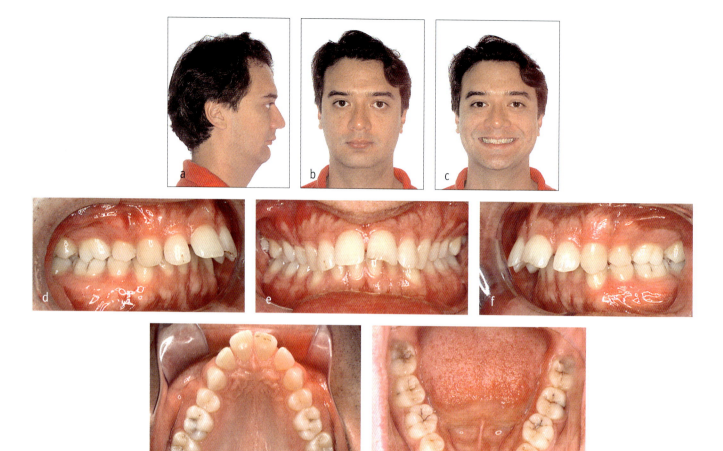

Fig 28-1 (a to h) Pretreatment photographs.

The ClinCheck can be useful in assessing the occlusal symmetry of the maxillary and mandibular arches. Use of the grid and superimposition tool can be helpful. Clearly, asymmetric movements can lead to asymmetric outcomes. Yet, there will be times when movements cannot be symmetric—for instance, when there are unilateral distalizations or single-tooth crossbites. Nevertheless, the default should be symmetric movements.

It is important for clinicians to remember that outcomes must not be based on the seductive videos of ClinCheck but rather on what is possible clinically. Surgical cases for which the use of a fixed appliance are planned provide the clinician a great opportunity to learn and use ClinCheck.

Case Report
Diagnosis

A 36-year-old man presented with a chief concern to fix an overjet. He had a history of orthodontic treatment in 1974 and 1975. He presented with a Class II retrognathic profile (Figs 28-1a to 28-1c). Intraoral photographs showed that molars and canines were Class II with an increased 12-mm overjet (Figs 28-1d to 28-1f). The first premolars had been extracted. The maxillary arch was constricted and V-shaped, the maxillary incisors were proclined, and 3 mm of anterior spacing was present (Figs 28-1g and 28-1h). The mandibular arch was U-shaped, and there was 3 mm of anterior crowding. Soft tissues were healthy; adequate attached gingiva was present. The panoramic radiograph was within normal limits (Fig 28-2). The initial cephalometric analysis (Figs 28-3a and 28-3b) revealed a Class II skeletal pattern with a retrognathic mandible and slightly retrognathic maxilla, proclined maxillary incisors, and an overerupted mandibular incisor.

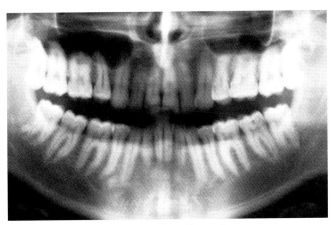

Fig 28-2 Pretreatment panoramic radiograph.

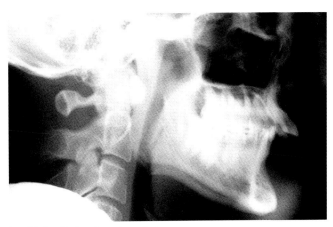

Fig 28-3a Pretreatment cephalogram.

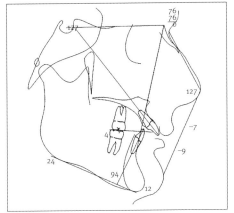

Fig 28-3b Pretreatment tracing.

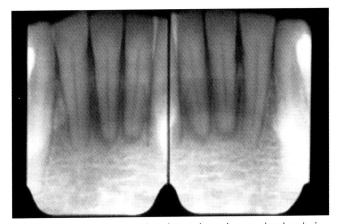

Fig 28-4 Minor root resorption due to intrusion mechanics during the pre-fixed appliance phase.

Treatment objectives

The skeletal objectives were to improve the profile via maxillary and mandibular advancement surgery. The dental objectives were to achieve Class I molar and canine relationships and achieve ideal overjet and overbite via surgery. The arches were to be coordinated, and the presurgical alignment was to be done with Invisalign. Presurgical alignment consisted of retroclining the maxillary incisors to close spaces and to level the curve of Spee by intruding the mandibular incisors. The movements in ClinCheck were programmed to move the maxillary incisors only by tip-back to improve the incisor position as well as to close the spaces. To preserve maximum anchorage, only the four incisors were moved; all other teeth remained stationary in ClinCheck. In the mandibular arch, the movements programmed into ClinCheck consisted of intruding the four incisors and keeping the remainder of the dentition stationary. Attachments were placed on the canines and premolars to aid in retention of the aligner during the intrusion.

Treatment progress and results

The initial examination was performed and impressions taken on January 28, 1999. A pretreatment orthognathic consultation was completed on May 21, 1999. Pre–polyvinyl siloxane (PVS) impression interproximal enamel reduction was done on June 23, 1999, and impressions were taken and sent to Align for ClinCheck fabrication. Treatment commenced on October 5, 1999 with bonding of attachments and delivery of the first aligner. The original treatment consisted of 28 maxillary aligners and 35 mandibular aligners. The aligners were initially made of pelethane, which was not retentive enough; the aligners were remade out of a different material (at the time polycarbonate was used). The new aligners were delivered on November 18, 1999, new attachments were placed, and treatment commenced. On May 5, 2000, progress records were taken. Some minor root resorption was present at the mandibular central incisors, which seems consistent with intrusion mechanics (Fig 28-4). On August 23, 2000, maxillary aligner 20 was given as a

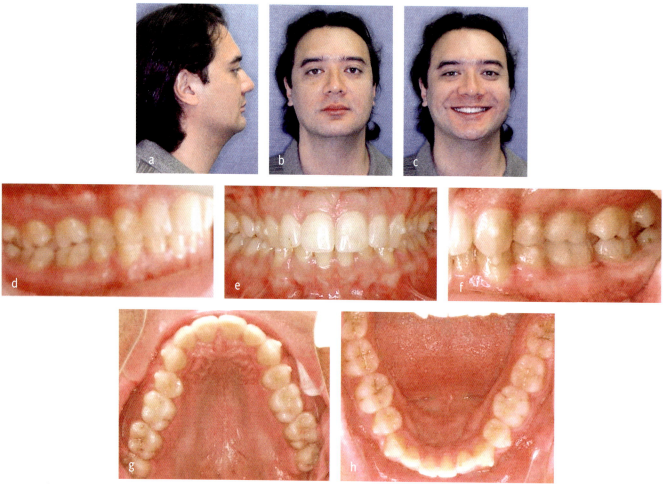

Fig 28-5 (a to h) Patient's appearance at the end of Invisalign treatment.

retainer, and the patient was instructed to wear it nights only. On November 29, 2000, Invisalign treatment was finished and photographs were taken.

After Invisalign alignment (Figs 28-5a to 28-5h), the maxillary spaces were closed. It can be seen from the maxillary superimposition that the maxillary incisor was tipped back 5 mm and retroclined about 30 degrees. The molar position was maintained. It is important to remember that ClinCheck moved only the four incisors. In the mandibular arch, the incisors were moved inferiorly 3 mm and advanced 2 mm. The mandibular molars remained in the same relative position.

Invisalign was used to achieve presurgical alignment. After about 1 year of Invisalign treatment, the patient was switched to a fixed appliance in preparation for surgery.

The patient was fully banded on December 13, 2000, and 0.014 NiTi wires were inserted. These wires were then changed sequentially to 16 × 22 NiTi on January 24, 2001, then to 19 × 25 NiTi on February 2, and finally to 19 × 22 stainless steel on March 21. Kobayshi hooks were placed

on May 10, and the date for surgery was set for June 21. The surgical procedure was maxillary and mandibular advancement. On July 11, the patient was seen postoperatively and was doing well (Figs 28-6a to 28-6h).

One week later, elastics were started from maxillary to mandibular canines and first premolars. On August 22, the maxillary teeth from second premolar to second premolar were repositioned and 0.016 NiTi delivered; then on September 4, a 19 × 25 NiTi maxillary archwire was placed. Photographs and study casts were taken on September 19; a panoramic radiograph taken on September 26 showed shorter anterior roots. On October 1, a 19 × 25 stainless steel wire was placed on the maxillary arch and finishing bends were placed for the next 3 months.

Impressions for retainers were taken on February 2, 2002, and the patient was debonded on March 27, 2002, with delivery of a maxillary Hawley retainer and a mandibular spring aligner. Class I molar and canine relationship was achieved with ideal overjet and overbite (Figs 28-7a to 28-7h). In addition to the advancement,

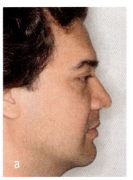
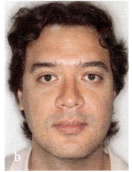
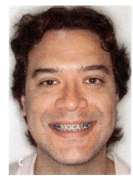
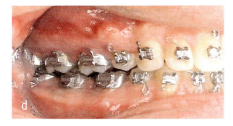
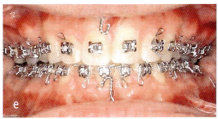
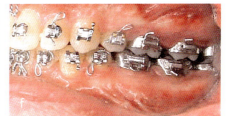
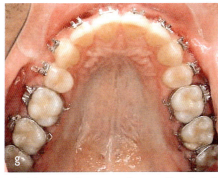
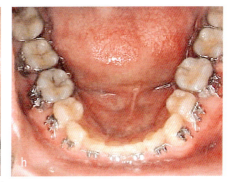

FIG 28-6 (a to h) Postsurgical images. Postoperative swelling is evident.

advancement genioplasty was performed (Figs 28-8a to 28-8c). The posttreatment cephalogram revealed that the maxillary incisors were retroclined and the curve of Spee leveled.

A maxillary black triangle between the central incisors was present at the end of treatment, and it was decided to correct this with additional aligners. New PVS impressions were made, five maxillary aligners were delivered, and interproximal reduction was performed between the central incisors. New maxillary and mandibular Hawley retainers were delivered to allow the posterior occlusion to settle. Retention photographs taken 1.5 years after the final photographs show that the correction of the black triangle is stable and also that the settling in the posterior occlusion resulted in good Class I relationship and occlusal interdigitation (Figs 28-9a to 28-9h). Minor relapse was noted in the mandibular anteriors.

Treatment summary

The patient's initial (January 1998) and final (March 2002) records were taken 3 years, 3 month apart, but first aligners were delivered November 1999. Treatment comprised three stages: (1) presurgical alignment achieved with aligners from November 18, 1999, to November 29, 2000; (2) presurgical treatment with fixed appliances from December 13, 2000, to June 21, 2001; and (3) postsurgical fixed appliances from July 11, 2001, to March 27, 2002, for detailing. Total treatment time was 1 year in Invisalign and 15 months in fixed appliances, for a total of 27 months of treatment.

This case illustrates the first completed surgical case treated with Invisalign and conventional fixed appliances. It documents that the combined treatment of Invisalign and fixed appliances can be used to achieve favorable esthetic and occlusal results, even though total treatment time may be slightly increased.

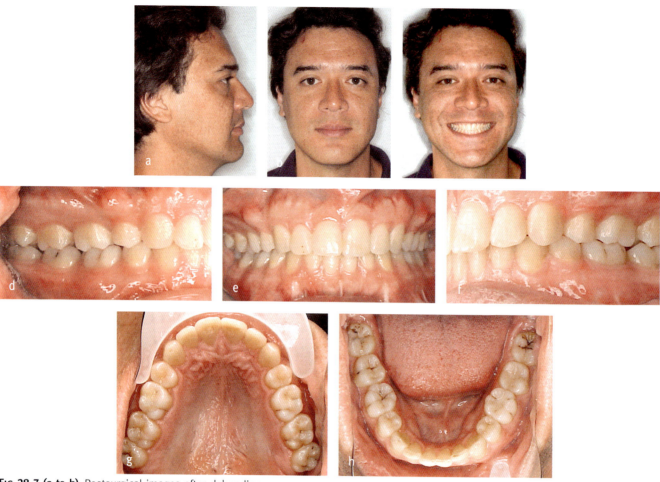

FIG 28-7 (a to h) Postsurgical images after debonding.

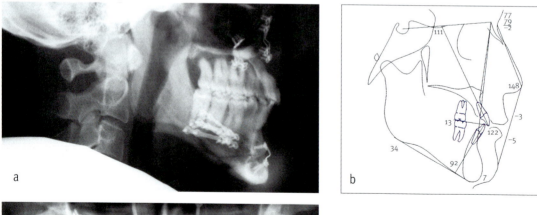

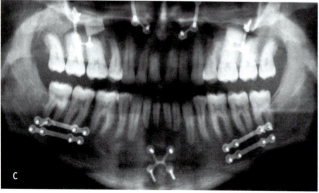

FIG 28-8 Post-debonding cephalogram (*a*), tracing (*b*), and panoramic radiograph (*c*).

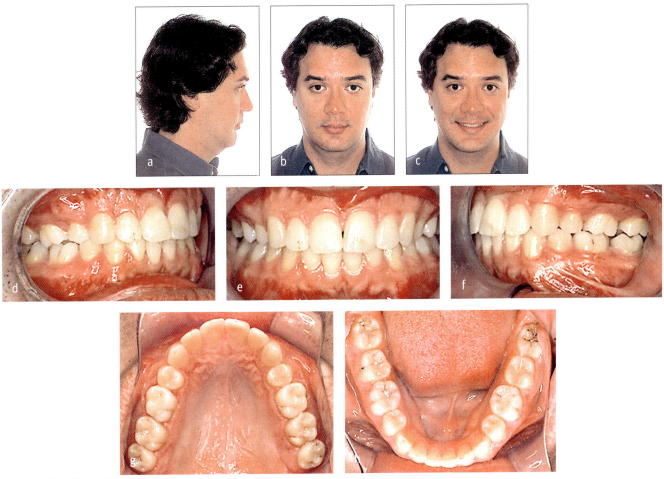

FIG 28-9 (a to h) Final records.

Conclusions

Advances in technology have increased the efficiency of orthodontics and improved the patient experience during treatment. Patients today have more options with the types of appliances they can choose, and orthodontists have various appliances, wires, and imaging tools available to them. It will be exciting and interesting to see the new advances and changes orthodontics undergoes in the future. As with any new technology, however, careful use and good judgement should always be used.

chapter 29

Feasibility Study of the Invisalign System in Treatment of Adolescents

by
Andrew Trosien, DDS and Robert Fry, DDS

Several articles have appeared in the literature to describe the effectiveness of Align Technology's Invisalign System since it was first introduced in 1997. Invisalign was originally offered to adult patients seeking orthodontic treatment with an esthetic appliance.

The first clinical study on the feasibility of Invisalign was performed on adult patients. Adults were chosen as the initial test sample for three reasons; (1) Adults have a static dentition, whereas adolescents and children have actively erupting teeth and growing jaws; (2) adults are generally regarded as the most compliant patient group. Children are thought to be somewhat compliant and adolescents are typically believed to be noncompliant. Studying the efficacy of aligners required that the patients wear them as directed; (3) from a business perspective, Invisalign treatment was targeted at adults who wanted orthodontic treatment but were reluctant to wear fixed appliances. The results gathered from the study of adults showed that aligners were effective at treating generalized crowding and spacing cases.

Shortly after the initial studies of Invisalign treatment began, 20 or so orthodontists around the country each began treatment on three patients as a beta test. Many of these patients were adolescents. The empirical data gathered from these clinicians showed that adolescents may be successfully treated with the Invisalign System. It was decided to initiate a formal study to determine if adolescents with permanent dentition (ie, second molar to second molar) could be treated with the appliance.

Study Design

In 2000, Align Technology and the orthodontists affiliated with the company's research and development department began working on a design for the study. At the time, very little was known about the capability of the Invisalign System. To focus specifically on the treatment of adolescents, many of the other variables had to be controlled. Because of this, a narrow scope of diagnosis was created for the inclusion criteria so as to remove variability of the treatment plans.

The primary objective of the study was to determine the efficacy of the Invisalign aligner in treating adolescent patients. The variables measured were tooth alignment, oral hygiene, patient cooperation, and quality of life.

Materials and Methods
Patient selection

Patients were recruited from the authors' private practices in Kansas City, Kansas (RF), and Tracy, California (AT). Twenty-one and 13 patients were recruited from each practice, respectively, with a total enrollment of 34 patients. There were 13 male patients (mean age: 15 years, 3 months) and 21 female patients (mean age: 15 years, 2 months) distributed between the two practices. Patients were included in the study if they were 12 to 18 years old and had maxillary and mandibular permanent dentition, mild to moderate spacing (1 to 6 mm), mild to moderate crowding (1 to 6 mm), and Class I posterior occlusion. Patients were excluded if they or their parents were unwilling to sign consent forms or if they had severe malocclusion. The selected patients and their parent(s) were informed of the study, asked to participate, and given a consent form. Patients were given a choice of Invisalign treatment or standard treatment with either fixed or removable appliances.

Records

Standard records were taken for each patient for the purpose of orthodontic treatment planning. In addition, for the purpose of the Invisalign treatment, polyvinyl siloxane (PVS) impressions of each arch and a centric occlusion wax bite were made. The PVS impressions, a prescription form, panoramic radiograph, lateral cephalogram, and photographs for each patient were submitted to Align Technology. Once received at Align, the cases went through the normal commercial process of pouring casts, three-dimensional scanning, and virtual treatment. All cases were treated under the normal commercial manufacturing guidelines for staging, speed, and attachments. The virtual treatments were based on the treating orthodontists' treatment plan in the prescription form. The final virtual treatment plan was presented in ClinCheck via the Internet to the treating orthodontist. The treating orthodontist reviewed the virtual treatment plan and either accepted or requested a modification in the treatment based on the desired treatment plan and goal. Once the treatment plan was accepted, aligners were fabricated and delivered. Intraoral photographs and progress casts were obtained every 6 months, and a panoramic radiograph was taken at the end of 12 months. At the completion of treatment, photographs, impressions, a panoramic radiograph, and a lateral head film were taken.

TABLE 29-1 Oral hygiene parameter coding used for scoring patients at each appointment

Score	Parameter*			
	Brushing	Flossing	Plaque	Gingivitis
1	Never	Never	None	Normal
2	Daily	Monthly	Some	Somewhat inflamed
3	2 × daily	Weekly	A lot	Very inflamed
4	3 × daily	Multiple times weekly	NA	NA
5	› 3 × daily	Daily	NA	NA
6	NA	2 × daily	NA	NA

* = Not applicable.

TABLE 29-3 Aligner wear parameter coding used for scoring patients at each appointment

Score	Parameter*			
	Aligner retention	Lost	Broken	Attachments
0	NA	No	No	None
1	Excellent	Yes	Yes	Yes
2	Good	NA	NA	Broken off
3	Fair	NA	NA	Removed
4	Poor	NA	NA	Rebonded

* = Not applicable.

TABLE 29-2 Change in oral hygiene habits parameter coding used for scoring patients at each appointment

Score	Change in hygiene habits*
n + 0	None
n + 1	Better (than last visit)
n − 1	Worse (than last visit)

* = Not applicable.
n = Current culmulative score in this category.

Data collection

Each patient was seen every 6 weeks after delivery of the first aligner. Data collection occurred at each visit. Collection was undertaken by either the treating orthodontist or a registered dental assistant. Neither the data collectors nor the patients were blinded as to the aspects of the study or the data collection. No calibration among data collectors was performed prior to the study. Training was limited to the instructions provided with each form.

At each visit, data were collected and recorded on an oral hygiene case report form and an aligner case report form. Five aspects of oral hygiene data were recorded: amount of plaque, degree of gingivitis, frequency of brushing, frequency of flossing, and change in oral hygiene habits. Scoring for these parameters is shown in Tables 29-1 and 29-2.

Retention, accuracy of fit, hours of wear per day, days of wear per aligner, and break/loss data were recorded on the aligner case report form. The criteria for scoring retention and break/loss data are listed in Table 29-3.

Every 6 months, data were collected on a new quality-of-life questionnaire. This questionnaire was adapted from the Dental Impact on Daily Performance scale by Leao and Sheiham.[1] It was used to measure the degree of satisfaction using the parameters of appearance, comfort, pain, performance, and eating restriction. The patient completed the questionnaire with no instructions other than those included on the form.

Progression of treatment

If, at any stage during treatment, the patient's teeth did not follow the prescribed path, the case was stopped and new PVS impressions were taken for additional aligners. During the time the new aligners were being fabricated, the patient was instructed to wear a clear vacuum-formed appliance to retain the current position of the teeth. Patients whose failure was due to poor compliance were, however, not retreated, but were instead cut from the study. After the last aligner was delivered, each treating orthodontist determined the need for additional aligners for minor adjustments.

Efficacy of treatment

Irregularity index measurements were made to quantify the alignment of the teeth before and after treatment. Measurements were made with a digital caliper on photocopied pictures of the pretreatment and final casts. The technique was adapted from Little.[2]

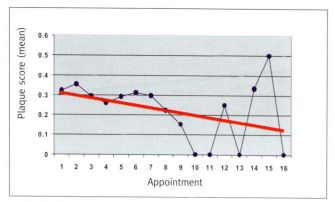

FIG 29-1 Mean amount of plaque found at each appointment. The trend line shows a slight decrease in the mean value of each patient's plaque score per appointment.

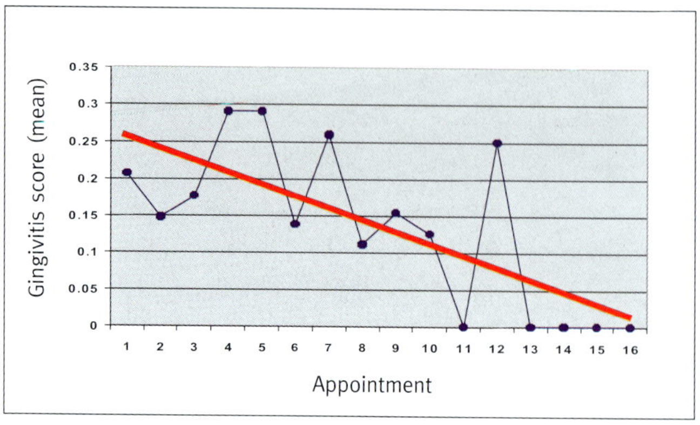

FIG 29-2 Mean degree of gingival inflammation found at each appointment. The trend line shows a slight decrease in the mean value of each patient's degree of gingival inflammation per appointment.

Results

Patient sample outcome

Five patients withdrew from the study and four were dropped, leaving 25 who successfully completed the study. Patients withdrew from the study if they moved away; patients were dropped as a result of poor compliance. Eighteen of the total 34 patients required additional aligners to complete their treatment.

Certainly, the attrition rate is notable. All of the patients who withdrew or were dropped from the study had been selected from a screening of an underserved population and were therefore given a 90% courtesy off of the treatment fee. This created a lack of financial commitment to treatment and may have been the cause of the failed appointments and cooperation.

Treatment length

The average number of aligners used was 19 maxillary and 21 mandibular. At the time the study was conducted, the staging methods used and the amount of movement per aligner were different than those implemented today. Contemporary staging of these cases would likely result in slightly fewer total aligners per case. Considering a 2-week-per-aligner wear schedule, the treatment would ostensibly result in a 40-week (10-month) treatment time. Eighteen patients required aligners additional to their original prescription.

The total number of aligners necessary for a given patient's treatment is significant in that it appeared to be inversely related to the cooperation of the patient. In other words, the shorter the treatment, the more likely the patient was to finish it successfully. The longer the treatment, the more likely the patient was to become noncompliant with

the wear schedule. Such a relationship is purely observational; data were not collected to measure this statistically.

Although all of the patients in the study finished their treatment in a reasonable amount of time, it was noted that the transition between active treatment and retention was ill defined. In traditional orthodontic treatment, there is a clear demarcation between active treatment and retention, as it is marked by the removal of the brackets. However, a single aligner by itself is essentially a retainer. In some cases, detailing of the final aligner was done over several weeks. This resulted in a prolonged transition into retention. From a practice-management standpoint, this caused a number of problems. The changing of the status of the patient, taking of final records, and celebration of the end of treatment were all difficult to pinpoint, since there was never a defined treatment endpoint. This discovery would suggest that a firm decision as to the end of active treatment and the beginning of retention be made in all cases, even if the retainer is an aligner.

Oral hygiene

Maintenance of good hygiene is an important factor during orthodontic treatment because it has been shown to affect treatment time and outcome. Research has shown that, in general, adults have significantly less plaque accumulation and healthier gingival tissues than adolescents during treatment.[3] Approximately 20% to 30% of the adolescents had inadequate plaque removal during treatment and lost significant periodontal bone support during treatment.[3] A longitudinal study showed that adolescents who had ineffective plaque removal during treatment also developed significant decalcification.[4] Studies have shown that the amount of plaque, gingivitis, and decalcification is higher in patients with fixed appliances than those without.[5-7]

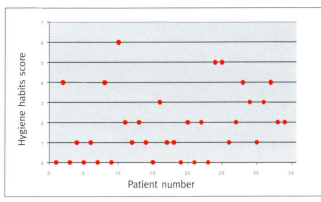

FIG 29-3 Oral hygiene habits at the end of treatment.

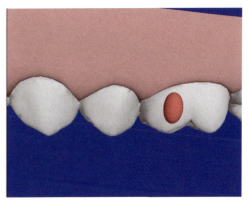

FIG 29-4 Shallowly erupted teeth provide little in the way of retention for aligners.

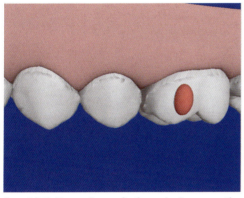

FIG 29-5 Retraction of the gingiva on the ClinCheck model provided sufficient undercuts for aligner retention.

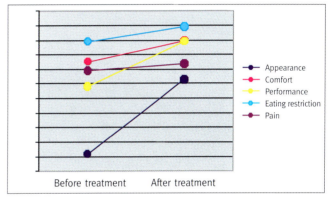

FIG 29-6 Comparison of quality-of-life parameters for before and after treatment (means for all patients).

In this study, the amount of plaque found on the teeth at each appointment decreased over the course of treatment (Fig 29-1), as did the degree of gingival inflammation at each appointment (Fig 29-2). Oral hygiene habits improved over the course of treatment (Fig 29-3).

Given the aforementioned deterioration in oral hygiene that is often seen in fixed-appliance cases, it is remarkable how well the hygiene was maintained in these cases. Certainly such good oral hygiene, and the improvement in oral hygiene habits, could have been caused by the oral hygiene instruction given at the beginning of treatment by the treating orthodontists. Although this instruction is also given to fixed-appliance patients in these practices, a lack of a control group does not allow a relative comparison. Even in the absence of such relative comparison, however, the salient point is that hygiene did not deteriorate over the course of treatment. Another potential bias is the fact that both the data recorders and the patients were aware of the study and were in no way blinded as to the appointment, data, or

purpose. Such a bias could have increased the recorded level of hygiene during treatment.

Aligner wear cooperation

Cooperation has been a high-visibility topic in orthodontics for many years. It is generally believed that cooperation with treatment is a key factor in achieving a successful result. This is certainly true with treatment that involves aligners. The fact that aligners can be removed easily could predispose poor cooperators to wear them fewer hours per day than prescribed. Also, the ability to remove aligners could lead to their being lost or misplaced. In this group, the aligners were worn, on average, 20 hours per day. With respect to individual aligner failure, 2.2% were lost and 1.6% were broken.

A component of cooperation is the comfort of the appliance being used. In traditional orthodontics, appliances such as removable thumb cribs and headgears are often worn a less-than-optimal amount of time simply because they are uncomfortable. In this study, we discovered that a similar discomfort could occur if the teeth were insufficiently erupted. In other words, if the teeth are not erupted far enough into the mouth to reveal the height of contour and the underlying gingival embrasure and undercuts, the aligners have nothing to "snap" over. In one study patient, the aligners would not stay tightly over the teeth (Fig 29-4). The addition of attachments did not assist in the retention of the appliance. However, reducing the gingival height of the ClinCheck model, thereby revealing the undercuts, solved the problem and resulted in excellent retention (Fig 29-5). This evidence suggests that younger patients with shallowly erupted teeth should be observed for treatment until they are older.

Quality of life

Means of all patients' quality-of-life data for the initial and final periods were calculated (Fig 29-6). Nonstatistical observation of the data suggests an improvement in appearance and performance. This makes sense, given that the patients' teeth were straightened during treatment. The malocclusions treated in this study were relatively mild, leading one to assume that there would not be a substantial change in a patient's quality of life over the course of treatment. One could postulate that a severe malocclusion would lead to significant changes in the quality-of-life data once the treatment was complete.

TABLE 29-4 Irregularity index measurements for 22 patients (pre- and posttreatment measurements of the anterior irregularity of study casts)

Patient	Maxilla			Mandible		
	Pretreatment (mm)	Posttreatment (mm)	% reduction	Pretreatment (mm)	Posttreatment (mm)	% reduction
1	3.70	2.83	23.51	4.65	1.36	70.75
2	6.91	0.45	93.49	7.90	0.93	88.23
3	3.94	1.56	60.41	4.89	3.29	32.72
4	3.99	1.58	60.40	2.54	0.54	78.74
5	7.35	1.59	78.37	6.82	1.48	78.30
6	6.41	1.96	69.42	2.17	0.64	70.51
7	3.37	2.46	27.00	4.28	1.39	67.52
8	5.35	0.70	86.92	4.53	0.64	85.87
9	6.70	2.94	56.12	6.71	0.65	90.31
10	8.28	0.80	90.34	12.17	0.88	92.77
11	4.92	2.59	47.36	4.32	1.48	65.74
12	4.54	3.96	12.78	2.37	0.54	77.22
13	3.03	2.51	17.16	3.18	3.54	−11.32
14	4.58	4.48	2.18	7.36	0.09	98.82
15	5.26	4.79	8.94	2.60	1.14	56.15
16	8.04	2.43	69.78	12.27	2.63	78.57
17	3.77	2.89	23.34	6.10	0.90	85.25
18	5.37	1.44	73.18	1.62	0.26	83.95
19	9.84	3.79	61.48	5.85	0.80	86.32
20	8.40	2.96	64.76	3.85	1.21	68.57
21	5.08	1.51	70.28	1.92	0.40	79.17
22	6.66	1.41	78.83	1.35	0.34	74.81
Mean	5.70	2.35	53.46	4.98	1.14	72.68

As mentioned, there was no blinding in the design of this study. This may have affected the data. The fact that 6 months passed between questionnaire assessments might have helped reduce this bias, as the patients may have forgotten their previous answers. In addition, the patients completed these questionnaires without assistance of the office staff, thereby eliminating additional bias resulting from the data collectors.

Treatment outcome

Irregularity index measurements showed an improvement in anterior alignment in each patient studied, with a mean reduction in irregularity of 73% in the mandible and 53% in the maxilla. The measurements for 22 patients are shown in Table 29-4. Initial review of the irregularity numbers indicates that the final results were not devoid of irregularity of the anterior teeth. In fact, the sensitivity of this metric is such that even a well-treated case will result in an irregularity index of greater than zero. That these numbers reflect a successful result is reflected in the posttreatment photographs and casts. Nevertheless, the simplicity of the cases in this sample limits the findings to simple cases. Furthermore, the lack of a fixed-appliance control group mitigates any direct comparison with fixed appliances.

References

1. Leao A, Sheiham A. Relation between clinical dental status and subjective impacts on daily living. J Dent Res 1995;74:1408–1413.
2. Little RM. The irregularity index: A quantitative score of mandibular anterior alignment. J Dent Res 1975;68:554–563.
3. Boyd RL, Leggott PJ, Quinn RS, Eakle WS, Chambers D. Periodontal implications of orthodontic treatment in adults with reduced or normal periodontal tissues versus those of adolescents. Am J Orthod Dentofacial Orthop 1989;96:191–198.
4. Boyd RL. Two-year longitudinal study of a peroxide-fluoride rinse on decalcification in adolescent orthodontic patients. J Clin Dent 1992;3(3):83–87.
5. Mizrahi E. Enamel demineralization following orthodontic treatment. J Dent Res 1982;82(1):62–67.
6. Huser MC, Baehni PC, Lang R. Effects of orthodontic bands on microbiologic and clinical parameters. Am J Orthod Dentofacial Orthop 1990;97:213–218.
7. Gorelick L, Geiger AM, Gwinnett AJ. Incidence of white spot formation after bonding and banding. J Dent Res 1982;81(2):93–98.

chapter 30

DATA MINING:
PRINCIPLES AND CONSIDERATIONS

by
Eric Kuo, DDS

Data mining is the process by which vast amounts of data are transformed into insight by finding trends and correlations that cannot be detected from individual case studies alone. In dentistry, data mining can be used to understand epidemiologic patterns, utilization of procedures, and demographics. Data mining uses software tools to query a large catalog of data. This approach can identify correlations and patterns that may go unnoticed when only a few individual data sets or data points are observed. For data mining to be successful, a defined information model and related infrastructure are required, since not all collected information will be relevant (Fig 30-1). Because the prediction is only as good as the model, one risk of this methodology is using an incorrect model and drawing erroneous conclusions from what could be noise inherent in any data system.

The Invisalign Metrics Analysis Program (MAP) is a data-mining pilot program developed to establish specific measurable quantities (metrics) to better understand key performance indicators, trends in treatment approach and outcome, key clinician and patient demographics, and treatment success and satisfaction with Invisalign treatment (Fig 30-2). It is an initiative that, once established, can grow into a robust orthodontic data management tool for scientific research and dental education. For the time being, it is used to design and develop better Invisalign product offerings and educational training materials.

In the Invisalign MAP model, specific case parameters are stored in a digital information warehouse. These case parameters can include demographic information such as patient age, clinical information (eg, treatment approach), and manufacturing information (eg, number of aligners manufactured for the case). This information can be useful to better understand how Invisalign is used by orthodontists, for what types of patients, and with what levels of success.

Case Study 1: Use of Reproximation with Invisalign

Reproximation (or interproximal enamel reduction [IPR]) is an alternative to extraction whereby a portion of the interproximal enamel is removed from one or more teeth to create arch length for alignment of crowded teeth. It is often used when the teeth should not be advanced or expanded buccally because of either poor periodontal health or inclination of the dentition. Moderately crowded

cases can also be treated with reproximation instead of extraction to avoid retraction of the anterior teeth and flattening of the profile, especially when the total extraction space significantly exceeds the total amount of crowding present. Reproximation, however, is technique sensitive, and understanding the impact of reproximation techniques on case complication is important to characterize (see chapter 26).

Reproximation can be built into the case in one of two ways. The clinician can create interproximal spaces prior to taking the Invisalign impressions, perhaps creating the space with interdental elastic separators for access. Alternatively, reproximation can be performed as the aligners are being delivered, using the reproximation form as the guide and interproximal space measurement gauges to determine accuracy (Figs 30-3 and 30-4).

The first approach may be more accurate, but unless a diagnostic setup is performed, it can lead to a certain amount of guesswork as to which surfaces require enamel removal. The latter approach reduces the guesswork, since the setup is reviewed alongside the reproximation plan; however, reproducing the exact amount of reproximation as indicated in the form is technique sensitive. Failure to deliver the exact amount of reproximation as indicated on the form can lead to either crowding at the end of treatment from inadequate space creation or interproximal spaces from overreduction. Usually, either of these scenarios can be corrected with additional aligners as long as the dental contours that follow the reproximation remain properly shaped. The need for additional aligners, however, can be a hassle for both the clinician and the patient.

Some of the questions that would be interesting to answer are:

1. To what extent is reproximation requested by clinicians?
2. Are reproximation cases more complicated than nonreproximation cases?
3. What is the effect of reproximation utilization on treatment convenience?
4. What is the overall trend in use of reproximation?

To answer these questions, a sample of Invisalign-treated cases was evaluated and categorized based on use of reproximation. Cases in which reproximation was performed prior to impressions were put in category 1. Generalized space-closure cases were also placed in this category since the physical appearance of both types was

FIG 30-1 Data-mining tools can identify trends and correlations within the information stored in the database, but the conclusions are relevant only if the information model is correct.

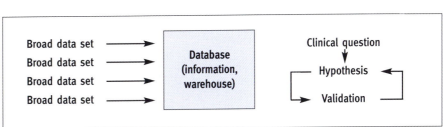

FIG 30-2 Align's data-mining infrastructure can store clinical parameters in an information database to test the validity of a clinical hypothesis.

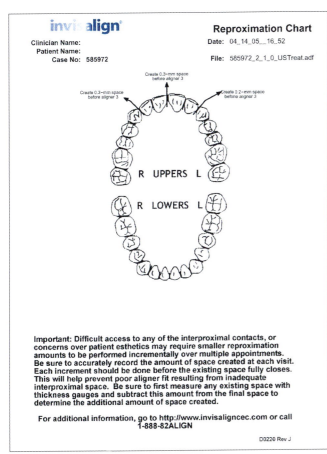

FIG 30-3 Reproximation form.

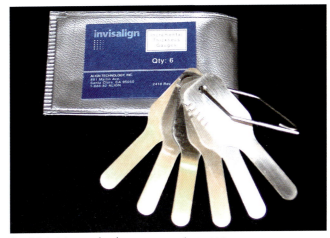

FIG 30-4 Interproximal measurement gauges.

essentially identical. Cases in which no reproximation was performed were placed into category 2. These were crowding cases in which the teeth were aligned without reproximation either before or after the impression. Cases that needed anterior reproximation during aligner delivery (postimpression) were put in category 3. Cases that needed reproximation distal to the first premolar during aligner delivery were put in category 4.

For this investigation, cases in which spaces were left for restorative work were omitted because such space closure could inherently lead to additional detailing work unrelated to the outcome specific to whether reproximation was used or not. Extraction and distalization cases were also not included, since it was believed that such cases could introduce complications that were unrelated to the use (or not) of reproximation.

The hypothesis was that cases requiring reproximation after impressions, especially of posterior teeth, were more likely to require additional aligners for treatment, since postimpression reproximation is technique sensitive, especially when trying to access posterior interproximal contacts. Performing reproximation before impressions, however, would probably be more accurate as long as the guesswork about which surfaces to recontour could be reduced.

For this study, 555 cases (1,005 treated arches) were randomly selected from all cases ordered between April

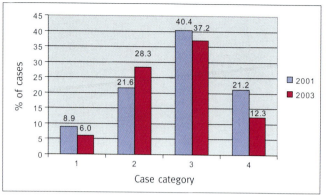

FIG 30-5 Distribution of treatment approaches for Invisalign cases with reproximation. Categories: (1) Preimpression reproximation/ space closure; (2) no reproximation; (3) anterior reproximation only, postimpression; (4) any posterior reproximation, postimpression.

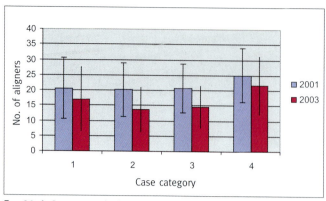

FIG 30-6 Case complexity as measured by mean aligner number per arch, the hypothesis being that more complicated cases require more tooth movement (and aligners) to resolve. Categories: (1) Preimpression reproximation/space closure; (2) no reproximation; (3) anterior reproximation only, postimpression; (4) any posterior reproximation, postimpression.

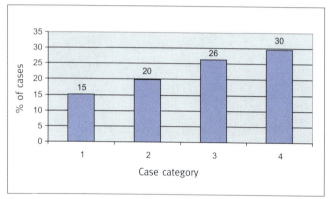
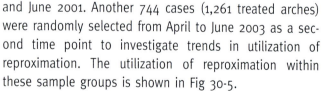

FIG 30-7 Percentage of cases in each category for which additional aligners were ordered to complete treatment. The data are consistent with the hypothesis that space management is critical to treatment outcome success. (Taken from 2001 sample; confidence level = 0.95.) Categories: (1) Preimpression reproximation/space closure; (2) no reproximation; (3) anterior reproximation only, postimpression; (4) any posterior reproximation, postimpression.

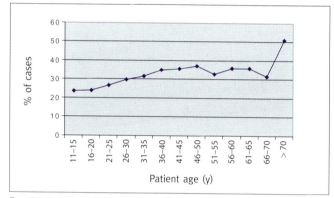

FIG 30-8 Rate of additional aligners ordered, by patient age. (Taken from 2003 data; n = 23,054 treated arches.)

and June 2001. Another 744 cases (1,261 treated arches) were randomly selected from April to June 2003 as a second time point to investigate trends in utilization of reproximation. The utilization of reproximation within these sample groups is shown in Fig 30-5.

Between 2001 and 2003, the use of reproximation decreased from 62% to 50% of cases. The increase in group 2 (no reproximation) and the decrease in group 4 (posterior reproximation) was statistically different between 2001 and 2003 (chi-square test, $P < .005$). One theory explaining this change is that as clinicians better appreciate the challenges associated with reproximation, they rely on it less to achieve their treatment goals, especially in the posterior dentition, where reproximation can be difficult to deliver with accuracy.

To determine the inherent complexity of each case, the number of aligners manufactured for each arch was used as an indicator (Fig 30-6). The critical assumption here is that this was a rough estimate of treatment complexity, since more complicated cases should require greater tooth movement and, hence, a greater number of aligners. The study results did not reveal a statistically different number of aligners among the different treatment approaches; however, cases planned with posterior reproximation, on average, had a higher number of aligners associated with the cases.

An analysis of the rate of additional aligner use for each category revealed that the more extensive the amount of postimpression reproximation, the higher the rate of additional aligners being ordered (Fig 30-7).

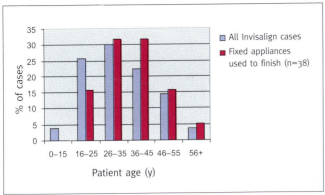

FIG 30-9 Distribution of treatment approaches for Invisalign cases with reproximation. Categories: (1) Preimpression reproximation/ space closure; (2) no reproximation; (3) anterior reproximation only, postimpression; (4) any posterior reproximation, postimpression.

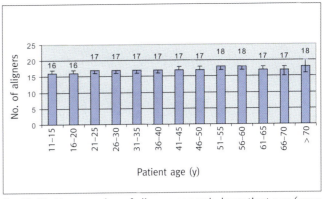

FIG 30-10 Mean number of aligners per arch, by patient age (2003 data).

The conclusion from this exercise was that the data were consistent with the observation and general belief that cases that require reproximation during the course of treatment, especially in the posterior dentition, were more likely to require additional aligners at the end of treatment, and that space-closure cases and cases in which space was created prior to impressions were less likely to require additional aligners. The fact that additional aligners were needed in 15% of space closure/preimpression cases (group 1), however, suggests that certain types of cases within this category may still require detailing at the end of treatment. Nonetheless, this information could be of interest to a clinician trying to assess treatment times as it relates to treatment approach. Pressed for a limited amount of treatment time, a clinician may elect to treat a case with either preimpression reproximation or no reproximation in an effort to reduce the need for additional aligners at the end of the aligner series. At the same time, not knowing how much to reproximate up front could also lead to additional complexity; hence, additional effort such as a diagnostic setup may be necessary to properly assess the treatment plan. The fact that there was not a significant increase in utilization of preimpression reproximation between 2001 and 2003, but an overall decrease in reproximation use concurrent with an increase in non-reproximation cases (see Fig 30-5), suggests that clinicians were becoming cognizant of the challenge of trying to deliver preimpression reproximation without a three-dimensional visualization of the treatment goal.

Case Study 2: Patient Age and Need for Additional Aligners

Invisalign is indicated for patients whose second molars are fully erupted. This guideline was established because erupting dentition and skeletal growth are not currently simulated by the ClinCheck software. Because of concerns about potential compliance problems with younger patients, it is important to characterize the effect of patient age on treatment.

To study this effect, all cases that included patient age were analyzed based on the use of additional aligners. If younger patients were not compliant in wearing the aligners, one would expect a higher rate of additional aligners being ordered for younger patients. As Fig 30-8 shows, however, the rate of additional aligners ordered was actually higher for older patients, not for younger patients. One possible explanation for the results is a greater acceptance of fixed appliances in younger patients in the event that they are needed for finishing. Adults may be less likely to accept fixed appliances and may prefer trying to finish their treatment using aligners. Survey data, however, did not show a higher utilization of fixed appliances for finishing in younger patients (Fig 30-9).

Another possible explanation for the higher rate of additional aligners in older patients is that older patients may have more complicated malocclusions, or their teeth may be less responsive to orthodontic movement; as a result, older patients may be more likely to require refinement. To test this hypothesis, the mean number of aligners per arch was calculated by patient age, with the assumption that the number of aligners is correlated to the complexity of the treatment.

Figure 30-10 shows that the mean number of aligners did increase with patient age, which means that the severity of malocclusion could be a function of patient age. This could explain why older patients exhibited a higher utilization rate of additional aligners for treatment. In other words, while compliance in younger patients may be an issue (this was not proven or disproven by the data), its effect appears to be overshadowed by the more significant effect of older patients needing more aligners to correct their more complicated malocclusions.

The assertion that younger patients are less likely than adults to be compliant with Invisalign, and are more likely to require multiple refinements to finish treatment, cannot therefore be supported by the data. Initially, this may be counterintuitive; however, given that Invisalign is still in its early stages of adoption and that many clinicians are still somewhat cautious in offering it to their patients, perhaps younger patients currently being treated with Invisalign are a well-selected population, who are determined to avoid wearing brackets and therefore more apt to be compliant. If this is the case, then the data make perfect sense. And based on these data, since the rate of additional aligner utilization in younger patients is no worse than in older patients, clinicians should be encouraged to treat younger patients with Invisalign, as long as the malocclusions being treated are compatible with the appliance's indications.

Concluding Comments

A successful data-mining program requires that the characteristics being studied are objectively parameterized. As demonstrated in the case studies above, much of what is being reviewed today in Align's research laboratories are still very basic parameters such as the number of aligners manufactured, treatment approach, and patient demographics. As such, the outcomes are only useful for assessing consistency with a given hypothesis, rather than for proving or disproving a theory.

A more rigorous but challenging approach could be to characterize cases based on traditional orthodontic parameters such as Angle classification, overjet, and amount of crowding. The reasons why the characterization approach is challenging is that the standards and definitions for these measurements can vary widely, and measurement processes need to be automated to be applicable to a large sample in an accurate and reproducible fashion. Poorly defined data in large quantities without any scientific hypothesis to test are not very useful, and do not lead to meaningful results. Large amounts of well-defined, quality data used to test specific hypotheses, however, are extremely powerful and can lead to interesting observations, which can in turn spark even more interesting questions and results. Align Technology's data-mining initiative holds great promise for better understanding how and why Invisalign treatment works and for identifying clinical parameters correlated with treatment outcome success.

SECTION V

OFFICE DESIGN AND TECHNOLOGY

chapter 31

INVISALIGN OFFICE DESIGN AND TECHNOLOGY

by

Orhan C. Tuncay, DMD; Marc S. Lemchen, DMD; and Agnes A. Kan

What is the function of the Invisalign orthodontic office, and how can it be designed to best deliver what is required of it? Other pertinent questions are, who uses the office, and what are these users' expectations? Patient needs and expectations are the two principal parameters, which suggests that the orthodontic office should seamlessly blend form with function. Unless the mission and objectives of the space are clearly defined, the architect will design a space that serves as a monument to himself or herself, or the builder will simply build a generic box. In the context of this chapter, "mission" is defined as tasks performed in the orthodontic office, and "objective" is defined as how these tasks are performed.

The mission of the orthodontic office may be listed as all of the following: patient waiting, reception duties and appointments, payment collection, patient data storage and retrieval, office work for correspondence and financial business, consultation of the patient with the clinician or clinical personnel, patient education, staff training, collection of diagnostic information, treatment, sterilization, and fabrication of orthodontic appliances.

It is necessary to break down these tasks to design a space that will permit the performance of these functions in a specific way. Orthodontic practices are high-volume establishments. In the absence of efficiency, they cannot reach their full potential of productivity. Efficiency is linked not only to high quality of treatment but also to income. The architectural design and incorporated technology must have a symbiotic existence. Retrofitting one element to suit another generally does not bring efficiency; it only adds one more element to an already crowded operation. This is an important consideration, as one can never know what kind of novel treatment techniques or additional equipment might be needed in the future. The design should prepare the space for easy conversion.

Functional Needs Fundamental to the Mission of the Orthodontic Practice

Patient waiting area

The waiting areas should never be used for waiting, but it is often hard to adhere to this principle. If waiting is to take place, what should be the design considerations for the waiting area? This question may best be answered by assigning a function for the space. This space can be

many things, but one element is certain: it should be relaxing. The space could be useful in helping to relax patients before their appointment. This relaxation benefit also applies to adults who are accompanying a child patient.

How does a waiting area invite people to relax? A person's experience of entry into the office is significant, as it is essential that he or she develop a positive first impression of the space. Some spaces are inviting, comfortable, and relaxing, whereas others convey a feeling of coldness or tension. The personality of a space and how it affects humans is called *feng shui* in the Chinese culture. The personality of a space is dictated not only by its layout but also by the harmonious interaction of its furnishings, color scheme, light, and materials. In terms of layout, factors that affect the waiting area must be considered first. The waiting area is located next to the reception area. Obviously, incoming patients stop at the reception desk first. The patient's approach to the reception desk, combined with his or her experience there, influences the "entrance" factor of the waiting area (Figs 31-1 and 31-2). Patients carry the mood of their day into the waiting area or to the treatment areas. Thus, whether it is the initial visit or a regularly scheduled visit, it is best to ensure that the patients are happy and in a good mood at all times when they are in the orthodontic office.

Receptionist's area

From the perspective of the patient or the parent, it is important to be "received." People who walk into an establishment—be it an orthodontic office or a restaurant—enjoy being recognized and accommodated. For the patient, the receptionist's area has a high impact value. It is essential, therefore, that the receptionist is in a position (spatially) to comfortably interact with the client, at eye level or lower. The client should have a comfortable stance and should not have to carry bags while trying to negotiate the appointment. (The staff should assist the patient in hanging coats or securing bags or briefcases in a coat closet). Nonetheless, the receptionist's area should distinctly separate the receptionist from the client. A traditional physical barrier (ie, a counter) is necessary (see Figs 31-1 and 31-2). Such a counter should have certain convenience features—most notably, a ledge on which the clients can place their handbags or briefcases. Above all, however, it has to "feel good" to be there. The materials used in the design of the receptionist's counter are as instrumental as the counter's design in promoting this feeling.

Many of the busiest orthodontic offices grow big without being noticed. In the early years of a practice, it is more important just to grow. More and more patients are brought into the practice, but the infrastructure is not modified. Many busy practices identify the receptionist's desk as a bottleneck area that interferes with rather than facilitates efficient patient flow.[1] Based on our data, 37 square feet per worker must be allocated for the reception area. The location of the reception desk needs to be sufficiently removed from other areas to provide a sense of privacy for the patient. Oftentimes, payments are made, financial matters are discussed, or appointment times need to be negotiated while the client is standing at the counter. Enough privacy to accommodate these conversations serves the office well. Thus, the reception counter is best isolated from the waiting area.

Areas for consultations, initial examinations, records, and patient education

It is recommended that areas used for patient-specific discussions be sufficiently isolated so as to not interfere with the flow of patient and staff traffic. It is beneficial, however, to locate the treatment coordinator in close proximity to where the initial examination will take place. Patients are better serviced when the treatment coordinator has ready access to everything he or she needs. This level of detail may not matter too much in a small boutique practice with only a few chairs; but even in a small practice, these functions must be isolated from the treatment area.

For larger offices, these areas are best located closer to the waiting area—but not along the way from the waiting area to the treatment area. Of course, these areas should all be easily accessible from the treatment area. The design of these areas cannot encourage excuses for not keeping them impeccably neat. These are areas of business where potential patients are educated about why they should choose this particular practice. Once the space is designed for this vitally fundamental function, the layout of the examination chair, radiographic equipment, and other imaging locations is nothing more than a "best fit" exercise. If the space is a serious problem, the clever use of panels made from transparent or semitransparent materials along with equally clever lighting layout creates exciting, clean, hi-tech spaces. Similar approaches can also be used in offices where space is not a limiting factor. Lighting makes or breaks a good design.

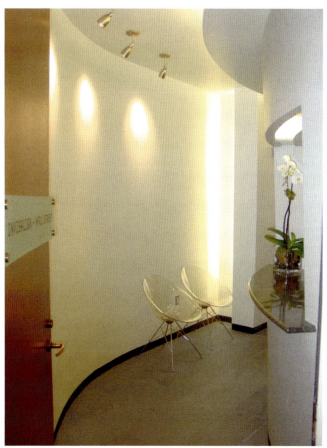

FIG 31-1 A foyer and receptionist's desk welcome the patient efficiently and purposefully. The clear Lucite chairs are more decorative than functional. Patients may use the chairs to rest their bags.

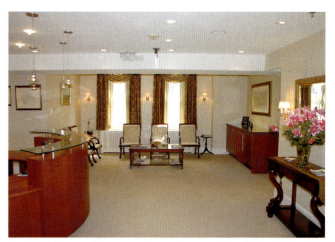

FIG 31-2 The waiting area in another practice is traditional in design, yet uncluttered. It is important to provide adequate space for the adults, as the location's patient population characteristics dictate. Computers are everywhere throughout the office, but they are unobtrusive in the living room–like waiting room.

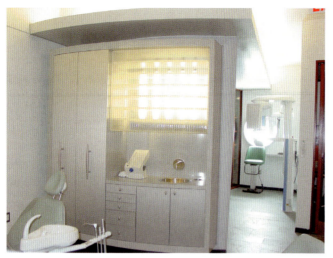

FIG 31-3 The back wall of a main clinic. It is equipped and laid out to take records in a compact space. Note the dramatic use of light fixtures. The first shelf of the cabinet above the sink is made up of slots to store the day's aligner trays to be delivered. Large boxes are stored elsewhere in the office.

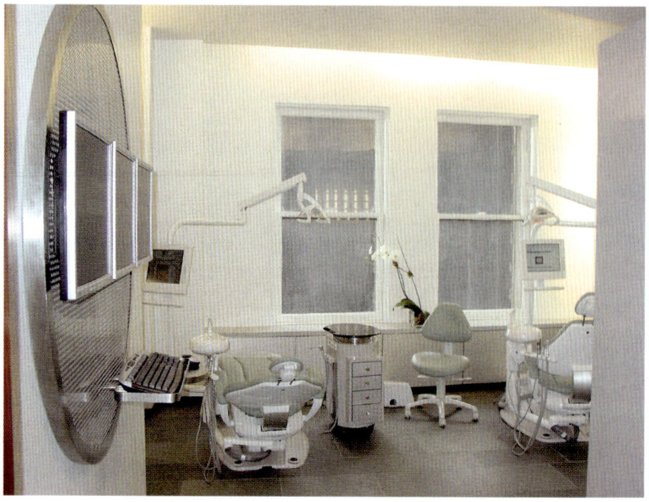

FIG 31-4 Main clinic. Mobile cabinets augment the cuspidor and flat-panel monitors.

Spaces for the staff

Construction of a staff lounge is a show of respect for the people who ensure the success of a thriving practice. Our data reveal that successful practices do not overlook the importance of a staff lounge. If space is limited, however, a staff lounge could be constructed with versatility in mind. A staff lounge could also be used, for example, as a space to conduct in-service training. The design of the staff lounge is best decided by input from the people who will use it. This gives the staff a feeling of belonging. Staff members who look at their duties as "just a job" cannot be good marketers of the practice.

Staff members use their lounge to change and hang clothes, eat lunch, take a coffee break, make private phone calls, and conduct other activities. If the staff members use the lounge to heat food or perform another activity that might generate odors not suitable for an office environment, the room needs to be well ventilated. The staff lounge is ideally located as remotely as possible from public areas. In a suburban setting, it may even have a separate entrance wherever possible.

Treatment areas

Treatment areas need to be constructed to perform two functions: patient treatment and support services. The treatment area is where the patients sit, and the support services area is where sterilization and consultation take place. Oftentimes, the support areas look and function as if they were an afterthought. In some cases, the treatment

areas are filled with distractions such as games, busy objects or paintings, and the like. Patients do not, and should not, sit in the treatment area long. Moreover, it is important to remember that, when they do, they mostly look at the ceiling. A television monitor is enjoyed by all patients, even though they only watch it briefly.

Whose comfort is most important in the treatment area? Clearly, it is the workers' comfort. Patients spend minimal time in the treatment area. Their time can be counted in minutes. As much as adult patients might recognize and comment on a luxurious treatment chair, a standard-issue chair does not elicit disapproving comments: patients are most forgiving. For example, if they have to get out of the chair and walk a few steps to the tooth-brushing area, they do not mind.

The unit treatment area should be viewed as a workstation, where everything is within easy reach for the clinical personnel (Figs 31-3 and 31-4). This includes not only how the clinical personnel can reach the items needed for a given procedure but also the ease of discarding used items. If the orthodontist has an existing practice and a new one is planned, it is useful to videotape the activities of the staff over various times of the day and for various procedures. In the videotape, weaknesses of the existing system will become apparent.

After a new office is built and the practice has had some time to function within it, almost everyone can identify elements in the office that they would do a little differently. To avoid such remorse, a videotape analysis can be useful. A camera mounted on a high tripod and placed

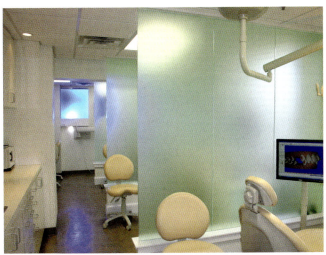

Fig 31-5 Glass paneling is used in such a way to suggest the Invisalign tray. In practical terms, it also provides privacy for conversations. Note that the monitor is visible to the patient to discuss treatment progress and to allow the patient to read the progress notes. This style of communication promotes better cooperation.

unobtrusively in a corner is all that is needed and can be of immeasurable utility before moving out of or renovating an existing office. Efficiency brings comfort no matter the setting; in this case, the comfort of the clinical personnel is the focus.

To achieve greater efficiency and convenience, it is necessary to design storage facilities that will enable the Invisalign boxes to be kept within easy reach. The delivery of aligners in a plastic bag should be smooth.

Finally, because Invisalign is an interactive experience for the patient, it is important to keep patients informed about their progress. Accordingly, a large monitor should be installed at each chair (Fig 31-5). Patients should see not only their ClinCheck images and progress photos, but also what is being written about them in the progress notes. This approach eliminates "you've never told me that"–type comments. Normally, with children, concerns are addressed to the accompanying parent. With adults, however, direct, one-on-one conversation must be standard operating procedure.

Sterilization area

An area that is often overlooked is the sterilization room. Obviously, its location should be near the clinic areas, but the way dirty instruments are brought in and clean ones taken out should be carefully planned. In a busy practice, even the smallest of traffic details matter. Our research data indicate that larger practices find the sterilization room setup inadequate. An opening into the sterilization room through which instrument trays can be passed is

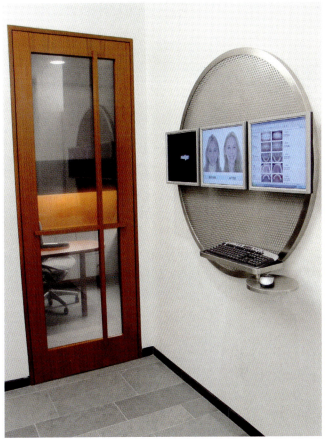

Fig 31-6 Data entry and patient education station is located in the entry of the main clinic. The side view of the three-panel arrangement can be seen in Fig 31-4.

preferred over walking the trays through the door. It also helps to furnish this area with high-speed sterilizers. Quick-turnover sterilization times reduce the need for a large inventory of intraoral instruments. High-speed sterilizers also do not generate a great deal of heat or steam. In close quarters, where a high-powered ventilation fan cannot be fitted, this strategy is preferred. Obviously, this is a problem encountered more often in older high-rise building locations. An architect who understands the flow of an Invisalign practice and its sterilization requirements can design the elements needed in this space sensibly.

Consultation room

The consultation rooms need to be substantial, as it is a key marketing area. In an Invisalign-exclusive practice, its function is slightly different. Education of the patient in Invisalign therapy takes place in this space. Patient education does not require separate quarters. Invisalign patients often have already been educated through their various dental experiences or prior orthodontic treatment. All that is needed for the potential patients is an explanation of the mechanism of the Invisalign System. As mentioned in chapter 19, for example, the clinician thinks in terms of distances over which forces are applied, rather than simply force magnitude.

The consultation room is also where payments are discussed. Privacy, therefore, needs to be provided in the design. Fundamentally, however, visual elements and equipment are critical (Fig 31-6). They must engulf the patient. The importance of the use of audiovisual equipment in this setting cannot be overstated. In this space, the potential patient is made to understand and see what the treatment entails. Unlike the conventional methods of explaining treatment with fixed appliances, patients see the intended treatment outcome and the stages by which it is achieved. This is done in an effort to eliminate misunderstandings. It is dangerous if patients fantasize about what their teeth will look like. Instead, they should see the intended result and how many aligners it will take to get there.

Finally, the consultation room is also used to educate the staff. It is useful to include seminars in the morning huddle. These seminars are structured such that the staff is educated about orthodontics, in a fashion not dissimilar to what a student of orthodontics is exposed to. The more the staff knows and understands, the better their performance and skills will be. Elements of ClinCheck, polyvinyl siloxane impressions, emerging technology, limitations of tooth movement, and similar topics should be covered.

Technology

The Invisalign System is a shift in the orthodontic paradigm. Clearly, it is technology dependent. The Invisalign office must be equipped appropriately to deliver Invisalign treatment. Imaging systems are the key. A network of computers in all areas of the office will be necessary to deliver the intended care. Invisalign is an interactive system. The clinical personnel interact with the patient at all phases of treatment. Because the patient is intimately involved in the process—because the appliances are removable—images need to be readily available in the treatment area. Thus, it is imperative that all chairs are equipped to facilitate this level of interaction. The equipment that is needed can vary in its configuration, either in the form of individual, networked central processing units (CPUs) or thin client terminals at each chair. These choices depend on many factors, but whatever system the office chooses, it cannot adversely affect the interaction with the patient. The most important equipment consideration is the mon-

itor the patient will see. A 19-inch monitor works best. It is cost-effective and big enough to engage the patient in his or her own treatment. With a 19-inch monitor at the chair, the patient will clearly see his or her ClinCheck and other images.

The Ideal Invisalign Office

Figure 31-7 presents a design for an optimized Invisalign office. As patients enter, they are not in contact with the rest of the office, and the seating areas for adults and children are separated. A concierge caters to people in the waiting areas for such matters as providing refreshments, arranging parking or reservations for lunch, and checking on train or airline schedules.

The most innovative element of this office is the conference center. This centrally located space may be used for staff meetings, continuing education, and meetings with patients. The clinician has a personal monitor, whereas the people seated across the conference table view flat-panel monitors mounted on the walls behind the clinician or the treatment coordinator. The outer walls of the conference center serve as countertops to support the clinic or waiting area.

In the treatment areas, chairs are divided by semitransparent panels to engulf the patient in the Invisalign experience. They also provide privacy. Images collected by the radiographic, scanning, or photographic equipment may be processed at the countertops.

This layout may be modified for computer support as outlined in this chapter.

Technology Requirements

The technology in the Invisalign office is the backbone of support and the central nervous system for efficiency. Indeed, adequate infrastructure for the implementation, maintenance, and upgrade of technology must be designed into a new office. These features include sufficient physical space; environmental controls for sound, temperature, and humidity; uninterruptible electrical power for present and future needs; and access to cabling within control areas to workstation locations. This will allow for the constant evolution of the office's technology backbone. The objective is to establish a technology platform that enables lightning-fast computer access, which is

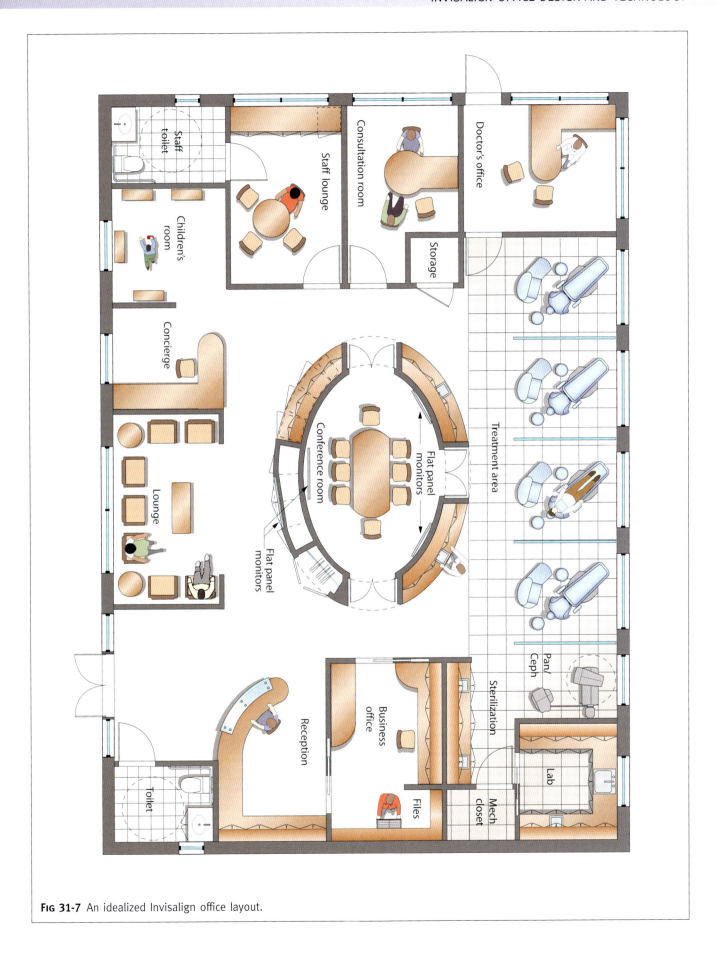

Fig 31-7 An idealized Invisalign office layout.

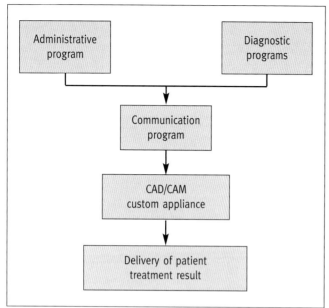

FIG 31-8 Flowchart of computer systems to deliver the desired Invisalign result.

essential for managing administrative, diagnostic (records, diagnosis, and on-line appliance design), treatment information (treatment cards), and inter- and intraoffice communication between clinicians, referrals, patients, and vendors. Not only does this technology enable the orthodontist to provide better treatment, but it allows greater patient participation in treatment choices. In return, this differentiates the practice to a whole new level and provides the "wow factor" to motivate both patients and parents to pursue their (and their children's) orthodontic needs.

Over the last 20 years, the role of computerization in the orthodontic practice has grown far beyond the seemingly elementary tasks of scheduling and billing. More than ever, orthodontists are empowered by this technology to do much more—and, conversely, paralyzed and able to do almost nothing when technology fails. There is a confluence of technology from the first entry of the new patient into the practice to the use of custom computer-designed and computer-manufactured appliances (of which Invisalign is only one of the first) (Fig 31-8).

It is helpful to first consider each of the areas most affected by the expression of this relatively new technology and then describe the physical requirements to implement and manage these programs effectively. Without question, the more orthodontists ask the computer to do in the office, the more powerful the system needs to be, the greater its requirements, and the more complex its maintenance.

Administrative programs

Administrative practice-management programs encompass the patient's first contact with the practice. This can be with the first phone call or visit to a website, the filling out of initial data, the check-in for the first visit, the scheduling of appointments, billing, and both hard and soft communications. All the information that is necessary for excellent patient care and practice growth is based on these management programs.

The whole concept of an Invisalign office has to do with state-of-the-art technology. This must start from the patient's first encounter with the office and follow through to the placement of the retainer and maintenance appointments. Keeping the use of technology as a point of focus will both facilitate treatment and differentiate the Invisalign experience from traditional orthodontic therapy.

Initial forms are completed and sent electronically to the office. In the ideal paperless office, these forms are never printed out, but just filed electronically. The perfect administrative program audits the patient's data, displaying warnings if pertinent data such as health histories, informed consents, or critical diagnostic records are missing.

Appointments are made either over the Internet or by phone. These appointments, and all subsequent appointments, are confirmed via e-mail. Ideally, notification of appointment confirmations and arrival of aligners should be done electronically prior to the patient's appointment.

Of course, no office can function without billing. There is nothing new about an accounts receivable program, but certainly its interaction with the clinical part of the management program is critical. Automated billing via credit card or direct bank withdrawal can dramatically simplify collections.

An additional feature of a practice-management program is the compiling and production of birthday cards, holiday greetings, thank-you letters for referrals, and other practice-building communications. These are coordinated by the administrative area of the practice-management program, either with traditional printed material or through e-mail, thus saving paper and postage costs.

Diagnostic programs

Paramount in an Invisalign office are the diagnostic programs. These programs organize and store diagnostic records, plan treatment, and monitor or modify treatment.

Image capture is managed by a program to capture, modify, and store digital images. These images include intra- and extraoral images and digital panoramic and cephalometric radiographs. The program also provides a method to digitize cephalometric images for diagnostic measurements using any number of standard analyses. The program must also provide a method of transmitting these images to other professionals and vendors. To complete the case submission for Invisalign, these data must be easily manipulated to enable the images to be uploaded to Align Technology.

Communication programs

Communication both within and outside of the office is a critical issue in any high-technology office, all the more so in one that must deal with a computer-designed and computer-manufactured appliance.

Within the office, paperless messaging and intraoffice communication may be done with a custom-designed program called V.Com. (Virtual Software Solutions). The system functions on several levels. It provides a banner across the top of the screen on each computer, which tells the clinician or staff where they are needed and for what procedure. The same system is also used for coded or text messages to tell the staff of phone calls, action instructions, and more.

V.Com has an additional message pad function. Messages can be entered on screen on a message pad form. If these messages relate to a patient, they are automatically noted in the patient's treatment card, as are any replies to the patient-specific message. For example, the clinician can call up the message pad from any computer, see all of the messages, and respond, with the responses going back to the sender or any other designee and being noted in the patient's chart. These messages can then be deleted from the message pad, archived, or printed.

E-mail messages can be sent to referring clinicians, consulting specialists, or even the patients themselves from within the patient's treatment card. Records, which consist of panoramic and cephalometric radiographs and digital photographs, can be uploaded to a host website (such as www.AnywhereDolphin.com, if the imaging program used is Dolphin Imaging). This also includes any messages or notes between the clinician and the person(s) to whom the records have been uploaded. An entry or comment made in the patient's treatment card can be sent by clicking the e-mail icon, which brings up a prompt that asks to whom the entry or comment should be sent. If, for exam-

ple, the patient's dentist is selected, that dentist will receive an e-mail stating that "on this date the following entry was made on (patient's name) treatment card." The fact that a copy of this entry was e-mailed to the selected party is automatically entered in the treatment card as well. The time saved by this feature is significant.

If an orthodontist wants to send a message that includes patient records, he or she can upload the records to AnywhereDolphin by simply clicking on the upload icon. The orthodontist is then asked to whom the records are to be made available and for any message that is to be attached. The intended recipient receives an e-mail with the attached message, a note stating that the records are available to them, and a link that brings them directly to the AnywhereDolphin site.

Computerized appliance fabrication

Invisalign, as well as a number of other new orthodontic appliance systems, now involves the transmission of patient data both to and from the orthodontic office before a computer-designed and computer-fabricated appliance can be placed for the patient. Other computer-designed and computer-fabricated appliances available or soon to be available include Orametrix's SureSmile wires and Ormco's Insignia bracket system, or the systems of OrthoCAD for bonding. Ultimately, the data will be entirely digital, provided by light, laser, or x-ray scans that produce the patient's three-dimensional data in what is known as *machine code* to be used to design and fabricate the appliance. At present however, a combination of digital and physical records sent to the appliance fabricator is used.

For Invisalign, digital images (extra- and intraoral photographs and digital cephalometric and panoramic radiograph images) as well as a physical set of impressions are sent. The impressions are digitized by a computerized axial tomography (CAT) scan process (see chapter 6). From this now-totally-digital data, a digital representation of the dentition is prepared. This is sent back to the orthodontic office over the Internet in the form of the ClinCheck. The ClinCheck allows the orthodontist to confirm that the treatment guidelines prescribed have been adhered to and that the result will meet or exceed expectations given adequate tissue response and patient compliance. The actual ClinCheck process is another topic (see chapter 11). What is important to note is the need for high-speed communication, which makes possible the transmission and reception of this data, as well as for powerful video hardware to be able to display and use this data to design the patient's appliance. Broadband Internet access is a must.

Computer room

To support the kind of hardware required to run these programs, carry data into and out of the office, back up data, and allow for maintenance and updating of this infrastructure, the construction of the hardware skeleton, or backbone, is required. An Invisalign office needs a "nerve center," or computer room, that communicates with a large number of workstations located throughout the office and in remote locations, as well. It is here that the traditional office has been sorely deficient. A new way of designing an office is required.

The use of computers in dental offices dates to the late 1970s and early 1980s. These first steps into the computer age usually involved word processing and billing. In the late 1980s, some use of scheduling programs and the very beginning of computerized treatment records and notes was seen. In the late 1980s, the computer began to store video images of patients. Some very early uses of computerized diagnostic tools also occurred. In the 1990s, digital imaging—both photographic and radiographic—became commonplace in the office. Currently, the era of instant transmission and sharing of patient records is at hand, which allows data to be viewed over the Internet by practitioners in different offices and different specialties.

The trend is clear. Over the past 20 years, what was thought to be cutting edge has become standard. The use of, and dependence on, computers in the professional office has grown at an ever-accelerating pace. Larger, more reliable, computer platforms are required in orthodontic offices to do everything from making appointments to generating appliances and prosthetics. Phone systems, if they do not do so already, will soon use the Internet to carry voices as well as data, while increasing the speed at which data can be transmitted. Even plaster casts, probably soon to become a tool of the past, are digitized and stored for retrieval electronically.

As professionals have embraced more and more technology, the use of the darkroom, and soon the file cabinet, has become a thing of the past. At first blush, this may appear to be a great way to save space in the office, as well as the labor of developing and duplicating radiographs and filing charts. This change is not without its requirements, however. No longer do orthodontists have a few computers in their offices, sitting isolated on desks, or even rudimentary networks sharing data on a peer-to-peer level. Currently, it is not unusual to find offices with 20 to 40 computers connected to powerful servers, uninterruptible power supplies (UPSs), sophisticated tape backups, and multiple smaller servers for everything from intraoral scanning to connecting multiple offices.

Decisions regarding the purchase of new technology are often made more difficult by the "FOO" factor. This "fear of obsolescence" is the most common reason for not integrating new technology. Paralysis can occur from always waiting for the next generation, the next fastest chip, or for the price to come down. It is necessary to accept the fact that the latest technology will be cutting-edge for little more than a day and that tomorrow inevitably brings something new or better. It is furthermore necessary to accept the fact that technology needs to be purchased only when it makes sense, either because of the need for increased efficiency or a more clearly defined return on investment. It is not reasonable to think that one system and one program can be installed and used without modification or upgrade for the next 5 years. The fact is that it will be necessary to upgrade hardware and software, perhaps frequently, to maintain a technological edge in both the diagnostic and management arenas. This edge often differentiates one practice from another.

Given the fact that hardware and software will need to be upgraded continuously, it is interesting that, up to this point, orthodontists have generally failed to build offices that facilitate the installation, maintenance, and upgrade of computer systems. An infrastructure that can allow computer systems to evolve, without inconvenient and costly reconstruction and modification of physical plants, is essential.

The issues that should be considered include the amount of physical space required, power requirements, ventilation, noise control, and access for wiring and rewiring. Ease of recabling, as well as space for phone equipment, should also be considered. All of these factors must be taken into account not only in relation to the systems currently in place but with consideration for the evolution that will undoubtedly continue to take place. These issues include additional software applications, larger storage devices for images with greater resolution, new diagnostic procedures such as intraoral scanning, and computer-driven appliance fabrication and treatment monitoring.

Constructing a data center in the orthodontic office is a science and should be treated as such. It is important to accept the fact that doing this correctly requires space.

The darkroom and filing area may be gone, but there is now a need for a dedicated computer room/closet that provides adequate ventilation, power, noise control, and—most important—access that allows neat organization of hundreds of cables that will run in and out of this space. While space is always at a premium in an office, this is now truly a required area, not a luxury.

Rack-mounted equipment

To go about making use of such an arrangement in an efficient manner, it is necessary to first make a commitment to using rack-mounted equipment. Rack-mounted equipment allows more devices to be packed into a smaller area in a more organized and maintainable fashion by using standardized sizing, both vertically and horizontally. Standard rack-mounted equipment is 19 inches wide, but varies in height. The height is listed as "U"s, meaning units of height. Each U is 1.75 inches. A server, for example, could be as small as 1 U in height (1.75 inches); a 2-U server would be 3.5 inches high by 19 inches deep. On a typical 7-foot Electronics Industries Association–compliant rack, there are 42 rack units. Generally, rack-mounted equipment sits on slides, similar to a drawer, that allow the unit to slide out for service. The cables are on extending arms to allow the machine to slide out without pulling out all the cables from the back.

The use of rack-mounted equipment allows for better cable management and easier maintenance, power handling, and ventilation. This is a significant leap beyond servers in floor-standing towers that are lined up along a wall or under a counter with a nest of poorly managed cables. In designing an office, it is important to note that not all racks are equal; there are some compatibility issues.

Size of the data center room

Room to move around the equipment racks on all sides and for adequate air movement is essential. It is also necessary to leave enough space to manage a lot of cables. There must also be room to grow as computer usage increases. Adequate space for phone equipment, which may tie into the computer, is also needed. Even if it is not rack-mounted, phone equipment should be included in the office's data center. Most everything will go on a rack, including servers, UPSs, switches to allow one keyboard and monitor to control multiple servers on the rack, a keyboard drawer, and monitor. A phone is needed on the rack as well, since it may be necessary to obtain technical assistance over the phone while doing upgrades and making modifications.

The data center need not be in the office. It could be in the basement or down the hall, since it should essentially be able to run as what is called a "lights-off" installation. In general, for a 4,000-square-foot office, a 6 × 10–foot room (60 square feet) should be adequate for present and future requirements. Ceiling height should also be considered. Smaller offices require less space, but it is important to keep in mind the rack's dimensions and the need to work comfortably around it.

Power requirements

It is best to provide the data center with two dedicated 30-amp lines, having available both 110 and 220 volts. These lines should be on a 24-hour circuit. Ideally, a backup generator will be available to handle the data center, including its heating, ventilation, and air conditioning equipment. Generators are not generally expensive or complicated to install. The UPS can be programmed to do an orderly shutdown of the server in the event of a power failure—another good precaution. These considerations are best regarded as insurance—a premium to be paid with the hope that the benefits will never be needed—that provides the comfort of protection.

Heating, ventilation, and air conditioning (HVAC)

Computers create a tremendous amount of heat and noise. The hotter the computer gets, the more likely it and its subsystems are to fail. Since reliability is a critically important factor, ventilation cannot be ignored. In addition, computer equipment, especially tape drives and hard drives, are particularly sensitive to dirt and dust. Since they all have a large number of powerful internal fans cooling them, the computers are pulling a good volume of room air over critical components. This, of course, pulls in any dust or dirt that is suspended in the air.

To protect computer equipment from heat and dirt, a controlled environment is critical. Ideally, the data center in the office will have adequate individually controlled air conditioning and good air filtration to remove particulate matter. Humidity should be controlled as well, to eliminate as much buildup as possible of static electricity, which can instantly "zap" hardware.

The following design criteria are often used by convention: temperature, 68°F to 77°F; and humidity, 50% ± 5. It is necessary to consult an HVAC contractor to find the best way of addressing these concerns.

317

Cabling

Choosing the type of cable to run is an important decision. Cables are categorized according to the amount and type of data they can carry and, importantly, at what speed. The category also indicates the type of shielding from interference that is in the cable. Cables are also rated as to their fire resistance; many local building codes now require that cables that run in the ceiling, floor, or walls be plenum rated. Cable requirements change continuously. Currently, at a minimum, category 6 cable should be used. Category 5 cables transfer data at a maximum of 100 MB/s, whereas category 5e and 6 cables transfer data at 1 GB/s. Whatever cable is run, however, will eventually be replaced to move more data more quickly. For this reason, how the cables are run is critical.

An early decision to make is where to run the cables. Cables can be run in the ceiling, beneath a raised floor with removable panels, or in the ceiling of the space beneath the office. In the ceiling, cables can be run in trays to keep them in one place, bundled together with nylon wire ties or wrapped with Velcro straps. It is important not to run the cables parallel with electrical cables and preferably not within 6 inches of an electrical cable. It is also best not to line the cables up too neatly, since this facilitates cross-talk between the cables, in spite of their shielding.

In big data centers, it is common to run cabling beneath a raised floor. These are often special floors made up of removable panels that look similar to a suspended ceiling. The sections can be removed for access. This would be great in a dental office, since all of the plumbing and electrical would be accessible as well. It is costly, however, since the floor has to be load bearing. It is also not necessarily attractive, unless covered with some other type of flooring, obviating some of its benefit.

As already noted, it is important to check local building codes. Whether in the ceiling, wall, or floor, according to code, cables are often supposed to be plenum rated for fire resistance. Additional codes requiring that all abandoned wiring be removed exist in some areas. This would be an issue when recabling. Removing abandoned cables certainly facilitates knowing which cables run where, but removing them from a tangled web in the ceiling is not an easy job.

Some computers are mounted on individual treatment units, and no longer just on a counter or stand in front of or behind the patient. This means there has to be a way of getting the cable to the chair, as well as up or down a wall into a wall jack if the computer is on a desk or counter. This is difficult even in a standard wall with plasterboard and studs; it is almost impossible in cement walls and floors or plaster walls. If there are areas in the office without suspended ceiling tiles, getting the cables through the ceiling is costly. More important, the need to recable relatively easily without having to redecorate with new floor covering, flooring, or wall covering must be considered. For this reason, once the cable leaves an accessible ceiling or floor and travels through any inaccessible area, it should be in a conduit to allow the old cable to be easily removed and a new one to be pulled.

Servers in the office

In today's professional office, there is likely to be more than one server in the computer center. For example, one author's (ML's) office runs:

1. A main server with dual 2.8 GHz Xeon processors, 4-GB RAM, 2 × raid controllers, 4 × 72–GB hard drives, and 2 × 36–GB hard drives
2. A second server running the terminal server, which allows access to the main server from remote locations (to allow clinicians to work from home) or access to all computer data from a second office location
3. An exchange server, which manages office e-mail
4. An old UNIX server, which is left over from an antiquated practice-management program but that is maintained for old, unconverted data
5. A dedicated server for Orametrix, a diagnostic and treatment tool that scans intraorally and fabricates custom wires

In contrast, another office (OT's) runs on a single server with mirrored hard drives and dual processors. A 1- or 2-year age difference is reflected in the equipment specifications.

Backup

Both of these authors' offices use a tape backup. This device has a library of eight tapes, which it rotates through in backing up critical data every night. Key staff members receive an e-mail from the server reporting that the backup was successful, or, occasionally, that it was not. Some imaging data is also backed up to a remote site managed by our imaging provider. Backing up data is a thankless task, unless disaster strikes. Conventional wisdom states that it is best to back up daily and take at least one backup copy offsite each week. It is also important to periodically attempt to restore data from the backup tape. It is not uncommon to find that the backup program indicates a successful backup, but that the tape cannot restore the data to your system.

Internet-protocol phone equipment

Phone equipment can also be tied into the computer system. This allows the addition of many interesting features, such as the ability to bring up a patient's chart immediately if his or her phone number is recognized by caller ID. Having the phone connected over the Internet also enables staff members who work from home, on insurance processing and word processing, to plug a special phone into their home broadband router and answer the office phones from home.

Broadband connection

Having the ability to transmit data requires a high-speed connection to the Internet. Some offices transmit almost all of their treatment notes, radiographs, and images to referring clinicians over secure Internet connections. One problem for offices that are so equipped is that some referring clinicians do not have broadband connections in their offices. Often, however, these professional offices are quick to upgrade when they see the many advantages of a broadband connection.

There are a number of broadband connections available. In our office, we use what is known as a T1 line. While it is relatively costly, we use it for our phone service as well, saving on the total cost. There is a tradeoff: when the phone lines take up part of the broadband bandwidth (referred to as a fractional T1 line), the rate at which data can be transmitted drops. With a new office location requiring data interchange with our main server, we have since reverted to separate lines for our phones, thus reclaiming our total T1 bandwidth. Other systems include DSL (digital subscriber line) over a phone line, which offers different speeds for uploading and downloading depending on price, or cable modems, which are fast and reliable but whose speed degrades as more people in an area use it. All of these technologies provide different speeds for uploading and downloading data. Because of the need in offices to upload images, which involve large amounts of data, upload speed is more important than it is for home broadband, for which downloading is the primary use.

Compromise

Because clinicians are not always able to fulfill their wish list because of space limitations, there are some smaller steps that can be taken to achieve a more manageable approach to computer installation. These steps include the following:

- Use a "short" rack system that can sit under a counter (although it will require more depth than a standard 24-inch cabinet); this will limit the number of devices that can be rack mounted. Two short racks could be used side by side. These racks are on wheels and can roll out to allow access to the cabling from the back. It is necessary to specify the correct vertical rails to accommodate computer equipment; there are several different kinds. Access is still best if you can move around the rack.
- Provide adequate 24-hour power.
- For ventilation, run an air-conditioning duct right down to the rack, and use an auxiliary blower in the duct to increase airflow. A good exhaust duct is a good idea as well.
- These machines and their cooling devices are noisy. Choose a spot where noise is not an issue or where you can provide sound insulation without interfering with the ventilation.
- Provide access for Internet connection (ie, cable, DSL, or T1).

Information technology support

As information technology (IT) needs become more complex, the need for 24-hour support becomes more evident. While it might be possible to run an orthodontic office if the imaging program, or even the scheduling or billing system, is down, the prospect of a total loss of all records during a computer malfunction now exists. We found it best to employ a full-time IT support person on staff. Between backups, program upgrades, hardware maintenance, and custom programming, he is kept busy. There is a significant cost factor here, which offsets some of the cost benefits of the digital practice. Before venturing into the high-technology world, the practitioner must be prepared to either spend an increasing amount of personal time working with the system, assign specific staff members to the task, have dependable outside local support, or have an in-house IT person. The importance of "local support" cannot be overemphasized. Even the best of the software vendors, with the best support, can only do so much offsite. A local, hands-on technician is a real requirement.

Summary

There is clearly no turning back. We have seen many new technologies evolve in medicine and dentistry. All of them seem to require more space, more equipment, and more technical support. It makes little sense to design and build a facility that does not take into account that more computer equipment is needed and that it is changing at an ever-increasing pace. It can only save time and expense to design into our offices the ability to keep pace with the rapidly expanding opportunities to provide our patients with the best possible diagnostic, treatment, and communication technology.

Reference

1. Lorino R. Design characteristics of the efficient orthodontic office [master's thesis]. Philadelphia: Temple University, 2004.

Recommended Reading

ABR'S E-Newsletter, May 11, 2001, no. 1, vol. 1. ABR Consulting Group website. Available at http://www.abrconsulting.com/Newsletter/05-11-01.htm. Accessed August 1, 2003.

ABR'S E-Newsletter, June 8, 2001, no. 1, vol. 2. ABR Consulting Group website. Available at http://www.abrconsulting.com/Newsletter/06-08-01.htm. Accessed August 1, 2003.

ABR'S E-Newsletter, August 24, 2001, no. 1, vol. 3. ABR Consulting Group website. Available at http://www.abrconsulting.com/Newsletter/08-24-01.htm. Accessed August 1, 2003.

ABR'S E-Newsletter, September 21, 2001, no. 1, vol. 4. ABR Consulting Group website. Available at http://www.abrconsulting.com/Newsletter/09-01-01.htm. Accessed July 31, 2003.

Types of cables. NetworkStuff.net–XDR2.com website. Available at http://www.networkstuff.net/WhatIsCable.htm. Accessed August 1, 2003.

What's the difference between CAT 5 and CAT 5e cable? CAT 5 Cable Company website. Available at http://www.cat-5-cable-company.com/faq-cat5-v-cat5e.htm. Accessed August 1, 2003.

Turner V, Pitt W, Brill KG. Industry standard tier classifications define site infrastructure performance [The Uptime Institute website]. Available at http://www.upsite.com/TUIpages/whitepapers/tuitiers.html. Accessed August 1, 2003.